MODULAR INSTRUCTION FOR INDEPENDENT TRAVEL
For Students Who Are Blind Or Visually Impaired: Preschool Through High School

BY

Doris M. Willoughby
and
Sharon L. Monthei

National Federation of the Blind
1800 Johnson Street
Baltimore, MD 21230

MODULAR INSTRUCTION FOR INDEPENDENT TRAVEL
For Students Who Are Blind Or Visually Impaired:
Preschool Through High School
By Doris M. Willoughby
and Sharon L. Monthei

[Note: Sharon L. Monthei was formerly known as
Sharon L. M. Duffy.]

Copyright 1998
National Federation of the Blind
1800 Johnson Street
Baltimore, MD 21230

Printed in USA
All rights reserved

Library of Congress Cataloging-in-Publication Data

Willoughby, Doris.
    Modular instruction for independent travel for students who are blind or visually impaired: preschool through high school / by Doris M. Willoughby and Sharon L. Monthei.
    p. cm.
Includes bibliographical references and index.
    ISBN 1-885218-09-5 (alk. paper)
1. Children, Blind–Orientation and mobility–United States. 2. Children, Blind–Rehabilitation–United States. 3. Visually handicapped children–Orientation and mobility–United States. 4. Visually handicapped children–Rehabilitation–United States. 5. Canes for the blind–United States.
I. Monthei, Sharon L., 1954- . II. Title.
HV 1596.5.W55 1998
371.91'1–dc21   98-9586
                                        CIP

In loving memory of

Dr. Kenneth Jernigan

Who inspired this book

And arranged its publication

TABLE OF CONTENTS

OVERVIEW AND GENERAL PRINCIPLES 1

Chapter A: HOW TO USE THIS BOOK (Scope and Style) 3
- THE MODULES 3
- INDEX OF SKILLS 6
- INDEX OF MODULES 6
- SKILLS LIST 7
- THE SCOPE OF THIS BOOK – SUMMARY 8

Chapter B: GENERAL PRINCIPLES AND OVERALL PLANNING (Monthei and Willoughby) 9
- MOTIVATION 9
- ATTITUDES TOWARD BLINDNESS 12
- FEAR 13
- BEFORE AND AFTER THE ROUTE 13
- WHO SHOULD TEACH? 14
- PROVIDING CANES 15
- TEACHING STRATEGIES 16
- WORKING TOGETHER 16

Chapter C: INTRODUCTION (Sharon L. Monthei) 19

MODULES 21

BASIC TECHNIQUES 23

- Module 1: DESCRIPTION OF BASIC TECHNIQUES (Including Stairway Technique) (Monthei) 24
- Module 2: INTRODUCING THE CANE (Including Stairway Technique) 30
- Module 3: POSTURE, GAIT, AND ARC (Level Surface) 39
- Module 4: HUMAN GUIDE 45
- Module 5: OBSTACLES: Noting Them and Proceeding 50
- Module 6: WALKING TOWARD A SOUND 57
- Module 7: SLEEP SHADES (Monthei) 60
- Module 8: POOR LIGHTING CONDITIONS: Independence at Night, In Dim Light, and With Glare 69
- Module 9: RIGHT AND LEFT 73
- Module 10: COMPASS DIRECTIONS 78

Module 11: ROUGH TERRAIN 81
Module 12: CARRYING THINGS 84
Module 13: IN A CROWD 88

AT HOME--INDOORS 91
Module 14: HOME – CONTENTS OF ROOM 92
Module 15: WHAT IS A "ROOM"? 94
Module 16: APARTMENT HOUSE OR CONDOMINIUM 98
Module 17: UNFINISHED BASEMENT, "CRAWL SPACE," OR ATTIC 103
Module 18: MORE IDEAS (For Lessons at Home, Indoors) 105

AT HOME – OUTDOORS 107
Module 19: BACK YARD BOUNDARIES 108
Module 20: BACK YARD (OVERALL) 114
Module 21: FROM HOUSE TO CURB 117
Module 22: HOME ADDRESS 120
Module 23: PORCH OR DECK 121
Module 24: OUTSIDE AND INSIDE THE HOUSE 123
Module 25: UTILITIES AND TRASH 125
Module 26: MORE IDEAS (For Lessons at Home, Outdoors) 128

AT SCHOOL – INDOORS 131
Module 27: ORIENTATION INSIDE NEW CLASSROOM 132
Module 28: ROUTES FOR NEW CLASSROOM (Early Elementary Grades) .. 134
Module 29: REST ROOMS AT SCHOOL 137
Module 30: FIRE DRILLS 140
Module 31: DOORS AND DOORWAYS 143
Module 32: DOORS CLOSED OR OPEN 147
Module 33: LUNCHTIME 151
Module 34: LUNCHROOM AND KITCHEN: Overall Layout and Procedures 154
Module 35: WALKING IN A LINE OF PEOPLE 156
Module 36: ERRANDS 161
Module 37: ALTERNATE ROUTES WITHIN A BUILDING 164
Module 38: ROUTES FOR NEW BUILDINGS AND NEW CLASSROOMS: Upper
   Grades Through High School 170
Module 39: MORE IDEAS (For Lessons at School, Indoors) 176

AT SCHOOL – OUTDOORS 179
Module 40: SCHOOL BUS 180
Module 41: MEETING A CAR 182
Module 42: PLAYGROUND 185
Module 43: WHAT'S OUT THERE? On the School Grounds 190

Module 44: EXTERIOR FIRE ESCAPE 194
Module 45: OUTSIDE AND INSIDE THE SCHOOL 196

COMMUNITY – OUTDOORS (BASIC) 199
Module 46: WALKING INDEPENDENTLY WHILE FOLLOWING SOMEONE 200
Module 47: SIDEWALKS 203
Module 48: AROUND THE BLOCK 206
Module 49: STREET CROSSING WITH LITTLE TRAFFIC 209
Module 50: DISTINCTIVE SOUNDS 214
Module 51: DISTINCTIVE ODORS 217
Module 52: ECHOES AND AIR CURRENTS (Including "Facial Vision") 219
Module 53: WALKING AT CURBSIDE 221
Module 54: STREET CROSSING WITH LIGHTS (Basic Skills) 223
Module 55: STOP SIGNS 229

COMMUNITY – OUTDOORS (INCREASING SKILLS) 233
Module 56: SIDEWALK FLAWED OR OBSTRUCTED 234
Module 57: VISUALLY CONFUSING APPEARANCE 237
Module 58: INCLEMENT WEATHER Including Ice Underfoot 240
Module 59: UNEXPECTED DROP-OFF OR STEP-DOWN 243
Module 60: WALKING ACROSS OPEN SPACE 246
Module 61: STREET CROSSING (Developing Flexibility and Competence) 250
Module 62: STREET CROSSING WITH OBSTRUCTION 257
Module 63: DRIVEWAYS, ALLEYS, AND STREETS 261
Module 64: NON-SQUARE 'BLOCKS' 265
Module 65: IRREGULAR STREETS 269
Module 66: COMPLICATED STREET CROSSINGS 272
Module 67: ASKING DIRECTIONS AND FIGURING IT OUT (By Doris M. Willoughby
    and Sharon L. Monthei) 279
Module 68: UNCONTROLLED INTERSECTIONS 283
Module 69: MORE IDEAS (For Lessons in the Community, Outdoors) 285

PUBLIC BUILDINGS – GENERAL 287
Module 70: GENERAL OVERVIEW – BUILDINGS 288
Module 71: STAIRS IN UNFAMILIAR BUILDINGS 293
Module 72: ELEVATORS 297
Module 73: ESCALATORS 300
Module 74: MALLS 302
Module 75: EMERGENCY EXITS In Various Buildings 310

PUBLIC BUILDINGS – EXAMPLES 311
Module 76: AN AUDITORIUM OR THEATER 312

Module 77: THE BANK 317
Module 78: A DOCTOR'S OFFICE 319
Module 79: A GROCERY STORE 321
Module 80: HOTELS AND MOTELS 324
Module 81: AN OFFICE BUILDING 326
Module 82: A RESTAURANT 328
Module 83: A SERVICE STATION 330
Module 84: VISITING A BLIND ADULT AT HIS/HER WORKPLACE 332

OUTDOOR LOCATIONS 335
Module 85: SWIMMING POOL OR BEACH 336
Module 86: BRIDGES AND OVERPASSES 339
Module 87: THE GREAT OUTDOORS 341
Module 88: RURAL ENVIRONMENT 347
Module 89: MORE IDEAS (For Lessons in Outdoor Locations) 351

PUBLIC TRANSPORTATION 353
Module 90: PUBLIC BUSES 354
Module 91: TAXICABS 364
Module 92: THE AIRPORT and Air Travel 366
Module 93: URBAN RAPID TRANSIT: Subways and Elevated Trains (Monthei) 370

APPENDIX 375
Appendix A: THE BLIND TRAVEL INSTRUCTOR (Monthei and Dunnam) 377

REFERENCES 381
BOOKS AND PERIODICALS 381
For Parents and Educators 381
Publications for Children and Young People 383
VIDEOTAPES, DRAMAS, FILMS 383
ADDRESSES 384

INDEXES 387
Index 1: INDEX OF SKILLS 389
Index 2: INDEX OF CHAPTER AND MODULE TITLES 393

OVERVIEW AND GENERAL PRINCIPLES

CHAPTER A

HOW TO USE THIS BOOK
Scope and Style

This book, *MODULAR INSTRUCTION FOR INDEPENDENT TRAVEL FOR STUDENTS WHO ARE BLIND OR VISUALLY IMPAIRED: PRESCHOOL THROUGH HIGH SCHOOL* (hereafter often called simply *Modular Instruction*), is a flexible, practical guide for teaching cane travel to students of preschool age through high school.

This book is designed to be used with the companion publication by the same authors:

> Doris M. Willoughby and Sharon L. M. Duffy. *Handbook for Itinerant and Resource Teachers of Blind and Visually Impaired Students.* Baltimore, MD: National Federation of the Blind. [Note: Sharon L. Monthei was formerly known as Sharon L. M. Duffy.]

The companion publication will sometimes be referred to as simply the "Handbook," for the sake of brevity. For the most part, material included in the *Handbook* (much of which is relevant to travel instruction) is not repeated in *Modular Instruction.*

The "References" section of *Modular Instruction* gives the full citation for the companion publication, as well as others which are especially relevant.

THE MODULES

Curriculum guides for science or language arts often contain recurring topics for emphasis – perhaps called "cycles," "threads," or "strands." Each teacher selects activities for a particular class, as appropriate for various circumstances. A Midwestern teacher might select activities to introduce basic concepts about ocean life; however, a Cape Cod class might enjoy advanced activities assuming much prior knowledge.

Similarly, these Modules sample recurring themes for emphasis. They facilitate integration into all aspects of living.

In most subjects (science, physical education, reading, etc.), there are a multitude of ready-made curricula and resource books. With cane travel, however, there are very few publications with concrete and varied suggestions such as these. The busy teacher or parent should not have to "re-invent the wheel" at every turn.

Examples

Examples are just that – examples. For instance, the Module called "Non-Square 'Blocks'" depicts the "Shady Lane Subdivision." "Shady Lane" is entirely fictitious, but is representative of a housing development with irregular street patterns. A concrete example with a map brings clarity to the discussion and makes the presentation more pleasant to read. Each instructor will apply the ideas and suggestions to actual places.

Some Modules, such as "Porch or Deck," appear to be quite limited in scope. Others, such as "Complicated Street Crossings," appear to be very broad. Again, it is a matter of bringing ideas and suggestions to the reader in a clear, organized way.

Depending on the student's age and skill, a given Module might be drawn upon in any of several ways, including:

  – Introducing a new skill

- Reinforcing and reviewing a particular skill
- Integrating progress in several skills together
- Detail and focus for emphasis
- Variety; practice without monotony
- Readiness and preparation for something to be mastered later
- Enjoyment and fun, to add zest to learning
- Demonstrating relevance to daily living
- Focusing on something which should not be left out, but may easily be omitted without an organized plan
- A different approach or manner

If a given Module or Example happens to fit a student's needs exactly, it may indeed serve as a virtually complete lesson plan in itself. More usually, however, it serves as a model from which the instructor draws plans. Modules are easily stretched, compressed, combined, or divided, to provide lengthy practice or a quick review. A given Module or Example may require many sessions over a period of time for one student, yet be mastered in a few minutes by another student.

To aid in this process, typical age levels are frequently indicated. Some Examples include detailed wording and procedures. All of these are guidelines and examples only. The particular skills taught and the approach used will vary greatly with individuals.

Modules are *not* necessarily placed in sequential order. They are *not* written as ready-made, complete lesson plans. Rather, *Modular Instruction* is intended as a resource from which activities and ideas will be selected according to students' needs and progress. The same is true of the Examples within Modules. They are *not* necessarily presented in the sequence of easiest-to-hardest, or typical first-to-last.

Various other considerations have dictated the sequence of presentation. Sometimes the example which is likely to be used most often is given first. Sometimes a general procedure is given first, followed by notes about younger students and special needs.

Detailed suggestions for related practice have been placed in some locations. For example, the Module "Stairs in Unfamiliar Buildings" has examples of practice in finding a seat within a room. There are many other Modules where this detail would have been equally logical; but for practical reasons, the suggestions were written up in certain chosen places. The Index of Skills helps in locating these kinds of things.

It is assumed that the teacher will examine the Modules that appear helpful at a given time, and that he/she will select and modify the appropriate portions.

The age and experience of the student are only two of the variables that affect how a Module (or an Example within it) will be used. A partial list of variables would include:

Age of student
Experience of student
General locale (e.g., rural or urban)
Climate
Location of school and home
Schedule of student and teacher
Kinds of opportunities for practice without the primary instructor
General health and stamina
Special security or safety precautions (e.g., high crime area)
Experience of teacher

Style of Writing

In some respects, this book devotes more attention to younger students. This is because many teachers have experience mainly with older students, and may not understand the needs of young children. Therefore, considerable detail is given for methods with young students. This does *not* imply that teaching cane travel to young students is difficult or unwise—only that appropriate methods should be used.

Some readers may wonder why a lesson would emphasize one particular thing, such as the flagpole or a tree. As discussed in "General Principles," such things provide necessary motivation, focus, and variety for a child of 8 or younger.

Older students should not need tasks simplified as for young children. Examples in the Modules include frequent indications of age level.

In some portions of this book, terms such as "he/she" are used to emphasize inclusion of both sexes. This is also done in the "Objectives" portion of each Module, so that the wording can be copied verbatim. However, in activities and examples we have arbitrarily used "he" for half of them and "she" for half of them, to avoid unwieldy wording.

Similarly, there is another literary convention which is not always used. In certain kinds of writing, it is now required that "people first" language be used without exception. This means that one must say "a person who is visually impaired," rather than "a blind person" or "a visually impaired person." This requirement has been helpful in doing away with unfortunate expressions such as "He is a severe muscular dystrophy" or "The doctor interviewed a retinal detachment." The person is indeed a *person*, not a physical condition.

In this book, however, we believe that we have met this standard in another way, while avoiding certain disadvantages which come with rigid requirements for specific "people first" wording.

This book brings out in every way the concept that students are regular, normal people who should be treated with respect and individual attention. However, we do use expressions such as "a blind student" or "blind people." Properly used, these expressions are analogous to others in the world at large. For example, people do not go out of their way to say "I took a picture of a woman who is a bank executive." They will probably say simply, "I took a picture of a bank executive." In discussing clothing styles and colors, people do not go out of their way to say "a woman who has red hair;" they often say "a red-haired woman."

The distinction seems to relate to talking about something "normal" and "ordinary" vs. something "abnormal" and "undesirable."

We believe that blindness is a characteristic like any other. Although a person does not choose to be blind, the fact of blindness can be an advantage, a disadvantage, or a "neutral," depending on attitudes, training, and the particular task at hand. The speech, *Blindness: Handicap or Characteristic* (see REFERENCES), brings this out eloquently.

In avoiding archaic expressions such as "She is a retinal detachment," it is also important to avoid remarks which make undesirable implications about blindness in general. The *Handbook*, pages 37-67, offers further discussion of expressions and attitudes.

Also, in speaking to students it is important to use vocabulary which will be understood. From time to time, the Modules include discussions about vocabulary and examples of suggested wording.

Names of persons portrayed are fictitious (unless indicated otherwise), as are the names of many places.

Unless specifically defined in context, the terms "visually impaired" and "blind" are used more or less interchangeably. Also, the terms "teacher," "instructor," and "educator" are used rather interchangeably, and include parents and others who take responsibility for instruction.

The terms "late-blinded" and "blind from birth" are used, rather than "adventitiously blinded" and "congenitally blind." The former terms are simple and clear.

We have tried to write with clarity and precision without being "dry," and to make this book pleasant and interesting to read.

Parts of the Module

Following is a brief outline of the Module structure, according to individual headings.

OBJECTIVE(S):

At least one Objective is stated for each regular Module. (Often, many objectives could potentially apply.) Only a "kernel" of wording is given; it is assumed that qualifying phrases and detail will be added for individual needs. Unless otherwise noted, this book assumes that the white cane and sleep shades will be used.

It is *not* assumed that a given Module is sufficient in itself to achieve the objective given. Two or more Modules often relate to the same objective, and it may be assumed that other instruction also takes place.

AGE:

A suggested age range is given, sometimes separately for each Example. This is a guideline only, and will vary with factors such as prior experience, special circumstances, and additional disabilities.

PRIMARY SKILL EMPHASIS:
ADDITIONAL SKILL EMPHASIS:

These lists are the major basis of the Skills Index for this book. (See SKILLS LIST, below.) For the teacher's convenience, they call attention to the skills that are most obviously involved. Usually, many other skills could also be integrated as desired. Emphasis can vary greatly according to needs.

TEACHER PREPARATION:

This calls attention to preparation especially relevant to the particular Module. It is assumed that the instructor will always make general preparation, by considering what locations and activities would be suitable for the student at this time.

STUDENT BACKGROUND:

In all subject areas, activities are introduced by providing or reviewing relevant background. When a kindergarten class plans a trip to the fire station, the children discuss the role of firefighters. When a mathematics class is about to study cube roots, they review square root. These Modules call attention to especially relevant concepts which should be discussed beforehand, sometimes with suggestions for specific prior activities. It is assumed that the instructor will always see that the student is properly prepared, both in general and specifically.

FIGURES:

Photographs, diagrams, and maps are sometimes provided for clarity. They are examples only.

REMARKS:
CAUTION:

A "Caution" note deals with something which could be dangerous or overtly harmful. A "Remark" is less urgent.

ACTIVITIES:
EXAMPLES:
VARIATIONS:

These headings indicate the main body of the Module. Depending on the activities, there may be more or fewer subheadings. They are not necessarily in chronological sequence.

RELATED PRACTICE:
FOLLOW-UP:

These point out activities which are particularly relevant afterward. It is assumed that the teacher will always provide follow-up and review over time as appropriate.

SEE ALSO:

The heading "See Also" refers to another place within *Modular Instruction* – usually another Module.

REFERENCES:

This heading refers to other publications.

****

NOTE: The first Module, "Description of Basic Techniques," is introductory. Rather than focusing on *how* to teach, it focuses on the techniques themselves. It is a reference chapter/module, designed to be used in conjunction with the other modules.

INDEX OF SKILLS

This Index is based on the Skills List, below. For the teacher's convenience, it calls attention to the skills that are most obviously involved in a particular Module. Note that *Module numbers* are given, and *not* page numbers.

INDEX OF MODULES

This Index gives the Modules in alphabetical order. It is similar to the Table of Contents in that it shows the page number where each Module begins. However, the reader looking for a particular Module title will find it more quickly here.

To a slight degree, this Index is "permuted" – that is, an entry can be found by looking for a significant word. For example, the Module "Description of Basic Techniques" is also listed as "Techniques, Description of Basic."

HOW TO USE THIS BOOK

SKILLS LIST

Following are the categories of specific skills, as used in this book. This is the main basis for the Skills Index at the end of the book. These skills are listed under the headings "PRIMARY SKILL EMPHASIS" and "ADDITIONAL SKILL EMPHASIS" at the beginning of each Module.

This list is intended only as a convenient guide. Emphasis can vary greatly according to needs. Other skills can also be integrated as desired.

Addresses
Air currents and echoes
[Arc – see "Posture, grip, gait, and arc"]
Attitudes toward blindness
Barefoot walking
Boundaries
Careers
Carrying things
Climbing, clambering, crawling, etc.
Communication and instructions
Compass directions
Corners, turns, and angles
Correcting a path
Daily living skills
Detecting step-downs or drop-offs
Doors and doorways
Elevators
Emergency procedures
Escalators
Etiquette
Examining things tactually
Finding a person
Finding a seat
Flexibility and confidence
Floor plans
General travel (indoors)
General travel (outdoors)
General travel
Hills and inclines
Human guide
In a crowd or a line
Interpreting odors
Landmarks
Maps
Meeting the public
Moving straight ahead
Obstacles in path
Open space
Orientation overall
Orientation within a room
Overhanging objects
Parallel and perpendicular
Posture, grip, gait, and arc
Public transportation
Purchase or transaction
Responsibility and citizenship
Right and left
Sidewalk
Sound direction and meaning
Stairs
Stowing cane
Street crossing
Street patterns
Structure of buildings
[Techniques – see specific topics]
Traffic movement
Understanding vision and partial vision
Varied terrain
Walking in company with others
Weather and temperature

THE SCOPE OF THIS BOOK – SUMMARY

This book DOES:

- Give many practical examples, often with considerable detail.
- Offer guidelines for age levels.
- Provide an approach that is appropriate for students with partial sight, as well as those who are totally blind, regardless of when the sight was lost.
- Anticipate common problems and concerns, and offer suggestions about them.
- Offer detail and simplification when it really is needed (notably for very young children).
- Include suggestions about matters closely related to cane travel (e.g., protecting oneself from crime when in public).
- Discuss appropriate vocabulary and approach for older and younger students, with some specific examples.
- Assume that the cane will be used at all times except during sports and when seated.
- Assume that blind students' abilities are in the same range as those of fully sighted students.
- Avoid unnecessary overdetail which slows learning.
- Explain human guide techniques, and how this method of travel interacts with the use of the cane.
- Provide a resource and a guide overall for teaching the use of the long white cane.

This book generally DOES NOT:

- Discuss aspects of general education which are not closely related to actual travel. (For example, although social conduct is mentioned frequently, there is little detail about actually teaching that area of skill.)
- Contain detail about other aspects of the education of blind children, such as Braille. (Readers are referred to the publication by the same authors, *Handbook for Itinerant and Resource Teachers of Blind and Visually Impaired Students.*)
- Discuss guide dogs, electronic travel aids, non-cane ("pre-cane") techniques, or history. (Human guide techniques, however, are discussed.)
- Provide detailed suggestions for students with severe multiple handicaps. (However, much of this book applies regardless, and there are some specific suggestions about additional disabilities.)
- Constitute a replacement for the teacher's receiving personal instruction and preparation, or a replacement for the teacher's preparation and planning for each individual student.
- Enumerate "dry" details at the expense of practical, easy-to-use information.
- Claim to have the final and complete answer to each and every possible problem.

Suggestions for further reading are listed at the end of this book and elsewhere. (References may be mentioned in some places by title only; complete bibliographical information is given in the REFERENCES section at the end of this book.)

REFERENCE(S):

Kenneth Jernigan. *Blindness: Handicap or Characteristic.*

Willoughby and Duffy. *Handbook for Itinerant and Resource Teachers of Blind and Visually Impaired Students.*

CHAPTER B

GENERAL PRINCIPLES AND OVERALL PLANNING
By Sharon L. Monthei And Doris M. Willoughby

MOTIVATION

Age 8 and Over (Approximately)

Envision yourself in a job or other circumstance which requires you to learn a completely new physical skill. (Sailing? Horseback riding? Driving a large vehicle? Climbing utility poles?)

Your instructor is pleasant and well-meaning, but sometimes seems to push you too fast or hold you back. Practice may be tiring or tedious. At times you feel quite nervous. Yet you know that the skill must be mastered, and will be mastered; you look forward to its becoming second nature. You set goals for yourself, and give yourself small "rewards" at milestones. This is an approximate parallel to the student's view of learning cane travel.

Below are some major factors which maximize progress. They apply to all age levels.

Students under 8, however, usually need additional factors as discussed below. Age 8 is not a magic line of demarcation, of course. And students who are "in-between" in age (approximately 6-11) are "in-between" in motivation also. Also, the older student who is particularly immature, or has additional handicaps or special problems, may need the kind of help suggested for younger children. Modules are written to facilitate adaptation for individual needs, including the matter of motivation.

All good teachers continually review the elements of motivation, trying to remove barriers and maximize positive factors. If you are used to teaching young children and start to work with someone older, you may need to revamp your approach. Consciously avoid "talking down" to the student and oversimplifying. Note your tone of voice. Work on age-appropriate activities in age-appropriate settings, even with a beginner.

Factors to Emphasize for Older Students

(Each item below has an example given in parentheses.)

- Independence in going from place to place (to the bank)
- Independence in daily living skills (finding a seat independently)
- Valued privileges (shopping without parent)
- Encouragement by family and friends (sister does not walk home with brother after he learns to go alone)
- Recognizing that alternative methods are respectable and normal (visiting a blind machinist at work)
- Dignity (no "babyish" activities; teacher does not "talk down" to student)
- Praise and approval given without "gushing"
- Variety (more than one route for practice)
- Age-appropriate activities, sometimes

including a preview of future learning (riding the subway)
- Skills immediately helpful (walking to rest room independently)
- Skills helpful in long run (rural student studying traffic in large city)
- Pacing of learning neither too fast nor too slow (busy streets introduced after student has gained some confidence, but before habits of avoidance build up)
- Small rewards from time to time (ice cream treat at end of unit)
- Documenting achievements (lists, charts, demonstrations)

Students Under Age 8

To a young child, learning to use a cane seems no different from the other things he/she is learning. Adults are continually reminding: "Brush your teeth....wear a coat....don't slam the door....wipe your feet....hang up your coat....write your name....sit quietly....get your coat....wash your hands....use a napkin...."

The younger the child, the less he/she will regard the cane as particularly "different" from anything else in life. It is just one more thing to learn. This is a great advantage, since feelings of embarrassment or stigma are unlikely. At the same time, this means the teacher must use the same general approach with which other things are taught to a young child.

If you are used to teaching relatively mature students, and find yourself with a young student (or an older one with special problems), you may need to revamp your approach. Consciously plan age-appropriate activities.

Ms. Fontana's previous students—all in junior high or above—had responded well. But Terri, in first grade, was increasingly uncooperative. "Do I have to do that AGAIN?" she would whine. Terri was inconsistent with posture and technique, and could not reliably walk anywhere outside her classroom. Ms. Fontana repeatedly explained the importance of practicing these skills. But lessons became more and more tense and unproductive.

Ms. Fontana invited Mrs. Pollock, a co-worker with several younger students, to teach a demonstration lesson.

"Do you like teddy bears?" asked Mrs. Pollock while greeting Terri. "I brought a teddy bear today, and I put it where we'll find it near the end of our work. When we find it, you may play with it, and then carry it during the end of the lesson....Now, this is kind of a treasure hunt. I will ask you to go to a certain place. I'll help you if you need it, but we might start over if I do need to help you....We'll go to five places, and then I'll tell you where the teddy bear is....First, please go to the water fountain...."

"Amazing!" exclaimed Ms. Fontana later. "I couldn't believe how enthusiastic she was. She did a lot better right away."

"That's the kind of lesson you want. Here are some more ideas," replied Mrs. Pollock as she jotted down several notes.

Many Modules in this book contain the kind of ideas that would help Ms. Fontana. High school instructors may be surprised at an entire session centered on "the flagpole," "trees," or "the public-address system." But this is precisely what provides interest and focus for a young child.

In the companion book, *Handbook for Itinerant and Resource Teachers of Blind and Visually Impaired Students,* by Willoughby and Duffy, there is much detail regarding age-appropriate expectations and programming.

[Note: Sharon L. Monthei, co-author of *Modular Instruction for Independent Travel for Students Who are Blind or Visually Impaired: Preschool Through High School,* is also the co-author of the *Handbook.* She was formerly known as Sharon L. M. Duffy.]

In the *Handbook*, see particularly pp. 157-198:
   "Travel with the Long White Cane"
   "Planning a Cane Travel Curriculum"
   "Orientation and Mobility for Children 8 and Under, and Those With Special Problems"
   "A Cane Travel Curriculum for Children 8 and Under, and Those With Special Problems"

Factors to Emphasize for Younger Children

- Length of session appropriate for age
- Frequent change of activity or focus during the course of a session
- Much variety; strenuous avoidance of monotony
- Age-appropriate fun and enjoyment, especially near the end of each session
- New skills introduced carefully (too much at once can easily overwhelm a child)
- Appropriate pacing – lessons neither too hard nor too easy.
- New experiences introduced carefully, to prevent fear
- Filling in gaps where sighted children learn through vision (example: touring the school kitchen, which sighted children see while walking past it at lunch)
- Integration with other areas of learning (for example, comparing the size of the school's pots and pans to those at home; discussing cooking and other daily living skills)
- Relatively frequent use of games and other diversions
- Appropriate lesson structure (During a given session, expect the greatest concentration and effort near the beginning. Activities near the end should be relatively less demanding and more "fun.")
- Praise and approval for accomplishment, and also for genuine effort
- Appropriate consequences for poor behavior ("What would we do if he refused to put on his shoes?" is a good question to provide perspective.)
- Overall planning so that overdependent behavior does *not* bring greater benefits. (Example: Terri assumes that if she does not find the clay when she walks across the room, a friend will help her and chat with her. But instead, Terri is expected to start over, try again, and delay the activity she enjoys.)

Motivation suggestions listed previously for older students apply to younger ones as well. However, the less mature the child, the less he/she will understand the value of independence, and the less he/she will have the self-discipline to strive for it. Adults must shape the environment so that independence (however slight) brings privileges the child currently appreciates. Below are a few examples.

The idea of "increased privileges" sounds like a simple concept. For an older student, it is not hard to think of examples. Walk to school...go shopping...go hiking with friends.......Ideas are easy to list.

But what about a four-year-old, or an even younger child? Sighted children of preschool age do not cross busy streets alone or shop independently. Depending upon age and situation, they may not even go next door alone. They should never be left without an older person nearby.

The following list gives some examples of age-appropriate privileges for young children. You will think of many more.

(1) When walking in the neighborhood, a toddler is not required to hold the parent's hand at all times. She may use her cane and walk near the parent.

(2) A four-year-old plays in the yard while others remain in the house.

(3) Mrs. Gallegos often takes three-year-old Maria along to the bank or on other errands. Formerly she required Maria to stay right beside her – after all, there were pillars, stairs, and other obstacles nearby. Now that Maria has a cane, however, Mrs. Gallegos is noticing that other small children often wander around the room while waiting and are not corrected unless they

(4) At preschool, Sam walks to the playground as a regular part of the group instead of holding someone's hand.

(5) While the family shops at a small store, the seven-year-old need not stay right with them. He may go to an area that interests him, make a purchase, or simply walk around.

(6) While her mother is in the hardware store, six-year-old Toni is allowed to walk next door and buy an ice cream cone with her birthday money.

(7) A first grader independently carries the lunch-count list to the kitchen during her turn at errands.

Note that in all of these examples, adults are close by, as is appropriate for the child's age. However, the child is gaining independence in the same manner as his/her sighted peers.

REFERENCE(S):

The *Handbook for Itinerant and Resource Teachers of Blind and Visually Impaired Students*, pp. 385-392, discusses motivation in detail.

ATTITUDES TOWARD BLINDNESS

Cane travel is one of the most valuable skills a blind person can attain. It not only means independence for the individual, but is more often the means of acceptance of blindness than any other skill. Learning Braille can be kept secret. Learning cooking hints is not a public event, but carrying a cane is. A blind person who uses a cane is not only making a statement to others that he is blind but (more importantly) is also acknowledging his own blindness. In dealing with the challenges that blindness brings, the first step must be this acceptance of blindness. The second is the ability to look at each problem unemotionally and logically to work out its solution.

Therefore, the most important concepts any travel teacher can teach are that it is respectable to be blind, that it is respectable to use a cane, and that it is normal for blind persons to use canes. Without these beliefs, no amount of training will ensure that a student will use a cane once training is complete. I have retrained a number of people who lacked these convictions. They either didn't travel after their initial training period, to avoid using a cane (attempting to hide their blindness), or they traveled without a cane as best they could. Either way, the initial training was a waste of time for the student and the instructor since the skills were not utilized. If the teacher looks at the training process as more than a technical exercise – considering the whole question of adjustment to blindness within the context of cane travel – successful training is much more likely.

I encourage my students to take their canes with them wherever they go, explaining the importance of identifying themselves as blind persons in terms of public awareness. Identifying oneself as blind can reduce the number of uncomfortable situations which would arise without it. The blind person who asks where something is – something in plain sight – spares himself and the sighted person embarrassment. Since the incidence of blindness is so low, a person probably would not immediately conceive that the individual asking the question is blind.

Many blind people mistakenly believe that they appear more "normal" if they don't carry a cane. The fact is that the public may not recognize that a person is blind, but does realize that there is something different – mental retardation, drunkenness, illiteracy – to name a few. Ultimately, it is more comfortable for blind people to identify themselves as blind, allaying the confusion that results from the misidentification that would otherwise inevitably occur. Many blind persons with residual vision report that a great burden was lifted once they began to admit their blindness. No matter how careful they were, they could not hide their inability to see things that others expected them to see.

Discuss these points openly with students. To the extent that a teacher succeeds in convincing a student to use a cane at all times, training is successful.

FEAR

Fear is an aspect of travel which must be reckoned with in training. A student who exhibits great fear may need to be taken more slowly than her actual level of skill might otherwise indicate. A student with no fear may need to be watched closely, because of dangerous, careless traveling habits. Peeking under sleep shades or walking quite slowly can be indicators of fear. Although it is often advisable to let students work things out for themselves, discussion can sometimes reduce fear as well as be instructive. Commenting on a student's reduction in fear symptoms can be helpful. If a student mentions her fear, take time to discuss it, but do not let a student out of class because of it. Discussing it in a direct manner can help reduce fear. Perhaps, give an easier route than planned, or perhaps work on the very thing that frightens her such as: lighted crossings, busy streets, escalators, etc. Perhaps, file the information away and decide to tackle it a little later.

I once had a student who said he would never ride "El" trains, because (he said) he had no desire to go downtown. I did not argue with him, but waited for the proper time, when he needed to get downtown, and we went. At the time he first mentioned this, he neither possessed the skill nor the confidence to ride on trains. Therefore, it would have been ridiculous to argue the point at that time. As he gained skill and confidence, he began to see that he could ride the trains.

A teacher must work to reduce fear associated with travel, because her success as a teacher depends upon it. For instance, if a student has beautiful technique but is afraid of getting lost, he is unlikely to go anywhere not specifically taught.

It is important to be aware of a student's particular fears. Here is a list of common fears: making a fool of oneself, asking directions, getting taken advantage of, getting hit by a car, noise, riding on buses or rapid transit trains, heights, escalators, falling downstairs, and getting stuck in elevators. Be alert for these and other fears and find ways of helping students overcome them. Send the shy student to find places at unknown locations. Send the student who fears being lost, on routes guaranteed to get him lost in areas where assistance from others is readily available. Send the student who fears dealing with store clerks on routes involving shopping for specified items, etc. All of these kinds of routes are good for most students to experience anyway, to build confidence and teach flexibility.

BEFORE AND AFTER THE ROUTE

When I send a student out, I want to give him maximum confidence and encouragement. I carefully explain the route; ask him to repeat it; tell him I think he can do it, even though it may be a very challenging route; ask if there are any questions; and send him out.

I never buy the argument (should a student propose it) that although he can't explain it, he can go there. Overwhelmingly, the reason for not being able to explain it is lack of a clear understanding of the route. [NOTE: If English is the student's second language, or there are other major barriers to communication, this may not be true. He might indeed understand the route but be unable to explain it clearly in English. The reverse can also occur – he may explain the route verbally, but fail to understand it.] I do not particularly encourage students to write routes down in Braille, because developing enough memory skill to follow verbal directions is most valuable in independent travel. Occasionally, there are exceptions: students with great fear; those who have an unusual amount of difficulty comprehending directions; and those with severe, physiologically-based memory problems.

When students return, it is necessary to discuss the experience. It isn't enough just to have students perform to a certain standard. How they think about it is of equal importance. Frequently, a student will say, "I did terrible!" when, in fact, she got into a tight spot and successfully got out of it. She needs to feel good about that, not dwell on the one imperfection of a route. Praise for good thinking and performance will keep a student trying. If a student really didn't do well, I simply say, "You learned a lot." That, by the way, is quite true. Then we talk about exactly what happened and why, so that the student can make a fresh try tomorrow.

For advanced students, I may require a description of how an entire route went. It can be useful to analyze a student's thinking and also to fill in any gaps in observation which may have occurred while I was observing other students. Beyond that, a reconstruction of the route can sometimes assist a student to figure out what happened and why, if there were any deviations from the route. This knowledge tends to give students more confidence in themselves, as they now know what happened and how to do it differently in the future.

A final reason for doing debriefings is simply for the purpose of letting a student unwind. Travel training can be very stressful, and talking about it often helps a student put things back into proper perspective and relieve tension.

Self-confidence is the goal of cane travel. It can be achieved through promotion of the respectability of blindness, teaching good technical skills, and challenging students to do what they did not believe they could do. Do whatever it takes to attain these ends. Challenge your students to achieve independence.

WHO SHOULD TEACH?

Everyone in the child's environment is his/her teacher. A child learns daily living skills from parents and siblings; social conventions from neighbors and relatives; academic and other skills from various schoolteachers; games and activities from young friends. Orientation and mobility is part of this large picture.

If a child does not develop increasing independence – including the use of a cane at an early age – he or she will expect continual assistance from others in getting around. If parents and school staff see that the child *does* begin cane usage early, then he or she will develop increasing independence appropriate for each chronological age.

Modular Instruction assumes that at least one person in the child's life (probably a teacher or parent) has made serious study of how the cane is used, and takes the lead in guiding others to facilitate learning. There are many ways to gain this knowledge; the National Federation of the Blind will be pleased to help you find a source.

When this book uses the term "teacher" or "instructor," it means whatever adult is working with the student in the activity.

Parents

The foundation of all learning occurs in infancy and very early childhood. The general development of infants and toddlers is beyond the scope of this book. However, many Modules contain suggestions which apply to toddlers and even infants.

Children walk with their parents to the neighbor's house; to cross the street; to go from the car into the drugstore. They go with the family to the grocery store; the doctor's office; the mall; the zoo. The Modules in this book give specific ideas for making each excursion an age-appropriate learning experience.

When an educator takes the lead in instruction, parents nevertheless continue to guide skill development outside of classes. Parents also monitor the instruction itself to assure that it is appropriate. And some parents, facing a lack of educators with appropriate knowledge, take the lead for instruction themselves.

Other family members – aunts and uncles, grandparents, siblings, and other relatives – share the responsibility. Often someone other than the parents (even a fairly young child) happens to have the best opportunity to teach a particular thing.

In a residential school, the houseparent is much like a part-time parent. Development of skill in travel is a part of this responsibility.

Specialized Teachers

Specialized teachers of blind students typically take the lead in cane travel instruction. The lead instructor should outline a curriculum to develop skills in an organized manner. He/she should ensure that the child learns what is currently needed (as by emphasizing street-crossing immediately for a city child). At the same time, he/she should make sure no major age-appropriate skill is completely omitted. (For example, a rural high school student should visit a larger town and work with traffic lights.)

The specialized instructor must not exist in an "ivory tower" in solitary splendor. Continual consultation with parents and with other teachers is essential. Specific practical suggestions, with demonstrations as needed, enable other adults to guide the child in integrated, consistent progress.

At times, the specialized instructor may play additional roles by default. If the parent, despite much consultation, never takes the child along to a store, the instructor should spend extra time with this. If the sixth grade teacher has promised to show the blind student the way to the rest room, but somehow this is not happening, the travel teacher may need to assist.

Similarly, there are many places around the school where the class may not go as a group, but which sighted students will understand through sight. The flagpole and the kitchen are two good examples. Sighted students see the flags flying and occasionally watch the custodian run them up and down. They see the kitchen when they walk by in the lunch line. But the blind 6-year-old may not know what a flag and its pulleys are actually like (he cannot reach the flag in the classroom either). He hears the clatter of the kitchen, but may not really understand what is there. When the travel teacher's lesson focuses on a single interesting location, it provides great interest and variety (vital for the young child) as well as filling in gaps in concepts.

Gaps in knowledge can occur at home also. The travel teacher may conduct many lessons near the home of a preschooler who is just learning to get around in a large yard and the nearby neighborhood. The teacher may help an older student walk between home and school, between home and the bus stop, between home and a nearby convenience store, etc.

Classroom Teachers and Activity Leaders
Many different teachers carry out activities which relate to these Modules. Day care providers, as well as school and preschool classroom teachers, are included. Leaders of Scout troops, religious groups, and other activities will also find this book relevant.

Routinely, preschool and elementary-school groups tour the dentist's office, the zoo, the grocery store, the City Hall, etc. Leaders will find these Modules helpful in making each excursion an age-appropriate learning experience.

When the specialized teacher introduces a skill, others must encourage and remind the child to keep it up. They must see that opportunities exist to put the skill into practice.

The Instructor Who Is Blind
The Module, "The Blind Travel Instructor," provides suggestions on alternative techniques. The parent or teacher who is blind or visually impaired will find this Module helpful. If the instructor has some other disability, these suggestions can provide a starting point for ideas. The National Federation of the Blind will be pleased to provide specific suggestions and the names of instructors who have disabilities.

The *Handbook for Itinerant and Resource Teachers of Blind and Visually Impaired Students* includes two examples of successful blind teachers.

Techniques Used by Blind Cane Travel Instructors, by Maria Morais *et al.,* deals with this subject in depth. (See REFERENCES at the end of this book for complete bibliographical information.)

PROVIDING CANES

The Module, "Description of Basic Techniques," includes discussion about the kind of cane and its length.

Even with something as inexpensive as a cane, the price is a problem for many parents—especially when a growing child needs a longer cane every few months. At the same time, school administrators (with budgeting problems of their own) often regard the cane as a personal item which should not be furnished.

An excellent solution is a "cane bank" or "cane exchange," now provided in many states by the

National Federation of the Blind and/or other organizations. Canes of various lengths are available for loan; when the child outgrows a cane, it is exchanged for a longer one. Organizations such as the Lions Clubs and the Delta Gamma sorority are often willing to pay for canes – either for a cane bank or for an individual.

TEACHING STRATEGIES

First, do not look at travel training as a series of exercises designed only to teach students to follow specific routes. What you want are travelers who will go wherever in the world they want to go. You want to liberate students, not make them dependent upon you forever more. I have had a number of students who requested such retraining. Had they been trained properly the first time, a change of location would not have presented a problem to them (as it does not to me).

Second, you want to arrange for the student to have frequent successes. Nothing will destroy confidence more than many consecutive failures. Although I do ask students to repeat routes from time to time, I rarely ask for a third try immediately. I may do something else for the next lesson or two and come back to it later if the particular lesson is necessary. Altering the route while teaching the same concepts can work also.

Third, ask of your students a little less than you believe they can actually do. Growing confidence will result from repeated successes. This does not mean that you should interfere in order to arrange for these successes. Good planning will work better, since every time you interfere, you project the message that students cannot do it by themselves. In the beginning this may be true at times, and you will need to teach thinking skills, how to handle traffic patterns, etc.

I generally believe my students can do much more than they think they can do. I know how their fears can be resolved, so that although I am aware of their fears, I do not let this knowledge obstruct training – instead, I use it in my lesson designs. I do not avoid situations that students fear. Rather, I work to reduce fear by arranging ways for students to face these fears in a way designed to yield positive results. The best strategy is to challenge students to do the very things they fear the most, in ways that they can handle.

Fourth, do not leave all of the hard or frightening things till last. If a student fears something and you wait a long time before tackling it, his fear alone may bar success in accomplishing it.

WORKING TOGETHER

Continual consultation with parents, educators, and the student is essential.

Mrs. Pollock had taught Chip to walk independently to the principal's office for errands. However, several weeks later she learned that he still went with another student at all times – usually forgetting his cane. She also learned he often got lost between the classroom and the rest room, despite having gone there "independently" for many months. Mrs. Pollock decided to send a brief list of specific questions to the teachers once a month.

The written form helped everyone to keep track more objectively and precisely. (Caution: Lengthy questionnaires tend to alienate busy teachers. Mrs. Pollock wisely wrote a simple checklist which could be answered in five minutes or less.)

Classroom teachers were asked to mark "A" for "Essentially Always," "S" for "Sometimes," and "R" for "Rarely," on items such as:

    Does Chip go to and from the rest room without help, in the same timeframe expected of others?

    Does he use his cane whenever he is walking around (except when actually engaging in a sport)?

    When he is seated, is his cane within easy reach yet positioned to avoid tripping others?

    Does he walk to and from the playground without help?

    In the lunch line, is he independent except for the kinds of help we discussed at our last meeting?

    Does he walk to and from the school bus

independently?

When errands to familiar locations within the school are assigned, does he go alone on the same basis as others?

Comments _____

Mrs. Pollock also arranged to observe regular class procedures herself occasionally, especially when students were moving around.

In the *Handbook for Itinerant and Resource Teachers of Blind and Visually Impaired Students,* the following chapters particularly analyze relationships among the various adults who are helping a child:

"General Classroom Arrangements and Study Skills" (pp. 225-238)

"Starting Anew Each Time" (pp. 363-376)

"Scheduling" (pp. 377-384)

"Working in Partnership With Parents" (pp. 393-400)

"Your Professional Role" (pp. 401-412)

"Paraprofessionals and Volunteers" (pp. 423-428)

"Working With Other Agencies and Organizations" (pp. 429-434)

If you are a teacher, follow standard procedures about parent permission before taking a child on an excursion. If you are a parent, talk with the school before planning to tour or visit. Whatever your role, ask permission before going onto private property. These things may seem obvious but are often slighted, causing ill feelings.

Introduce yourself. Talk about the student's progress, and about the weather (but not too long, and not at a time that is bad for the other person). Attend meetings, formal and informal. Ask for and give feedback. Don't be a fragmented, isolated person apart.

A college professor arrived to observe a student teacher in an itinerant position. The importance of being well-acquainted had been discussed often. The professor recorded a compliment even before the lesson began. "When I asked for you at the office," she smiled, "they KNEW WHO YOU WERE!"

REFERENCE(S):

Willoughby and Duffy. *Handbook for Itinerant and Resource Teachers of Blind and Visually Impaired Students.*

Richard Mettler. *Cognitive Learning Theory and Cane Travel Instruction: A New Paradigm.*

Maria Morais *et al. Techniques Used by Blind Cane Travel Instructors—A Practical Approach: Learning, Teaching, Believing.*

CHAPTER C

INTRODUCTION
By Sharon L. Monthei

[*Note: Sharon L. Monthei was formerly known as Sharon L. M. Duffy.*]

A friend of mine described the travel lessons of her childhood like this: "The teacher would take me to a place within a building using sighted guide. Then, she would give me directions to go down the hall and find the third door on the right and return to her. After that, she would take me back to class using sighted guide."

This book is intended to help teachers know how to avoid such meaningless exercises by setting out specifics regarding how cane travel can help a blind youngster become independent in every setting. Traveling with a cane should be an integral part of life for a blind child, and, with good training and encouragement from supportive adults, can help enable her to be as independent as any sighted child of the same age.

Unfortunately, independent travel for blind children isn't the norm yet; however, my hope is that this book will help to make it the norm—that blind children will have the freedom that I only acquired after training as an adult.

I was thirteen when I got my first cane, but I didn't learn to use it effectively until I was required to have it with me at all times and to have regular practice in using it. Originally, I was so negatively inclined toward my cane that I believed I would quit using it when my training was over. But after I'd used it for about three months, it became such a useful tool for my independence that I have never seriously considered putting it down—even though at age 23 I had eye surgery which improved my vision to 20/400 in my left eye. My lack of depth perception and my understanding of the need to let people know that I am a blind person have kept me using my cane faithfully to this day.

Not only have I continued to use my own cane, but I have spent a considerable portion of my career training other blind people to use a long white cane. I have taught blind children and adults in many and varied settings: in Des Moines, Iowa, and rural communities nearby; in Boise, Idaho, and in rural areas there; in the Chicago metro area; in Alamogordo, New Mexico; and in Minneapolis.

I am now working as an independent contractor, working mainly with computers. Although I no longer teach travel regularly, I remain committed to seeing that blind people receive what may be their most important skill for independence. In my experience, independent cane travel is something anyone can learn with proper training, if the person has reasonably good health and is within the average range of intelligence or higher.

Like most things worth having, good travel skills require concerted effort and considerable practice, but they are eminently achievable. I hope the readers of this book will make it come true for the blind youth of this country.

MODULES

BASIC TECHNIQUES

MODULE 1
DESCRIPTION OF
BASIC TECHNIQUES
Including Stairway Technique
By Sharon L. Monthei

ABOUT THIS "MODULE":

This chapter, or Module, consists of a *description* of basic techniques in the use of the cane. There are many illustrations.

Since the topic is so broad, many of the elements given in most Modules are not given here—Objectives, for example. Other elements are placed or handled in a different way—for example, the "See Also" references to other Modules are at the beginning of each subtopic.

The topics included in this chapter/module are as follows:

> THE CANE AS A SYMBOL
> THE LENGTH OF THE CANE
> WHICH CANE TO USE
> THE TOUCH TECHNIQUE
> SLIDING TECHNIQUES
> LANDMARK LOCATION
> STAIRWAY TECHNIQUES
> ESCALATORS
> REVOLVING DOORS
> CONCLUSION

This chapter/module concentrates on how a person holds and manipulates the cane itself. A number of things which are "basic" in some respects are not discussed until later Modules—for example, street crossing. The Index, the Table of Contents, and comments within the various Modules will help the reader locate specific topics.

This chapter/module is intended as a reference. It is assumed that the instructor will refer to other Modules for detailed suggestions about *how* to teach each technique. When the instructor is reading one of the other Modules, he/she can refer to this chapter/module for more detailed description of the techniques themselves.

AGE OF STUDENT: All Ages

PRIMARY SKILL EMPHASIS:

Posture, grip, gait, and arc
General travel
Doors and doorways
Obstacles in path
Detecting step-downs or drop-offs
Landmarks
Moving straight ahead
Stairs
Attitudes toward blindness
Escalators

NOTE: The techniques described in this chapter are relevant to the practice of virtually any skill.

SEE ALSO (Other Modules):

> (References to other Modules appear at the beginning of each subtopic.)

FIGURE(S):

FIGURE 1-1: Hand Position
FIGURE 1-2: Touch Technique
FIGURE 1-3: Going Up Steps
FIGURE 1-4: Going Down Steps

THE CANE AS A SYMBOL:

Many people resist using a cane, because they imagine that it represents dependence. They are ashamed of being blind (or of their relatives being blind, in the case of family members). However, the cane is actually a symbol of independence since it is the means for a blind person to travel safely by himself.

Most adolescents are sensitive regarding any difference that they may have from the average—weight, relative height, ethnic origin, blindness, etc. It is not surprising, then, that a junior high age student may object strongly to carrying a white cane, because she feels this advertises this difference. It does do this; however, it is most unlikely that other children are unaware of a classmate's blindness anyway. It isn't a deep, dark secret, although many blind teenagers wish it were.

It is very important for a teacher to deal directly with these negative feelings about canes, and also about sleep shades (a very similar issue). It is respectable to be blind; and this must be said and expressed in every action, because society's attitudes about blindness are generally so negative.

One of the best ways to combat negative public attitudes is for the student to get to know a number of blind adults who use canes regularly, and, if possible, establish an ongoing relationship with competent blind people. The National Federation of the Blind is an excellent vehicle for this.

Ken did not think it was "macho" to carry a cane until he became friends with a blind man whom he admired. After that, he perceived other people's negative comments about the cane as ignorant, and, in fact, felt more "macho" at being able to maintain his position that carrying a cane was a good idea.

THE LENGTH OF THE CANE:

There is some debate about the appropriate length of the cane. Blind people have found through experience that the length of the cane is an individual matter, depending upon the length of stride, walking speed, and reflexes of the student. To consider the length of the cane, hold it vertically in front of the individual: ordinarily it should reach somewhere between the armpit and the nose. Shoulder height is a good length for a first cane. A cane reaching only to the sternum (breastbone) is not long enough for the average student to assume a normal walking speed with safety. The cane must be long enough to allow a student two steps to stop.

Generally speaking, a traveler will want a longer cane as speed is developed, and this should be left up to the student who is an experienced traveler. The desire for a longer cane should be viewed as a positive sign.

One way to check whether a cane is the right length is to observe where the foot steps in relationship to the cane touch which would cover it (i.e., the place where the cane last touched on that side). If the foot touches approximately the same place the cane did, the cane is the right length. If the foot touches in front of where the cane touched, the cane is too short. If the foot touches significantly behind where the cane touched, the cane is too long. (Or, occasionally, the stride may be found to be much too short.)

The cane also must reach two steps ahead on stairs. Although shoulder height is a good length for an adult's first cane, this tends to be too short for a young child. For children, generally the cane should reach as high as the nose when held vertically.

Since children grow, it is necessary to change cane lengths periodically. Some National Federation of the Blind state affiliates have cane banks for kids, so that canes in children's sizes are available on loan and can be traded in when necessary. Since it would not be unusual for a child to change canes ten or more times from early childhood through adolescence, this is a considerable saving.

WHICH CANE TO USE:

The best cane currently on the market is called the "NFB straight cane." It is hollow fiberglass with a rubber and metal tip and plastic cylindrical handle. This cane is the most sensitive because it is light and flexible, is made in one piece, and has a metal tip which provides information both through touch and sound. It also weighs only a few ounces so that small hands do not become tired using it. Because of its construction, it can be used with either hand or switched from hand to hand when convenient. It is available in children's sizes (with handle and shank properly proportioned for small hands) from the National Federation of the Blind at the National Center for the Blind.

In my opinion, the next best cane on the market is sometimes called a Rainshine™ cane after the company which manufactures it, and also sometimes called the Iowa cane. It is solid fiberglass and is otherwise much like the NFB straight cane. It is not quite as sensitive or as light as the NFB straight cane. Some people prefer this cane because it is virtually indestructible.

Many other straight canes are rigid, have nylon tips which do not slide easily, and provide little information about substances touched. They wear in such a way as to make the cane either left- or right-handed. (This problem is partly due to the "golf grip" handle often used.)

Collapsible canes have one main disadvantage – they *do* collapse. They are not very sturdy because they are held together either by nylon cord or by telescoping joints. The movement of the cane shakes the pieces apart. Because they are not one solid piece, they do not telegraph information as accurately. Many blind people buy them so that they can collapse them when they don't want people to know they are blind. Use of a collapsible cane encourages avoidance of facing the real issues of blindness.

If a collapsible cane is used at all, the best use is as an extra to be kept in reserve. For example, it might be kept in the desk at work in case something happens to the regular cane.

THE TOUCH TECHNIQUE:

SEE ALSO (Other Modules):

Introducing the Cane
Posture, Gait, and Arc (Level Surface)
Obstacles (Noting Them and Proceeding)
Sleep Shades (Occluders)
In a Crowd (Including Stairway Technique)
AT SCHOOL – INDOORS

This basic technique is sometimes called arcing the cane, or the foot cane technique. It is used in most situations. It is achieved by holding the cane in the dominant hand with the index finger pointing down the shaft, and the thumb and other fingers curled around the cane – a position analogous to shaking hands with the cane (Figure 1-1).

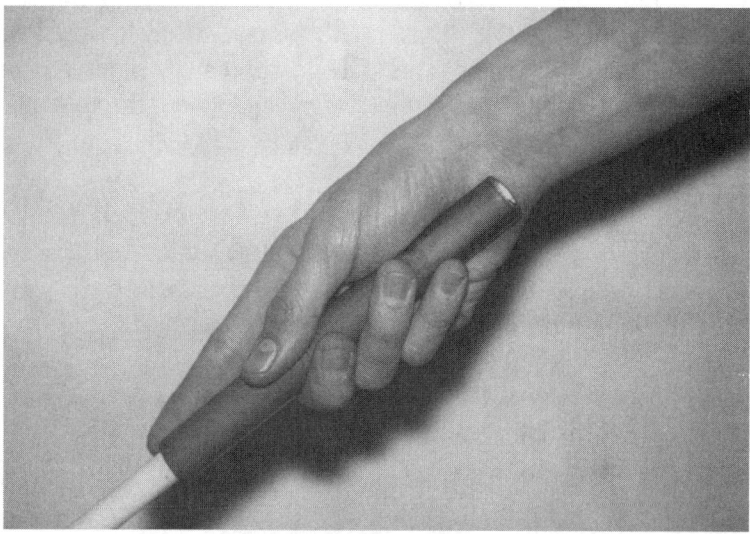

Figure 1-1
Hand Position

The cane is swung from side to side and should cover the ground approximately the width of the traveler's shoulders. When the right foot is forward, the cane should touch on the left side, and when the left foot is forward, the cane should touch on the right side – one tap per step. The hand should be centered in front of the body with the primary action in the wrist. (Keeping the forearm against the waist or hip helps to center the hand and prevent fatigue.) The elbow may be bent comfortably. (Figure 1-2).

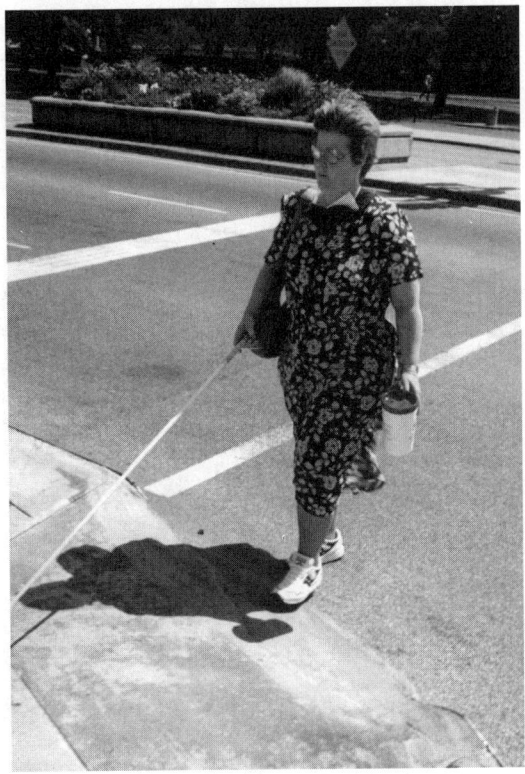

**Figure 1-2
Touch Technique**

The reason the cane should touch on the opposite side from the forward foot is to maintain a two-step warning for objects and steps encountered. A traveler who is out of step is clearing only one step ahead and may miss some objects altogether until they are encountered with the body.

The arc of the cane should be even on either side. If a traveler tends to drift either left or right, observe that the traveler is probably arcing farther in that direction than on the other side. Also, if the hand does not remain centered, a variation in the arc may occur, and the traveler will have more difficulty developing good distance perception with the cane. Distance perception can also be thrown off by changing the length of cane.

In crowded areas, the cane can be moved into a more upright position, causing some variation in grip and slowing of walking speed. Normally, a cane traveler should be able to walk as fast as a sighted person in similar physical condition.

SLIDING TECHNIQUES:

Sliding the cane rather than tapping it may occasionally be desirable. For example, when traveling next to a parking lot, there may be a substantial crack or ridge between the sidewalk and the parking lot. The cane may be slid across from one side to the other until it encounters the crack or ridge. This technique is of limited value since a crack or ridge may not be detected easily.

Ordinarily, the cane should be tapped rather than slid, to avoid sticking and the premature wearing out of cane tips. Also, the sound of the tap provides information about the surface touched and (by means of echo) the proximity of buildings, etc. Many good travelers vary cane techniques to suit the travel situation.

LANDMARK LOCATION:

SEE ALSO (Other Modules):

Obstacles (Noting Them and Proceeding)
Right and Left
Doors and Doorways
Sidewalks
AT SCHOOL – INDOORS
AT SCHOOL – OUTDOORS

Locating doorways, perpendicular sidewalks, etc., can be done by arcing the cane as usual but extending the arc a little farther to one side to contact the side of the building, the side of the hallway, or the grass. The touch on the opposite side should be in the usual place. It will be necessary for the traveler to walk close to the grass or the wall.

Note that when one is *not* looking for a doorway or a perpendicular sidewalk, one should *not* hug the wall or the edge of the grass.

STAIRWAY TECHNIQUES:

SEE ALSO (Other Modules):

    Introducing the Cane (Including Stairway Technique)
    Carrying Things
    Routes for New Buildings and New Classrooms
    Exterior Fire Escape
    Unexpected Drop-off or Step-Down
    Visually Confusing Appearance
    Stairs in Unfamiliar Buildings
    General Overview (Buildings)
    AT SCHOOL – INDOORS

To go upstairs, the cane should be held in an upright position, with the tip just below the second step above the traveler, approximately in the center of the body. After a quick sweep at the start to measure the width of the stairs, the traveler should proceed with the hand held still and with the cane tip encountering each successive step. At the top of the flight of stairs, the traveler will have two steps' warning. (Figure 1-3)

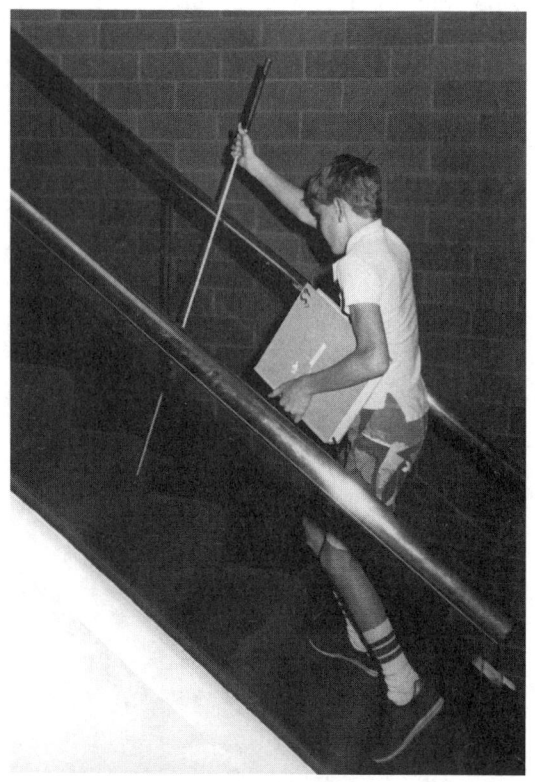

Figure 1-3
Going Up Steps

In descending the stairs, ordinarily the cane should not be tapped from side to side. The arm may be relaxed at the side of the body. The cane tip should extend just beyond the second step below the traveler, approximately centered in front of the body, and the tip should slide down each succeeding step. (See Figure 1-4) Again, the cane will give two steps' warning. Using this technique, it is not necessary to hold the handrail.

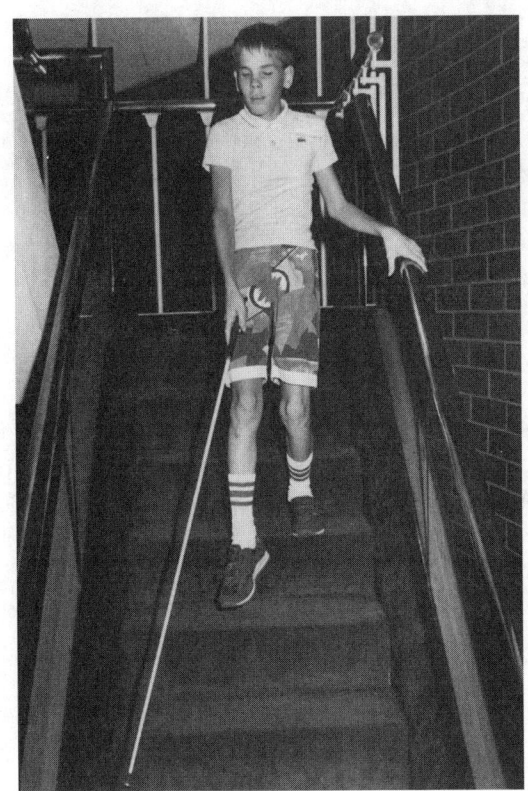

**Figure 1-4
Going Down Steps**

ESCALATORS:

SEE ALSO (Other Modules):

Escalators
Malls
The Airport (And Air Travel)

Escalators frequently make a low-pitched noise or a squeak and thus can be located by sound. The cane should contact the moving stairs and the student may put a hand on the rail before actually stepping on. Thus the direction of the escalator is easily determined.

After the traveler steps on, the cane should rest two steps ahead.

When the stairs flatten out or the cane is bumped by the stationary step, it is time to step off.

REVOLVING DOORS:

SEE ALSO (Other Modules):

Doors and Doorways
General Overview (Buildings)
PUBLIC BUILDINGS – GENERAL
PUBLIC BUILDINGS: SPECIFIC
    EXAMPLES

There is no right or wrong way to negotiate revolving doors. I prefer to put my cane out and make contact with the revolving door to judge where it is and step in. It may be slightly safer to approach from the left in order to minimize the likelihood of smashing the cane in the door.

The Module, "General Overview (Buildings)," contains detailed suggestions for teaching a beginner to use a revolving door.

CONCLUSION:

The preceding are suggested techniques, not to be confused with absolute rules. I know a man who holds his cane in an unusual way and moves his hand continuously. However, he manages to touch his cane in the right places for optimum safety and has excellent distance perception and is overall an excellent traveler. Variation of any technique should not be discouraged unless it does not work, presents a really bad appearance, or provides unnecessary danger to others.

Two things make a good cane traveler – a positive attitude about traveling, and effective techniques. This chapter has provided a list and description of time-tested techniques. The progress of the student, together with the curriculum plan, will determine just when each is taught.

MODULE 2
INTRODUCING THE CANE
Including Stairway Technique

NOTE: The Module, "Description of Basic Techniques," has detailed description of the techniques themselves. This Module, "Introducing the Cane," is oriented toward actual lesson planning. Also note that the Module, "Stairs in Unfamiliar Buildings," describes additional practice.

OBJECTIVE: The student will state the purpose of the cane. He/she will demonstrate basic technique on level ground, with obstacles, and on stairs.

AGE OF STUDENT: This Module is divided under three major subheadings:
(A) Preschool/Kindergarten
(B) Primary Grades
(C) Fourth grade and above.

PRIMARY SKILL EMPHASIS:
Posture, grip, gait, and arc
General travel
Attitudes toward blindness
Obstacles in path
Stairs

ADDITIONAL SKILL EMPHASIS:
Detecting step-downs or drop-offs
Right and left
Sound direction and meaning
Sidewalk
Stowing cane
Landmarks

SEE ALSO (Other Modules):
OVERVIEW AND GENERAL PRINCIPLES (introductory chapters)
Description of Basic Techniques (Including Stairway Technique)
Posture, Gait, and Arc
Obstacles
Sleep Shades
Stairs in Unfamiliar Buildings
Sidewalks
Rural Environment
Doors and Doorways

(A) PRESCHOOL AND KINDERGARTEN:

TEACHER PREPARATION: Look for a safe, convenient place where there are easy-to-detect changes of terrain and easy-to-find obstacles. An example is a playground which has contrast between hard surface and grass, and also has various play equipment.

Select a cane of appropriate length.

FIGURE(S):
FIGURE 2-1: Here we go!
FIGURE 2-2: I can do it myself!

REMARKS: This description assumes the child is very young (kindergarten or below) and has had no previous experience with a cane.

It also assumes that the teacher has already built rapport through other activities. If this is not true, it is wise to schedule at least one get-acquainted session beforehand, in which nothing new is taught. Familiar activities should be enjoyed while initially building rapport.

Sleep shades should also be introduced beforehand in a manner appropriate for a young child. (See the Module, "Sleep Shades.") They should be worn during each lesson with the cane.

It is usually not advisable to attempt to teach "keeping in step" at first with a very young child. Help her to move the cane from side to side but do not expect her to keep in step.

ACTIVITIES:

EXAMPLE 1: *INITIAL LESSON WITH CANE*
(Preschool/Kindergarten)

"Today I'm going to show you something very interesting. Let's sit down and look at it. This is a nice new white *cane*. It even smells new!"

Encourage the child to reach for the cane. Try to note hand preference, though many young children have not developed a clear preference.

Help the child examine the cane – its handle, shaft, and tip.

"This white cane is for you. It can help you walk faster and not get bumped. I'll show you how it works."

Help the child put on the sleep shades if they are not already on. Place the cane in her hand and gently place her fingers around it in essentially the standard grip. Take hold of her and move her through the motions of taking a few steps on level ground, while talking about how handy the cane can be. (I prefer to walk slightly behind and to the right of the child, with my left hand on her left shoulder, and with my right hand on her hand to help her hold the cane.)

"We're walking on the sidewalk now. Notice how the cane makes a nice tap, tap on the hard sidewalk. Now, soon we're going to come to something softer. Let's see if you can tell me when the cane taps something a lot softer than sidewalk." (Help the child recognize when the grass is found.)

Practice for a short while as she repeatedly walks a few steps on one surface and then recognizes the other surface. Let go of her at least part of the time, allowing her to walk alone and hold the cane herself, even though technique may be very imperfect at this time. Point out that the cane reaches ahead and recognizes the surface before her feet actually get there.

"Now let's look at another thing the cane can do. Sometimes, when we walk along, we find something in the way. If we don't know it, we may get bumped. But the cane can tell you what's there, so you won't get bumped."

Holding onto the child, as above, walk her toward a piece of playground equipment. Help her strike it firmly with the cane several times to aid in understanding. Discuss what the equipment is, and have the child feel it with her hands as a confirmation.

Repeat as the child finds other obstacles with her cane. Again, part of the time she should walk by herself and hold the cane herself; imperfect technique is acceptable at this point, as long as the cane is in front with the tip touching the ground.

You may choose to "steer" the child toward obstacles so that they are quickly encountered.

"So, what are two kinds of things the cane can find?....Yes, it can find the swing or monkey bars. And it can tell you if you're walking on something hard or soft. You know, some people say the cane can talk! It tells you what is there, ahead of you. It's a good thing to have."

In conclusion, allow the child to play on the equipment.

VARIATION(S):

For an especially immature child, a single session should include only one kind of task – e.g., only detecting the change of surface.

If the initial lesson is done indoors, carpet and tile are a good surface contrast. Walls and furniture provide obstacles. If a good setting is not conveniently available, move furniture or boxes to create one.

Some teachers prefer to introduce the cane by using one themselves (an adult-sized cane) and having the small student walk more or less under it, holding on as the cane is moved by the adult. This technique is shown in the video, *Kids With Canes*. (See REFERENCES.)

For some very young children (especially aged three and under), it may be helpful to slide the cane back and forth rather than tap it. Speed of walking will be slower, but the constant contact with the surface can be helpful. This technique can be phased out after awhile.

REMARKS:
(1) If the child is relatively mature, the lessons should be approached much as described for the primary grades.
(2) Discuss with the parent (and/or classroom teacher) beforehand to consider when the child should take the cane along after the first lesson. An immature preschool child may only gradually reach the point of using the cane regularly. A kindergartner, however, may be ready and eager to keep the cane after only one lesson. (Classroom teachers and parents should be prepared to supplement instruction. Perfect technique would not be expected immediately. But the cane could be used in a limited way immediately, and the expectation of regular, normal use would be established at once.)

EXAMPLE 2: *INTRODUCING STAIRWAY TECHNIQUE*
(Preschool/Kindergarten)

With an older student, stairway technique should be introduced almost immediately. It is a more individual matter with a very young child, for several reasons:

- Very small children with no disabilities are often assisted on stairs, especially where there are no railings. A standard-sized step is very large compared to the legs of a three- or four-year-old.
- A young child learning one technique (e.g., arcing the cane on level terrain) may be quite confused if quickly introduced to another one.
- In many environments, there are no steps. The steps in the home (if indeed there are any) are so familiar that it is difficult to demonstrate the value of the cane.
- For a very young child, constantly closely supervised anyway, it is acceptable to gain independence in one respect while lacking it in another.

For reasons such as these, a child of this age may build cane skills on flat terrain for several weeks or months before the stairway technique is taught. If steps are encountered while the cane is being used, the child might (1) simply carry the cane on the steps, rather than actually using it, (2) continue arcing it, more or less as she would do on a flat surface, while moving up or down stairs – in effect, using a somewhat non-standard technique.

Before a great many months have elapsed, however, the standard technique for stairs should be introduced.

Before introducing the cane on stairs, determine how the child has previously dealt with stairs. This example assumes that her parents have warned her of steps and held her hand. On occasion she has walked alone while holding the rail, with an adult close by.

Some young children form the habit of holding the rail with *two* hands and moving sideways. Work with the family to eliminate this, even when the cane is not used. Holding the child's free hand is usually the simplest approach (to be phased out later when the habit has been overcome). Hold the child's hand when the cane is used, also: keep your hand around the hand that holds the cane, while the child's other hand is on the railing.

With a young child, it is usually best to begin by *adding* the use of the cane to the method already familiar to the child – e.g., holding onto an adult's hand and/or the railing. Then, gradually, the child can begin to use the cane alone.

"Here we are at the stairs near the Laundromat. You've come here with your mother lots of times. I'll take your hand like your mom does, and you show me how you can go up and down stairs..."

"Great! We went up and down two times now. I see you really know how to go up and down stairs..."

"You've been just kind of carrying your cane, and that's OK. But now I'm going to show you how your cane can really help on stairs. We'll go up again, and this time I'll hold onto you a little differently, and I'll make your cane do something new...."

INTRODUCING THE CANE

With close physical assistance, help the child to walk up the stairs with the cane in approximately the standard position. If there is a railing, this may be done by helping her to keep one hand on the rail while using the cane with the other.

It may be wise to work only on going up during the first such lesson, with the child going back down in her former manner.

Proceed in a similar manner to introduce walking downstairs with the cane touching each step in approximately the standard way.

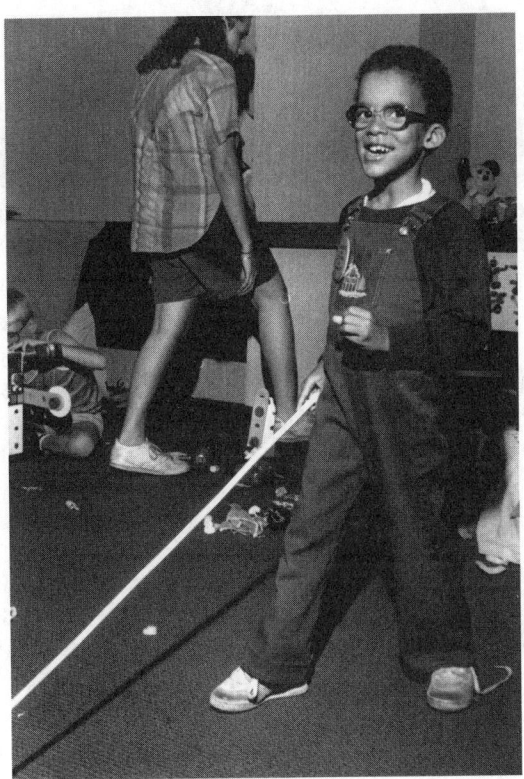

Figure 2-2
I can do it myself!

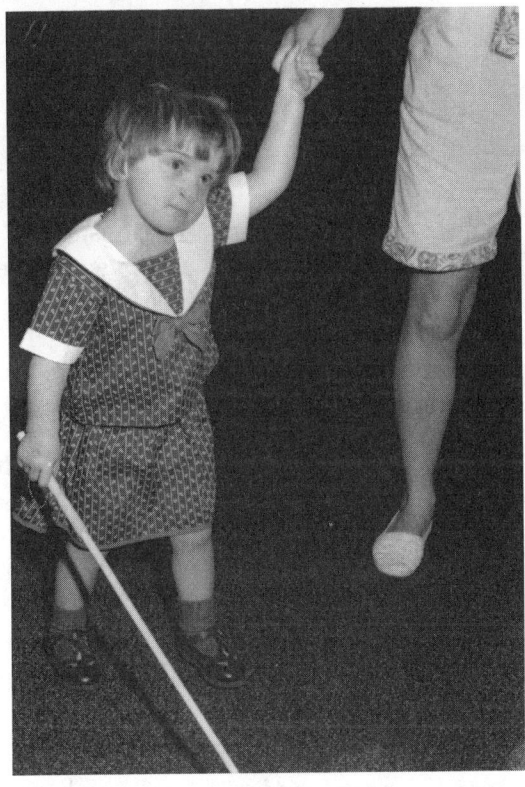

Figure 2-1
Here we go!

(B) PRIMARY GRADES:
(Grades 1, 2, and 3 – approximately ages 6-9)

REMARKS: This description assumes a primary-grade student of average maturity. It is suggested that the activities below be spread out over several sessions. However, see also the descriptions for older and younger students; avoid arbitrary assumptions about ability based on age alone.

TEACHER PREPARATION:
Be well informed about the student's current understanding of the purpose of the cane, and his/her experience (if any) in trying one out and observing cane usage by other people.

Talk beforehand with parents and classroom teachers. Develop an organized plan for when the student will begin using the cane outside of lessons, and how others will help her build skill. See that other students learn what the cane is for, so that they do not move it or interfere with it.

EXAMPLE 3: *INTRODUCTORY LESSON*
(Grades 1-3)
Locate a safe, easy area for the first lesson.

Taking into account the child's age, previous experience, and knowledge, explain the purpose of the cane in an appropriate manner. Be sure the student understands that skills will be taught gradually. (A child could misunderstand and believe she will instantly be expected to take on many new tasks alone.)

Help the child put on sleep shades. [They have been introduced before the actual lesson with the cane. See the Module, "Sleep Shades."]

It is important to discuss the purpose of the cane and sleep shades. Avoid, however, cajoling the student in such a way that she might regard the work as optional. If the decision for cane lessons has already been made by the adults, the lesson should be approached in a manner similar to any other – math, reading, physical education, etc. Each teacher tries to make the lesson pleasant and relevant, but makes it clear that the student will do what is expected.

Help the student examine the cane and name its parts. Verify its length as appropriate.

Help the child grasp the cane and begin to use it. Combine explanation with physical guidance. A typical progression for the first lesson would be:

- Tap the cane from side to side several times, without walking.
- Walk on level terrain, while continuing to arc the cane.
- Discuss the width of the arc: "The cane needs to tap back and forth in front of each foot. Then it will protect you from things that might bump you on either side. If I stand behind you, I should see that the tip goes just a little bit to each side, just a little bit past your feet."
- Approach an obstacle and note when the cane finds it.
- Walk onto a different surface – as, from carpet to bare floor – and note how the cane indicates this.
- Continue walking around in the chosen area, finding obstacles and changes of surface.

Unless the student is particularly mature with good coordination, it is best not to mention at first that the cane should be tapped in front of the foot which is not leading. Instead, first merely explain that "the cane tip should go back and forth, in front of your feet," and demonstrate. (See the Module, "Posture, Gait, and Arc," for continuing explanation.)

At the end of the lesson (if not before) sit down briefly and show the student how to lay the cane on the floor. Discuss what has been learned. Anticipate increased independence and privileges.

Unless the student is particularly immature (see Preschool/Kindergarten, above, and other Modules), she should take the cane with her after her first lesson and expect to begin using it. At this point, it is expected that she will have help with stairs and other situations which she may not have learned to handle independently. In easy settings, she will begin to walk independently with minimal help. She will stow the cane appropriately when seated, playing a game, or in her own home.

EXAMPLE 4: *STAIRS*
(*Grades 1-3*)

Discuss how the cane has been used since the last session. What successes have occurred? Have there been problems or questions? Do classmates and others understand the use of the cane and not interfere with it?

Some children enjoy giving the cane a humorous name such as "Snoopy."

Review the grip and stance. Work briefly on any postural errors, but do not expect perfection.

Review walking on the level. Find easy obstacles such as walls and large objects. Note terrain underfoot.

Approach a stairway which goes up. Physically show the student the technique for going up stairs. (See also the Modules, "Description of Basic Techniques, Including Stairway Techniques" and "Stairs in Unfamiliar Buildings.") It is helpful to go up first, since walking upstairs usually seems easier for the beginner.

After walking up one or two flights, have the student walk some distance away from the stairs. Then, with close guidance, help her approach the stairs and note how clearly the cane detects a step-down. Repeating this (that is, walking away from the stairs and then returning to detect the step-down) may be helpful. Show the student the technique for going downstairs, and proceed down at least one flight.

Depending on maturity, the student may need much assistance at first on stairs. It is acceptable, if needed, to hold onto her and guide her constantly. She will probably benefit from holding the rail at first, if there is one. (However, strongly discourage the tendency of some young students to hold the rail with *both* hands.) With a less mature student, consider this a "readiness" lesson for stairs, to give some familiarity with the technique without expecting independence at this time. Some students need considerable help on stairs for many months, but meanwhile gain greatly in skill on level ground.

With a student who is particularly nervous or immature, it may also be helpful to work on a very short flight of steps at first, if available (e.g., three steps leading up to the front door).

Show parents and classroom teachers the techniques for stairs. Encourage them to help the student improve.

EXAMPLE 5: *SIDEWALK*
(*Grades 1-3*)

Review general posture and grip. Discuss progress so far.

Go outdoors to a sidewalk which is rather typical, without curves or other major irregularities. Note the sound made by the cane on the hard cement. Have the student walk for some distance (at least a block), practicing all aspects of posture.

Help her understand when the cane tip encounters grass at the side. Pause to examine the grass with the cane the first time it is found; the student may also want to touch the grass with her hands or step onto it, to verify what the cane is indicating. After the first instance, however, the student should expect to use the cane alone to determine the terrain.

Proceed along the straight stretch of sidewalk. Part of the time, help the student walk fairly straight. Guide her with a hand on her shoulder if necessary, to help her experience walking normally on a sidewalk.

Part of the time, she should walk alone. Help her make an appropriate correction when she touches the edge of the walk. (See the Modules, "Description of Basic Techniques (Including Stairway Technique" and "Sidewalks.")

At the end of the block, find the curb, noting that the street is there (but probably not crossing the street at this time).

REMARKS: At this point, the student has been introduced to all the most common techniques, though they are not yet mastered. Talk with parents and teachers about how much to expect. Help them to foster growing independence without frustrating the child by unrealistic expectations. Plan how to keep others informed of new skill levels as you note they are achieved. (Example: You will write a note to the teachers, with a copy to the parents, every two weeks during the year. You will summarize any new learning; any skill being particularly emphasized and reviewed; any problems or difficulties. Every nine weeks there will be a conference for complete discussion.)

Arrange continued contact with other blind persons who make good use of cane travel skills.

(C) INTERMEDIATE GRADES AND UP: *(Age 10 and over)*

TEACHER PREPARATION:
Be well informed about the student's current understanding of the purpose of the cane, and his/her experience (if any) in trying one out and observing cane usage by other people.

Select a location with opportunity for easy walking.

REMARKS: It is important to discuss the purpose of the cane and sleep shades in a matter-of-fact and positive manner. Avoid, however, cajoling the student in such a way that she might regard basic procedures as optional. If the decision for cane lessons has already been made a part of the student's program, the lesson should be approached in a manner similar to any other–math, reading, physical education, etc. The teacher tries to make the lesson pleasant and relevant, but makes it clear that the student will do what is expected.

When the student is in her early teens or younger, if adults have made the decision for cane travel and present it in a positive way, it is usually possible to proceed even if she does not yet really see the merit. Valued privileges (such as going to various places alone) can be conditioned upon a certain level of skill. If a student is extremely uncooperative, negative consequences may be applied as they would for any other subject in the curriculum. (See pp. 385-392 in the *Handbook* for detailed discussion of motivation and philosophy.)

With an older teenager, however, it is essential to have at least partial agreement on the part of the student. If an older teenager strenuously disagrees with the idea of cane travel, it may not be possible to succeed with instruction. It may be necessary to have further discussions involving the student, parents, and others before proceeding.

A student 18 or over has the power to make decisions about her own education. Lessons would not begin without the student's approval. If at any time the student of this age raises serious questions about whether instruction should proceed, it should be fully discussed at once.

EXAMPLE 6: *INITIAL LESSON*
(Age 10 and over)

Review the purpose of the cane and sleep shades. Often this will have been done previously at some length, during a conference or other meeting, and a brief summary will suffice.

Ask the student to put on the sleep shades (assist as necessary). Examine the cane and verify its length. Show the student the appropriate grip and stance. Although less physical assistance is necessary than with a young child, some physical assistance is needed to prevent lengthy attempts at verbal description.

Ask the student to tap the cane back and forth a few times without starting to walk; discuss the width of the arc. Direct the student to practice walking in an easy location, with solid footing and few obstacles, and with no step-downs. Good examples include a long hallway; an empty part of a large room; a schoolyard or sidewalk. A student of this age should readily understand how the cane finds walls and other obstacles.

Explain how to keep in step–i.e., tap the cane in front of the foot which is not forward. Note that this provides the maximum amount of information–the cane taps as far in front of the respective foot as possible. Many students grasp this easily and need only occasional reminders. If it is hard for the student to keep in step, or if the attempt results in unnatural or very slow steps, disregard this part of the skill for a short while.

After a few minutes of practice, review the grip, stance, and general posture. If any unnatural or awkward motions have appeared because of inexperience or tension, work on correcting them. Emphasize the idea of normal posture, with the cane serving as a natural extension of one's own senses.

Approach a stairway from the bottom. Physically show the student the technique for going up stairs. (See the Module, "Description of Basic Techniques–Including Stairway Technique.")

Walking up usually seems easier for the beginner than walking down.

After going up one or two flights, ask the student to walk some distance away from the stairs. Then help the student approach the stairs; note how clearly the cane detects a step-down. (Repeating this – walking away from the stairs and then returning to detect the step-down – may be helpful.) Introduce the technique for going down stairs, and proceed down at least one flight.

At this point the student will probably feel more confident while holding the rail. Expect soon, however, that the student will not require this.

If the student has not yet walked outdoors, practice briefly on the cement. Note that the cane can detect the edges of the sidewalk and other changes in the surface.

After the introductory lesson, discuss what has been learned. Talk about what the student hopes to gain as skills are learned: added privileges, independence, comfort, confidence, etc. Ask for suggestions on what to work on in the next few lessons.

The student should take her cane with her and expect to use it henceforth (as well as she is able at any particular time).

Talk frequently with parents and other teachers as the student begins to use the cane. Watch for misunderstandings and difficulties which might interfere with a smooth beginning.

FOLLOW-UP: Arrange continued contact with competent blind persons who use canes regularly.

REMARKS: For less mature students of this age, see suggestions for younger age levels.

CAUTION: Some physical contact between teacher and student is necessary in demonstrating cane usage. However, the teacher must consider carefully just where and how the student should be touched. Avoid any appearance of touching in an overly personal manner.

REFERENCE(S):
Kids With Canes (video).

Future Reflections magazine.

Richard Mettler. *Cognitive Learning Theory and Cane Travel Instruction: A New Paradigm*, pp. 107-120.

MODULE 3
POSTURE, GAIT, AND ARC
Level Surface

NOTE: The Module, "Description of Basic Techniques," includes detailed information about the selection of a cane and the mechanics of basic cane usage, including stairway technique.

OBJECTIVE: 1. (*Preschool*) When walking on a level surface, the student will hold the cane appropriately and tap it from side to side in an arc slightly wider than his/her body.

OBJECTIVE: 2. (*Elementary grades and up*) When walking on a level surface, the student will hold the cane appropriately and tap it from side to side in an arc slightly wider than his/her body. He/she will "keep in step," so that the cane touches on the side where the foot is not forward.

AGE OF STUDENT: Preschool and up (See Objectives and Examples)

FIGURE(S):
FIGURE 3-1: Hand Position

PRIMARY SKILL EMPHASIS:
Posture, grip, gait, and arc
General travel
Obstacles in path
Detecting step-downs or drop-offs

ADDITIONAL SKILL EMPHASIS:
Moving straight ahead
Right and left
Corners, turns, and angles
Varied terrain

SEE ALSO (Other Modules):
Description of Basic Techniques
Introducing the Cane
Obstacles: Noting Them and Proceeding
Unexpected Drop-Off or Step-Down
Sleep Shades
In a Crowd
Doors and Doorways
Right and Left
Sidewalks
Rural Environment

TEACHER PREPARATION: When introducing the cane, try to determine hand preference. Children 8 and under may not be able to state this verbally, and the youngest children may not have developed a clear preference. Ask parents and teachers, and/or observe how the child performs various tasks—e.g., throwing a ball, brushing teeth, using crayons, eating, etc.

With a child of kindergarten age or below (or an older child whose maturity is in this range), carefully plan how to build rapport. At least one "get-acquainted" session, with familiar activities only, is important before starting instruction. Also, at this age it is best to introduce the sleep shades separately beforehand, in conjunction with a familiar activity. See the Modules, "Sleep Shades (Occluders)" and "Introducing the Cane."

DESCRIPTION OF BASIC TECHNIQUE:

The technique used in most situations is called arcing the cane, or the foot cane technique. It is achieved by holding the cane in the dominant hand with the index finger pointing down the shaft, and the thumb and other fingers curled around the cane—a position analogous to shaking hands with the cane. (See Figure 3-1)

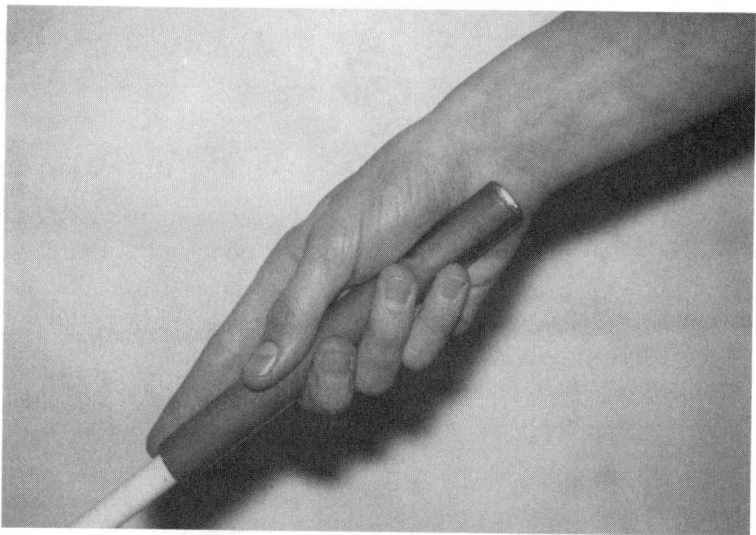

**Figure 3-1
Hand Position**

The cane is swung from side to side and should cover the ground approximately the width of the traveler's shoulders. When the right foot is forward, the cane should touch on the left side, and when the left foot is forward, the cane should touch on the right side – one tap per step. The hand should be centered in front of the body with the primary action in the wrist. (Keeping the forearm against the waist or hip helps to center the hand and prevent fatigue.) The elbow should be bent comfortably.

The reason the cane should touch on the opposite side from the forward foot is to maintain a two-step warning for objects and steps encountered. A traveler who is out of step is clearing only one step ahead and may miss some objects altogether until they are encountered with the body.

The arc of the cane should be even on either side. If a traveler tends to drift either left or right, observe that the traveler is probably arcing farther in that direction than on the other side. Also, if the hand does not remain centered, a variation in the arc may occur, and the traveler will have more difficulty developing good distance perception with the cane. Distance perception can also be thrown off by changing the length of cane.

In crowded areas, the cane can be moved into a more upright position, causing some variation in grip and slowing of walking speed. Normally, a cane traveler should be able to walk as fast as a sighted person in similar physical condition.

Sleep shades should be worn if the student has any sight at all – even light perception. Even a small amount of sight can hamper the learning of good technique.

Techniques for use on stairs are described in the Module, "Description of Basic Techniques."

ACTIVITIES:

EXAMPLE 1: *PRESCHOOL AND KINDERGARTEN*

The Module, "Introducing the Cane," gives detailed suggestions for helping a very young child begin. In almost every respect, it is best to take hold of the child and show her physically, rather than trying to explain verbally.

The student should be in an appropriate location and wearing sleep shades. Place the cane in her hand and gently place her fingers around it in essentially the standard grip. Take hold of her and move her through the motions of taking a few steps on level ground, while talking about how handy the cane can be. (I prefer to walk slightly behind and to the right of the child, with my left hand on her left shoulder, and with my right hand on her hand to help her hold the cane. This description assumes, of course, that both teacher and student are right-handed. The position is easily adjusted according to hand preference.)

Practice for a short while as the student repeatedly walks a few steps on one surface and then recognizes the other surface. Let go of her at least part of the time, allowing her to walk alone and hold the cane herself, even though technique may be very imperfect at this time.

It is usually not advisable to attempt to teach "keeping in step" at first with a very young child. Help her to move the cane from side to side but do not expect her to keep in step.

She Can't Learn It All at Once

Very young students often cannot grasp very much at once. It may be necessary to spend several lessons in teaching the basic position and motion. Nevertheless, actual travel with the cane should be begun while the technique is still imperfect, with more and more elements of the standard form being gradually added.

Suppose, for example, that a beginner is still learning how to hold the cane and keep the tip down. She should nevertheless walk with the cane and find obstacles, even if she is not yet tapping in an appropriate arc. Part of the time the teacher might take hold of her and move her through the standard motions. But part of the time the child should move on her own, however imperfectly, as long as the cane is finding obstacles. If this is not done, the child probably will not understand the purpose of the cane, and lessons will also be impossibly boring.

I use the following sequence of skills when the child is too immature to learn them all at once:

(1) Begin to understand the purpose of the cane.
(2) Keep the tip down.
(3) Hold the handle with one hand. (Note: See exceptions under "TROUBLESHOOTING," below.)
(4) Keep the cane hand centered at waist level, with the arm against the body and the elbow comfortably bent.
(5) Tap the cane from side to side.
(6) Use correct grip and finger position.
(7) Make the arc consistent on each side.
(8) Keep in step.

Note that this is a process of refining and improving techniques which are very imperfect at first. Some instructors say that this is wrong—they believe the cane should never be used except with perfect form. Their concern is inconsistent with the way other developmental tasks are handled. Recall the analogy to using silverware: The progression (for a sighted or blind baby) ordinarily is something like this:

(1) Begin to understand the purpose of silverware.
(2) Hold the handle.
(3) Insert spoon into mouth (with food having been loaded onto spoon by someone else).
(4) Lift the food to the mouth, keeping the bowl of the spoon upright (again, spoon having been loaded by someone else).
(5) Direct the bowl of the spoon into the food and proceed (receiving some help in loading the spoon).
(6) Scoop some food from the bowl and proceed independently.
(7) Consistently use correct grip and finger position.
(8) Avoid messiness.

Build on Experience

Any number of other skills are gradually refined and improved with maturity and experience: drawing, writing, walking, bathing, etc. Withholding a cane completely from a young child is no more logical than totally withholding the washcloth because she flops it around.

"Improving and refining" includes developing more and more independence. At first we place the child's hand on the cane in the proper position. Later she holds the handle correctly when reminded. In time she will remember by herself.

As the child progresses, introduce new elements of technique. Simply proceed for awhile with a given level of skill, and then say, for example, "Now you're going to learn how to move the cane just the way a grownup does." Avoid waiting unduly long between refinements, lest the immature technique become too established. The ultimate example of "waiting unduly long," however, is to delay starting with the cane at all. Then the habits to be changed include shuffling feet, outstretched hands, slow motion, irregular gait, and crippling fear.

EXAMPLE 2: *PRIMARY GRADES*

Help the student examine the cane and name its parts. Verify its length as appropriate.

When the sleep shades are on, help the child grasp the cane and begin to use it. Combine explanation with physical guidance. A typical progression for the first lesson would be:

- Hold the cane with essentially the correct grip and stance.
- Tap the cane from side to side several times, without walking.
- Walk on level terrain, while continuing to arc the cane.
- Discuss the width of the arc: "The cane needs to tap back and forth in front of each foot. Then it will protect you from things that might bump you on either side. If I stand behind you, I should see that the tip goes just a little bit to each side, just a little bit past your feet."
- Approach an obstacle and note when the cane finds it.
- Walk onto a different surface—as, from carpet to bare floor—and note how the cane indicates this.
- Continue walking around in the chosen area, finding obstacles and changes of surface.

Unless the student is particularly mature with good coordination, it is best not to mention at first that the cane should be tapped in front of the foot which is not leading. Instead, first merely explain that "The cane tip should go back and forth, in front of your feet," and demonstrate. When the student can do this easily, you may wish to talk about "tapping once with each step," but not emphasize precise correlation.

If the student learns quickly, or asks about correlation, explain the exact pattern during introduction. Also, if the student should develop a consistently *wrong* correlation (i.e., tapping the cane in front of the *leading* foot always), this should be corrected.

Some students may appear to understand keeping in step, but persist in making exaggerated or slow steps. In this case, it is best to insist that for awhile the student *stop* trying to keep in step. Otherwise, awkward and slow motion may become ingrained.

When a student is not able to grasp keeping in step at first, introduce it at a later time as a further refinement. It may be phased in: at first require it only for a short while during each lesson, and then gradually increase.

Many primary-grade students are still unable to keep in step well even after several months during which the cane is used well in other respects. Periodically, try again. If a student reaches age 9 or 10 and still cannot keep in step, make a concerted, continued effort; consider consulting a physical education teacher or physical therapist. A student over age 8 with normal coordination should be able to learn this skill. With a younger student, however, it is often wise to teach the rest of the technique and wait awhile about keeping in step.

EXAMPLE 3: *INTERMEDIATE GRADES AND UP*
(Age 10 and Over)

Review the purpose of the cane. Often this will have been done previously at some length, during a conference or other meeting, and a brief summary will suffice.

Similarly, review the purpose of sleep shades, and help the student put them on.

Examine the cane and verify its length. Show the student the appropriate grip and stance. Although less physical assistance is necessary than with a young child, some physical assistance is needed to prevent lengthy attempts at verbal description.

Ask the student to tap the cane back and forth a few times without starting to walk; discuss the width of the arc. Direct the student to practice walking in an easy location, with solid footing and few obstacles, and with no step-downs. Good examples include a long hallway; an empty part of a large room; a schoolyard or sidewalk. A student of this age should readily understand how the cane finds walls and other obstacles.

Explain how to keep in step – i.e., tap the cane in front of the foot which is not forward. Note that this provides the maximum amount of information – the cane taps as far in front of the respective foot as possible. Many students grasp this easily and need only occasional reminders. If it is hard for the student to keep in step, or if the attempt results in unnatural or very slow steps, disregard this part of the skill for a short while.

After a few minutes of practice, review the grip, stance, and general posture. If any unnatural or awkward motions have appeared because of inexperience or tension, work on correcting them. Emphasize the idea of normal posture, with the cane serving as a natural extension of one's own senses.

EXAMPLE 4: *TROUBLESHOOTING*

Some beginners are better off using *two* hands on the cane for awhile. They may center the handle better and may overcome a tendency to reach out with the free hand.

Also, very young beginners may find it easier to slide the tip back and forth rather than tapping it. Furthermore, there are some situations where any traveler may find it desirable to slide the cane. For example, when traveling next to a parking lot, there may be a substantial crack or ridge between the sidewalk and the parking lot. The cane may be slid across from one side to the other until it encounters the crack or ridge. This technique is of limited value since a crack or ridge may not be detected easily.

Ordinarily, the cane should be tapped rather than slid, to avoid sticking and the premature wearing out of cane tips. Also, the sound of the tap provides information about the surface touched and (by means of echo) the proximity of buildings, etc. Many good travelers vary cane techniques to suit the travel situation.

Appropriate challenges: The best motivation for good technique is a continual increase in variety and challenge, appropriate for the child's age. If obstacles or step-downs are never encountered unexpectedly (because the child is in a very restricted environment and/or always led by the hand) there is little motivation for a safe arc. But if the child is expected to move quickly (with independence appropriate for her age) in a varied environment, the advantages of a good arc will be apparent.

See that obstacles and step-downs are *not* always directly ahead.

Humor can help: "Remember – don't fall in the ocean!" I sometimes say. I explain that one of my travel instructors began his training in California, a few blocks from the Pacific, and this was a superb motivator for good cane usage. (I do not, of course, say this to a child too young to understand that there is no ocean actually nearby.)

I also sometimes say in a school hallway, "Remember the mop buckets!" – having discussed the unpleasantness of a possible collision with a janitor's pail of water.

One of the best ways to get a point across is to demonstrate the *wrong* approach, sometimes in exaggerated form. Often, for example, I have a student who tends to tap the cane on one side only. I may say, "Let me show you something. I'm going to put my hand on your hand and make your cane tap in a certain way. You tell me if it's the right way or not." Then I make the cane tap for awhile on the right only; the left only; both sides correctly; in the middle only. Each time I ask, "Is this good? Why?" Younger children usually find this amusing as well as instructive.

(NOTE: When humor is used with an older student, be careful not to seem sarcastic.)

Checking the width of the arc: Explain that the arc should be shoulder-width, to avoid finding things with the shoulders instead of with the cane. (A rather large woman once replied, "I'm aiming for something wider than my shoulders!") The instructor can easily check the width and symmetry of the arc by walking behind the student. A sighted teacher should see the tip appearing just slightly beyond the student's body on each side. A blind teacher should hear each tap clearly and consistently, not muffled by being in front of the student's body.

What is crucial? Some students, especially those with additional disabilities, have great difficulty keeping in step. One student with a mental disability swung her cane twice as fast as necessary. This technique is safe. Less than every step is not safe. A traveler is relatively safe if the cane swings once per step even if not perfectly in step.

It is essential that the arc "cover the steps," that is, reach beyond the shoulder on each side. This is very difficult to achieve if the handle is not centered in the middle of the body. Teach your student to rest the wrist against the body at about waist height, with the elbow comfortably bent; this keeps the hand centered and prevents fatigue.

The precise recommended grip, with the forefinger extended, is not crucial. It is taught because it helps to direct the cane and keep track of where it is. Wrapping all fingers around the handle, however, is acceptable.

If the cane is too short, the student will not have enough time to stop or change direction when encountering an object. The cane should be at least shoulder height when held vertically, and often considerably longer. The desire for a longer cane is a sign that the student is moving more quickly and confidently. For a growing youngster, the length should be checked at least every three months.

FOLLOW-UP: The student's overall posture and the width of the arc are important facets that easily degenerate. Remind your student frequently, in creative ways that are not just nagging. Provide increasing challenges that demonstrate the value of good technique.

REFERENCE(S):
Richard Mettler. *Cognitive Learning Theory and Cane Travel Instruction: A New Paradigm*, pp. 107-120.

MODULE 4
HUMAN GUIDE

OBJECTIVE: The student will walk with a human guide in selected circumstances, using appropriate techniques.

AGE OF STUDENT: All ages

PRIMARY SKILL EMPHASIS:
Walking in company with others
Human guide
Posture, grip, gait, and arc
General travel
Attitudes toward blindness

ADDITIONAL SKILL EMPHASIS:
In a crowd or a line
Etiquette
Flexibility and confidence

FIGURE(S):
FIGURE 4-1: Human Guide
FIGURE 4-2: Blind Person as Human Guide

SEE ALSO (Other Modules):
    Carrying Things
    In a Crowd
    Walking Independently While Following Someone
    Walking in a Line of People
    The Airport
    Lunchtime

REMARKS: It is important to discuss the subject of human guides during the first few lessons and to review it periodically. One of the greatest barriers to independence is the incorrect belief (on the part of the blind person as well as his friends and family) that the cane is only useful when the person is walking "alone." This is false for two main reasons: (1) most of us are rarely completely "alone," but we act independently in many ways while in the company of others; and (2) if the cane is to be used only when the person is "alone," it will be unfamiliar and unavailable even at those times.

This text uses the term "human guide," rather than "sighted guide," because the guide may be a competent blind person.

ACTIVITIES:

EXAMPLE 1: *INTRODUCTION*
Some students may be unfamiliar with efficient techniques of walking with a human guide. (Figure 4-1) Review or teach briefly as necessary:

The blind person takes the elbow of the guide. (A small child will probably take the hand of an adult.) The blind person is attuned to the body movements of the guide, while walking about a half-step back in relation to the guide.

With most students, this posture can be reviewed or introduced while the student continues to use his cane. If the student is very young or has difficulty grasping concepts, it may be best to practice for a few minutes without the cane before demonstrating the combination.

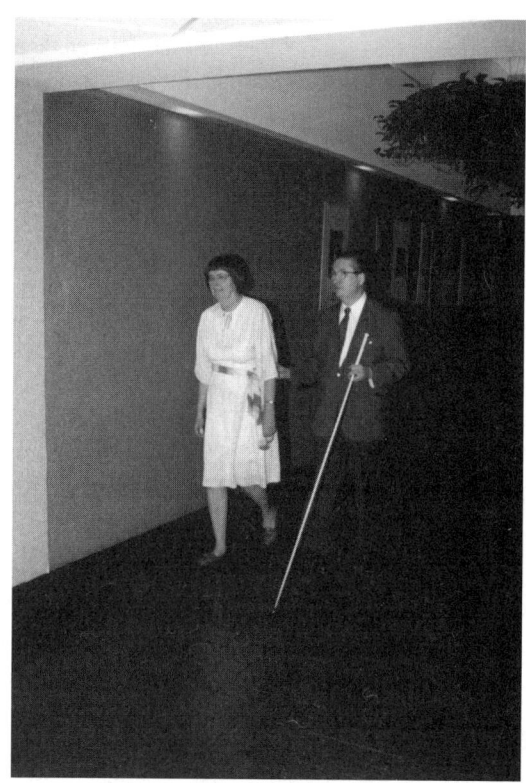

**Figure 4-1
Human Guide**

EXAMPLE 2: *DISCUSSION OF PURPOSE*

It is important to discuss why the cane is used in combination with a human guide. There are two aspects to this discussion:

Why use the cane if the guide is available?

and

Why use a guide at all if the cane is so helpful?

Depending on the maturity of the student, discuss the points below, with concrete examples. Intersperse discussion with actual practice.

A preschool-aged child may simply be told, "Sometimes you will walk with your cane by yourself. Sometimes you will walk with someone so you can stay together. But you still will use your cane. Then the other person won't have to bother telling you about things in your way. You can take care of yourself, but still stay together."

A more mature student needs explanation on his own level, with the opportunity to discuss fully.

Following is a discussion guide in outline form:

A. Why use a human guide at times even though the student has cane skills?

- It is easy to stay together in a crowd.
- If the other person is showing you where to go, sometimes direct guidance is more efficient than spoken direction.
- In a noisy location, it may be very hard to hear spoken directions.
- For social reasons, two people may prefer to walk together.
- Especially for a younger student, it is sometimes necessary to walk with someone else because of age and safety reasons.
- There may be situations where the student's cane skills are not yet adequate, or where there are particular advantages to the use of a human guide.

B. If the human guide is there, why use the cane at all?

- A young child may rarely be more than a few steps from an adult – especially in public – because of age and safety reasons. If the cane is only used when no adults are near, the child will gain hardly any experience.
- The youngster who does not use his cane when walking with others will fail in a transition that other youngsters make naturally: walking alone more and more as he gets older. Instead of gradually going farther alone in the mall, in public buildings, in stores, and on the street, he simply stays with others. No one may give much thought to this, but independence simply does not increase.
- If the human guide is entirely depended upon, the blind person is at a loss when the guide becomes unavailable. For example, the blind person may want to go into the rest room, shop in a different aisle or store, etc. Also, the guide could be unreliable or become ill.
- The more the human guide is depended upon, the less experience the student

will gain, and the less effectively he will use the cane when he does choose to do so.
— Accompanying an independent blind traveler requires little or no effort on the part of the guide. It should be essentially no different than accompanying any other person of comparable age and general ability. However, accompanying a dependent blind person is an effort and a responsibility. If the guide is forgetful, the dependent blind person will trip, fall downstairs, bump into doorways, etc. However willing the guide may seem, this is a burden.
— Guiding a dependent person is also time-consuming. The person guided cannot anticipate changes in terrain – steps up or down, slopes up or down, uneven dirt, etc. The guide often must pause to avoid jolting him. But if, instead, the person guided is using his cane, he *can* anticipate such changes for himself. Both persons can move along smoothly.
— The attitudes of the guide and the guided are shaped by the behavior of the person guided. It is the difference between accompanying any person (as in showing a stranger the way, enjoying the company of a friend, etc.) vs. assisting a helpless individual who cannot take responsibility for his own movement.

EXAMPLE 3: *PRACTICE IN VARIOUS SETTINGS*

Walk with the student, with yourself as the human guide, and with the student using his cane.

Walk in a flat, unobstructed area. Note the width of the arc – the student may need practice to protect his steps adequately when beside someone else. If this is done skillfully, ordinarily the cane will not trip the guide. However, it may take some practice to avoid becoming tangled.

Approach a curb or other step-down. Again, depending on the student's maturity, you may choose to give a warning at first. Also, at first it is helpful to hesitate slightly before stepping off. An experienced traveler, however, should be able to detect the curb with the cane before the guide steps off, and follow along smoothly without hesitation.

Approach a step-up such as a curb. Practice in a similar manner.

Approach an obstacle, such as a table. Walk past it in such a way that the student needs to alter his path slightly and "squeeze" past. Depending on the student's ability, you may or may not choose to announce the obstacle at first to give practice. Soon, the guide should be able to proceed without announcing obstacles, and the cane should detect them. (Caution: Since the two persons are side by side, if the guide hurries past an obstruction at very close range, it will be hard for the other person to avoid it in time. A mature blind traveler should be able to react quickly, let go of the guide's arm momentarily, and proceed behind the guide in a tight place. But ordinarily, if the guide remains aware that there are two people together and allows enough room, both people can go around the obstacle together.)

Practice on a flight of stairs. Unless the steps are very wide, it is usually best to let go and proceed single file while actually on the steps. Practice going up and down. Approach from some distance away, each time.

Help the student practice in the above ways with at least one family member. Discuss the reasons for using a cane with a guide.

EXAMPLE 4: *A BLIND PERSON AS A GUIDE*

As a part of the student's experiences in becoming acquainted with blind adults as role models, have the student walk with a blind guide. Emphasize that a guide need not be sighted, but must be a responsible and mobile individual.

If possible, also give the student himself experience in guiding someone who is younger or less able. It is *not* essential that the person being guided have less sight than the guide. The younger person may be totally blind, partially sighted, or fully sighted.

Often a guide who is blind assists someone who needs help only in knowing where to go, but needs no help with the act of walking. For example, the older blind student might show a new student around. The person guided might be a fully sighted student, or a blind student (totally blind or partially sighted) who uses a cane well. In such an instance, the blind guide will act as leader. He will use his cane to protect his own steps, but will not expect to keep the other person from tripping or bumping objects.

Sometimes, however, a blind guide will assist a person who cannot walk safely without actual help. The other person might be a very young child, a mentally handicapped person, or a blind person who has not learned cane skills. (Figure 4-2) In such a case, the blind guide must arc more widely to protect the steps of both himself and the other person. He must detect stairs and obstacles in front of *either* person, and help as necessary. Ask a competent blind adult to demonstrate this. A student should not be expected actually to assist another person in this way unless he is quite mature and able; however, a younger student should learn that it is possible.

(Note: Most of this text assumes that the teacher is sighted. If the teacher is blind, this part of the lesson will occur naturally. However, it is wise to call attention to it at times.)

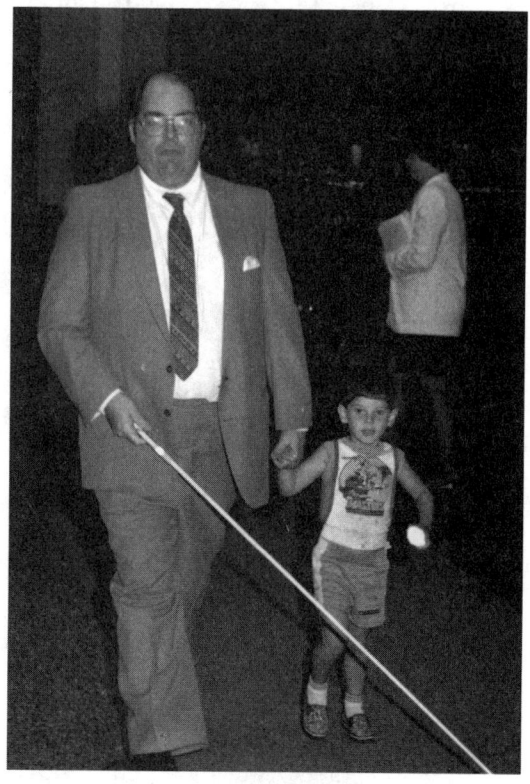

**Figure 4-2
Blind Person as
Human Guide**

If the school has several blind or visually impaired students, particularly avoid an insidious pattern: partially sighted students continually acting as guides for totally blind students. Responsibility should be on the basis of skill, not sight. Also note that a partially sighted person who relies on sight alone is likely to be a poor guide, exposing the other person to hazard; the guide should use a cane if his sight is not really adequate.

Whenever possible, insist that each student travel individually rather than being assisted.

If it should happen that all the relatively mature students happen to have partial sight, and all those who need assistance happen to be totally blind, arrange for a totally blind adult to come in occasionally and demonstrate ability to lead.

EXAMPLE 5: *CONTINUED DISCUSSION*

Analyze situations where it would be efficient to use (1) the cane without another person physically guiding; (2) the cane with a person guiding; and (3) a human guide alone. Practice as many examples as possible.

Below are a few examples – by no means an exhaustive list.

Use of a cane alone, without holding onto another person:

Preschool or kindergarten:
- Walking in familiar areas at school, finding obstacles and steps independently
- Walking around within a narrow range while remaining near adults, in a safe and simple situation (at a picnic in a park; visiting a friend's home; in a store that is not extremely crowded; etc.)

Elementary school student:
- Walking on the street in non-complicated areas where parents permit him to go
- All around school, including unfamiliar areas where the student might go on an errand
- Shopping (parents may be nearby but not immediately present)

High school student:
- All above
- Shopping at mall, when family or friends are elsewhere
- Walking on the street in complex locations
- Errands in public buildings
- On public transportation

All ages:
- Walking toward a sound, or following a person by listening, but without holding onto anyone.

Using the cane while holding someone's arm:
- Staying together while shopping
- Holding parent's hand (young child)
- When touring a complex area, starting at a new school, going to a meeting at a hotel, etc.
- When complex verbal directions would be much more cumbersome than taking someone's arm
- Unusual situations, such as walking to a picnic in a large, open park area

Use of human guide only (without cane)
- If a preschool child uses his cane only part of the time, and is not using it at a given time
- During participation in sporting events, when walking a short distance from one area to another. (If walking a considerable distance, it would probably be more efficient to have the cane available and use it.)

REFERENCE(S):
Willoughby and Duffy, *Handbook for Itinerant and Resource Teachers of Blind and Visually Impaired Students,* pp. 160, 180-181.

MODULE 5
OBSTACLES
Noting Them and Proceeding

OBJECTIVE: The student will detect an obstacle in his/her path, proceed around it, and continue in the desired direction.

AGE OF STUDENT: Preschool and up

PRIMARY SKILL EMPHASIS:
Obstacles in path
Correcting a path
Flexibility and confidence
Moving straight ahead
Orientation overall
General travel
Posture, grip, gait, and arc
Landmarks

ADDITIONAL SKILL EMPHASIS:
Compass directions
Right and left
Overhanging objects
Detecting step-downs or drop-offs
Maps
Stairs
Corners, turns, and angles

SEE ALSO (Other Modules):
    Introducing the Cane
    Doors Closed or Open
    Unfinished Basement, "Crawl Space," or Attic
    Sidewalk Flawed or Obstructed
    Street Crossing With Obstruction
    Alternate Routes Within a Building
    Back Yard (Overall)
    In a Crowd
    Walking Independently While Following Someone
    Description of Basic Techniques

"AHA!" not "OOPS!":

Jenny, age 6, was learning to find her way in the school hallways. Whenever her cane touched a box or other object, her teacher said "Oops." Jenny walked slowly.

Ian carried his cane in a gingerly manner. It seemed as though he were carrying a tray of dishes instead of a cane – trying not to bump it into anything.

Jenny and Ian were victims of a common error often made by educators and family members: unconsciously viewing the cane's touch as a "collision" (not really desirable) rather than a "discovery" (desirable). This rubs off on the student, who unconsciously learns to proceed slowly and gingerly, and fails to take real advantage of the potential of the cane.

This Module emphasizes attitudes and techniques which help ensure the use of the cane as a *tool*. Cane usage is an alternative technique with its own characteristics – not just a weak attempt to imitate the methods used by the sighted. The goal is *not* to proceed with as little sound as possible, touching as few things as possible. Rather, the goal is to proceed quickly and efficiently. Some sound is expected and desirable, as the cane tip touches objects and the surface underfoot. Proceeding confidently – as opposed to a timid, even cringing approach – is part of the overall attitude that it is respectable to be blind.

When Jenny and Ian became Mrs. Vrbek's students, she quickly helped them change patterns of attitudes and techniques. With Jenny, she began by saying "Aha!" in a pleased voice each time she observed Jenny's cane finding an obstacle. Jenny soon picked this up and began saying "aha" also, instead of the "oops" she had acquired from her previous teacher. Soon she was bouncing down the hall at twice her previous speed, from time to time murmuring "aha" as she went around something.

Mrs. Vrbek asked Ian (age 9) to put on sleep shades, and she went with him to the playground. She faced him toward a chain-link fence and asked him to walk forward quickly. After a few steps, the cane tip encountered the fence and Ian stopped short. Mrs. Vrbek could "see the wheels going around in his head" as he internalized the idea he should have grasped long ago: "Now I really understand what the cane can do! It can find things before I get to them, when I can't see them, or when I can't see them well enough to tell what they are."

"Now he realizes," Mrs. Vrbek said afterward, "that the cane is *supposed* to touch things, to give him information."

This Module, as well as many others, emphasizes the attitudes and techniques which make the cane an effective tool. There are two major aspects: (1) recognizing the presence of an obstacle, and (2) proceeding in the desired direction.

ACTIVITIES:

EXAMPLE 1: BASIC INSTRUCTION
(*Elementary grades and above*)

Children age 6 and over, and many who are younger, ordinarily grasp the general idea of going around an obstruction during the first lesson. It then becomes a matter of practice and refining techniques. Particularly, the student needs to build skill in (1) arcing the cane consistently and reacting quickly, so that the object is immediately detected, and (2) maintaining orientation in order to continue in the desired direction.

A child in the earliest grades, or a student with special problems, may need emphasis on concept building as described for preschool (below), though in an age-appropriate manner.

The Modules, "Sidewalk Flawed or Obstructed" and "Street Crossing With Obstruction," have suggestions for various ages.

If educators and family members over-anticipate obstacles for the student, the child will learn to depend on verbal cues and/or physical guidance, rather than developing independence. The Module, "Walking Independently While Following Someone," describes a student following me through a parking lot. He was amazed to encounter utility poles, traffic islands, and concrete barriers, because he had always been guided around them.

Sleep shades are essential. If the student sees objects visually, however fuzzily – or thinks she can – she will not learn what the cane can do.

Remember: When the student's cane encounters an object, the comment is "Aha!" [found it!] or perhaps "Hmmm" [let's think], and NOT "Oops!" [a mistake!]

EXAMPLE 2: BASIC INSTRUCTION
(*Preschool*)

In the Module, "Introducing the Cane," one Example has detailed suggestions for initial instruction with a very young child.

A child of preschool/kindergarten age will need physical guidance as well as verbal explanation with appropriate vocabulary. If you say, "This cane can detect obstacles," she will probably not understand. But she will understand if you say, "This cane can find things so you don't get bumped," and if you move her through plenty of physical demonstration.

Understanding that the cane can tell the difference between a clear path and an obstacle is perhaps the most basic concept in actual mobility. Without this understanding, the child will not really move "independently." She may move, with verbal assurance and/or physical assistance – and she may be learning. But until she actually realizes what the cane can tell her, she is not really using the cane to get information.

For a very young child, gaining this understanding is a developmental process – it comes gradually, and continually increases.

Following is a representative list of specific experiences which aid in developing understanding and skill:

– Often use a very large "obstacle." Face the child toward it at fairly close range, and direct her to "Find the ___." [wall, fence, sofa, etc.] When she finds it, sometimes let her examine it tactually (and sit on it, in the case of a sofa).

Occasionally, humorously scrunch yourself and the child up against the wall or fence while saying, "Whew! We can't go on ahead here, can we? This wall is REALLY in the way."

– Seek out situations where there is an obstacle in just the right place for the child's current level of understanding. Set up situations if they do not occur naturally. Place a chair in the hallway; scatter boxes across the middle of the room; leave a large toy on the sidewalk. (*Note:* Always consider possible inconvenience to others. For example, if objects are placed in a common hallway, they should be removed immediately after the student has practiced. Also, as necessary, talk with other staff about the reason for the obstacles.)

– When the child knows she is headed toward a desired location, there is an eminently "teachable moment." She is particularly ready to perceive that the obstacle is "in the way," and that she must go around it and resume her desired path – or she will not reach her destination. Examples include a desk between her and the toy shelf; a coffee table in front of the couch; a large box in the hallway. Sometimes, give her a running commentary for added emphasis: "So, now we're walking toward the toy shelf....Hmmm, here's that desk. You found it with your cane...and you're going around it....Good! Now you've gone around the desk, and you're walking on toward the toy shelf....Yes! Your cane found the wooden shelves, and now let's see what toys we have today...."

– Some of the time, a young child needs to be physically guided through the pattern of (1) encountering an obstacle, and (2) going around it and proceeding in the desired path.

I often place a hand on her shoulder, gently helping her along. Guiding the child from *behind* is distinct from the usual human-guide posture where the guide is a half-step ahead. The purpose is entirely different; guidance from behind is much more analogous to the traditional help to a beginning *swimmer*. The helper gently assists while the learner proceeds on her own power. Assistance can easily be gently faded in and out as the situation demands.

If this kind of thing is never done, the child may not move quickly enough or consistently enough to understand. However, if this is done too much, she never has the experience of correcting her own path and making decisions herself. Thoughtful judgment provides help an appropriate percentage of the time.

– Verbal directions often are not sufficient with a young child. Saying "Go to your right," for example, is not enough if the child still cannot tell left from right. Give her a physical nudge in the correct direction, while explaining verbally.

– Sometimes stand beyond the obstacle, so that the child is guided onward by walking toward your voice. This provides help without physical assistance, and it also develops the concept of a fixed destination. A similar idea is to have some other sound at the destination.

– Except for the initial lesson and other planned exceptions, do not anticipate for the child what her cane will tell her in a few moments anyway. Urge parents to follow this policy also. If you always tell her everything, she will never learn to trust her cane (and neither will the adults in her life).

– The Module, "Doors Closed or Open," gives detailed suggestions for developing concepts.

– The Module, "Street Crossing With Obstruction," gives examples of natural and contrived obstacles.

Remember: Say "aha" – not "whoops" – when

the child finds something with her cane. An in-between comment (as, the "hmmm" above when the desk was in the way between the child and the toy shelf) can be helpful also. A worried "whoops" should be reserved for times when the child actually bumps into something painfully, or knocks something over (presumably because the cane was not used skillfully).

EXAMPLE 3: *TROUBLESHOOTING*

If a student has particular difficulty with obstacles, analyze the problem according to three aspects: (a) detecting the object, (b) going around it and resuming the desired path, and (c) overall independence and attitude. Below are suggestions (not exhaustive) for approaching the problem according to cause.

Detecting the Obstacle

- The cane may be too short for the student's stride or individual style. Experiment with longer canes. The traveler needs to have time to react before her body encounters the object.
- If the handle is gripped poorly or too loosely, information will not be received as it should. If the grip is too tight and tense, this too interferes with receiving information.
- A common problem is an uneven or inadequate arc. Especially when the student is looking for something on one side (such as a door), or when she believes she knows where obstacles exist, the cane may simply not reach where it should. Insist that it be tapped evenly on both sides.
- Similarly, if the student believes she can see obstacles visually, she will not pay attention to information from the cane. Sleep shades are essential. If the student travels well under sleep shades but has great difficulty when not wearing them, consider having an occasional special lesson without the shades for integration of techniques.
- Guard against letting the student expect warning of obstacles. This warning may not always be the obvious one of someone's saying, "Watch out for the pole." Other forms include hearing someone walk around the obstacle; hearing a change in tone of voice (if someone is talking to the student while walking along); hearing the teacher stop to watch; etc.

If I am not giving close physical guidance, I make a point of walking in an unpredictable path which is not related to the child's. ("Don't pay attention to where I go," I explain. "I'll just walk around all over, watching you and maybe doing something else too. I may go somewhere different from where I asked you to go.")

If the child is so young that I continually talk to her, I consciously avoid accidentally giving hints through my tone of voice.

- Walking very slowly interferes with all aspects of travel. A slow traveler tends to have generally slow reactions and to wobble and waver. Brisk movement encourages speedy reactions and straight movement.
- Although it is a less common problem, sometimes a student walks too fast for her current level of skill or for the environment. An immature or overeager youngster may need to be told to slow down. (Caution: family members and others are all too ready to assume that any blind traveler is going too fast. Walking too slowly is much more common.)
- Nervousness and inexperience interfere with all aspects of travel. This problem is to be expected at the beginning of instruction, but can also show up later. Is a new setting causing nervousness? Is some other problem (e.g., illness in the family) distracting the student?
- Many blind persons tend to grope with the free hand to search for obstacles. This tendency is fostered by the school of thought which discourages cane use indoors, and by the use of folding canes,

which tend to be folded instead of used. See that your student (a) uses the cane at all times except when in her own home; (b) looks for obstacles and doorways with the cane, rather than with her free hand; (c) carries something in the free hand in situations where she is tempted to explore with that hand. With a young beginner, consider having her hold the cane with both hands at first.
- Isolate the task of *detecting* the object from the task of proceeding onward. Occasionally, ask the student to "freeze" when she encounters an object, and to announce "Here it is" before she proceeds.
- If the student is very young or has special problems, recognize that it may take time to develop concepts and to put understanding into practice. See the suggestions for young children.
- A young child may want to touch and explore the object. In this regard, she may be rewarded for plunging ahead and *not* responding to the cane's information. Therefore, the teacher should sometimes pointedly allow the child to touch and explore, and at other times insist that she proceed without doing so. Lessons should be structured so that detecting objects correctly with the cane results in more opportunity for "fun" exploration, not less. ("Until you get to Mr. Pierson's office, don't stop to look at things. If something is in your way, just go around it quickly. But after we get to the office, then you may ask to go back and touch any special thing.")
- If the student walks in a hesitant, gingerly manner and cringes slightly when her cane touches something, she is probably the victim of the "oops" syndrome discussed throughout this Module. Emphasize that the cane's striking an object is desirable and informative. Also, consider whether someone is unduly fearful that the child will get hurt.

Continuing in the Desired Direction

- The student must develop "mental mapping" skills. Help her keep in mind a picture of where she is and where she is going. Other Modules which emphasize this include "Back Yard (Overall)," "Alternate Routes Within a Building," "Routes for New Buildings and New Classrooms," and "Walking Across Open Space."
- Actively avoid the approach of memorizing specific, isolated routes. Instead, emphasize overall understanding and flexibility. Make frequent use of simple tactual maps.
- From time to time, interrupt the student with a deliberate "distraction." For example, pull her out of the way of an imaginary janitor's cart, face her in an indeterminate direction, and expect her to recover. (Explain that you will be doing this now and then for practice purposes.) Gradually, make distractions more challenging.
- If the traveler walks very slowly, she wavers. It is hard to maintain a consistent path, with or without obstacles. Help your student walk faster. Sometimes place a hand on her shoulder and gently move her along as she becomes accustomed to faster movement.
- A young student may resist moving along because she wants to stay and examine the object. Direct the student firmly, and see that age-appropriate opportunities to examine objects do occur in the course of the lesson.

Overall Independence and Attitude

- A student having difficulty may not really be convinced that true independence is possible. Or, she may not be motivated to achieve it – due to fear or other conflicting emotions. A common feeling (usually not expressed) is,

"Well, yes, I saw a couple of people getting around pretty well with the cane. But they are so *exceptional.* I know *I* could never do that." See that your students often observe competent blind travelers. Help them to regard good travel skills as normal rather than "an unusual exception."
– Similarly, parents (and other adults) may feel conflicting emotions.
– It is vital that the cane be used *at all times,* except when the student is in her own home or actually engaging in a sport. Otherwise, it will not become a normal part of things – an "extension of her senses."
– Sleep shades must be worn during lessons. Otherwise, the student will not really learn how to rely on the cane, and she will tend to regard any success as being due to residual vision.
– A student of any age can become bored. Plan appropriate challenges of gradually increasing difficulty. See the heading, "Making Lessons Interesting" (*Handbook,* pp. 191-193), for detailed suggestions for younger children.
– Be familiar with the typical level of understanding for each age. Consider whether the student is genuinely immature in concept development or experience. If there are special problems of additional disability, extreme overprotection at home, etc., these must be taken into account.
– A young child may focus on the desire to touch and explore the object encountered. She may be too distracted to think about continuing around it. According to the child's level of maturity, the teacher must alternate appropriately between (1) insisting that the child note the obstruction and go around it without examining it, and (2) pointedly allowing her to explore it. Encouraging the child to examine an object at leisure should be a kind of reward for achievement (e.g., having found other obstacles and gone around them quickly).

The *teacher* should decide when and if the student may pause to explore. However, it is unwise to insist that a young child always refrain from touching things she knows are interesting. One option is to say, "We will come back and look at this soon, after you have finished ___."

EXAMPLE 4: *OBSTACLES NOT DETECTED BY STANDARD CANE TECHNIQUES*

Objects Overhead

If something hangs overhead and does not extend downward near the traveler, the cane will not find it. The most common example is a tree limb. Other examples are pipes hanging from a low ceiling in a basement, and extra-low doorways in historical ruins.

Help your student anticipate where this problem is really likely – wooded areas, old basements, caves, ancient ruins, etc. If the situation clearly calls for it, the traveler may choose to keep one arm up for a short while. Also, a cap with a bill is an excellent aid. See the Modules "Rural Environment," "The Great Outdoors," and "Unfinished Basement, 'Crawl Space,' or Attic."

Occasionally a sign or other structure is much wider above the ground than at ground level. If the difference is not extreme, a good arc with the cane will probably find the object.

Do not allow your student to wave her free hand in the air continually in fear of tree branches. Help her to assess where this kind of problem is really likely, and to consider various solutions (such as a cap with a bill). If she bumps her head or shoulders on walls and other things which *do* extend to the ground, re-emphasize a wide and consistent arc.

A Small, Very Low Object

Some objects are so small and low that they may not be detected when the cane is lifted slightly in the center between taps. With a loose object, such as a bit of trash, the effect is usually negligible – the pedestrian may kick the object or step on it, hardly noticing (unless it is the proverbial banana peel).

But if the object is attached and solid, it can easily trip a person. Examples include:
- *A water valve sticking up an inch high in the middle of the sidewalk
- *A ridge in the sidewalk, with one section of cement slightly higher than another
- *A rock sticking up from a dirt surface
- *An unfinished pipe, sticking up an inch from the basement floor

If there is reason to expect such problems, the traveler may choose to slide the cane from side to side rather than tapping it.

If an object does catch the traveler's foot and trip her, it is hoped that she will either (a) "dance" a bit and then recover her balance, or (b) trip and fall but not be significantly injured. (The sighted pedestrian, it should be noted, is also likely to trip, because these kinds of objects are unexpected and hard to see.) We live in an untidy world. An occasional skinned knee or elbow is a small price to pay for moving freely and quickly.

EXAMPLE 5: *A STEP-DOWN*

A step-down is not an "obstacle" in the sense meant by most of this Module. However, any instruction which emphasizes obstacles above ground should also keep in mind the opposite: sometimes the surface drops down. Step-downs are discussed in detail elsewhere, especially in the Modules "Unexpected Drop-off or Step-Down" and "Rough Surfaces."

REFERENCE(S):

Willoughby and Duffy. *Handbook for Itinerant and Resource Teachers of Blind and Visually Impaired Students,* pp. 175-198.

Richard Mettler. *Cognitive Learning Theory and Cane Travel Instruction: A New Paradigm,* pp. 107-120.

MODULE 6
WALKING TOWARD A SOUND

OBJECTIVE: The student will walk toward a sound, while using appropriate cane techniques.

AGE OF STUDENT: Preschool and up

PRIMARY SKILL EMPHASIS:
Sound direction and meaning
General travel
Finding a person
Moving straight ahead
Parallel and perpendicular
Street crossing
Traffic movement
Landmarks
Moving straight ahead

ADDITIONAL SKILL EMPHASIS:
Air currents and echoes
In a crowd or a line
Right and left
Walking in company with others
Open space
Corners, turns, and angles
Correcting a path

SEE ALSO (Other Modules):
   Distinctive Sounds
   In a Crowd
   Auditorium or Theater
   Walking in a Line of People
   Meeting a Car
   Walking Independently While Following
      Someone
   Echoes and Air Currents
   Rural Environment
   Swimming Pool or Beach
   Right and Left

REMARKS: Going toward a sound is a skill that should be practiced continually and naturally from babyhood.

An infant begins to turn her head toward a sound. (Babies localize sounds toward the side first, and slightly later toward the front or the back.) The older baby learns to reach, wriggle, and crawl toward a sound.

Nevertheless, from time to time a concentrated lesson is helpful as the student learns to integrate various skills.

This kind of practice also serves a vital purpose for the teacher: demonstrating how the student hears and interprets directional sound. A hearing impairment may be unrecognized, incompletely analyzed, or poorly documented. The travel teacher needs to learn immediately about any problems with directional hearing. Any difficulties should be discussed with an audiologist.

TEACHER PREPARATION: Consider the child's abilities (to the best of your knowledge) in walking independently with the cane and in determining the direction of a sound.

Select an area where appropriate concentrated practice can be accomplished.

As in other lessons, the student should wear sleep shades for these activities. Otherwise, she may not actually rely on her hearing.

ACTIVITIES:

EXAMPLE 1: Go to a classroom at a time when the class is not present. The student stands still while you go to another part of the room. (You may or may not try to walk silently.) Then speak or make a sound (see below) and have the student walk toward you. The cane enables the student to walk comfortably around obstacles as necessary.

You may choose to work in a gym or other large area without obstacles.

Sometimes have the student merely point or face toward you. This helps to distinguish problems of directional hearing from problems of mobility.

This may also be done outdoors, where a much wider space may be used. Depending on the student's experience, an area can be chosen with various surfaces underfoot, and with or without trees and other obstacles.

VARIATION(S): For preschool and the primary grades, frequently include humorous amusement. Consider the following:

>Sing or whistle a tune. The child names the tune.
>Recite an amusing poem or limerick.
>Tell a riddle. (Repeat it as often as necessary until the child arrives. Alternatively, talk about some other subject also.) When the child arrives, she tries to guess the riddle.
>Tell a story, with another installment each time you move. (If the child is slow to arrive, keep repeating the same installment. The next segment will be told at the next location.)
>A noisemaking toy, recording, or other device is turned on at each location. When the child arrives, she may keep the device turned on for a few moments and enjoy it.
>The child goes out of the room while you "hide" a noisemaking device. She re-enters, listens carefully, and tries to walk directly to the object.
>When the child arrives and the cane touches your foot, shake hands ceremoniously and say "Howdy do!"
>Each time the student arrives, *she* may tell *you* a riddle or joke.

EXAMPLE 2: With an older student, walking toward a sound can be helpful when he/she needs extra practice with a certain terrain underfoot or with certain obstacles. For example, in a theater or auditorium you might stand in various places (with or without naming your location aloud), and ask the student to come toward you as you speak.

EXAMPLE 3: When getting acquainted with a new student of any age, it is important to do a directional exercise early in training. Having a student follow you or go toward a sound is informative and may save a lot of frustration. For example, have the student follow you around inside a building and then do the same outdoors. This can be done very naturally while you talk about the surroundings.

EXAMPLE 4: When beginning to work on street crossings at any age, ask the student to listen and point to analyze traffic. A student in seventh grade or above should be able to:

- Indicate which way traffic is moving
- Tell when she first hears a car approaching (with little traffic)
- Face so that she is parallel to traffic, or perpendicular to traffic (the words "parallel" and "perpendicular" may need to be explained)
- Point toward cars which are turning in various directions (in a non-complicated situation)

These tasks give the teacher a further evaluation of the student's directional hearing. They also help the student concentrate on characteristics which are essential in street crossing.

If the student is in sixth grade or below, she may not be able to do all of the above tasks at first, even with excellent hearing. The same may be true if the student is extremely nervous or lacking in experience. However, ordinarily even a kindergartner can indicate when she hears a car approaching and tell which way it is going.

REMARKS: Always consider the general knowledge and ability of the student, together with directional hearing ability.

A hearing impairment brings some limitations. However, avoid assumptions which lead to unnecessarily low expectations. For example, many students assume that veering off the desired path is caused by their hearing loss. Actually, this problem is often due to inexperience and can be improved greatly with practice.

CAUTION: One situation in which it may not be advisable to use sleep shades is when a student has a substantial hearing loss which causes directional hearing problems, and is actually crossing streets and dealing with traffic. The same student, however, should wear sleep shades in other situations. (See the Module, "Sleep Shades.")

MODULE 7
SLEEP SHADES
(Occluders)
By Sharon L. Monthei

OBJECTIVE: [Note: The use of sleep shades is usually stated as a "condition" for other objectives, rather than being an objective in itself. Typical wording is: "Given a long white cane and wearing sleep shades, the student will ...."]

AGE OF STUDENT: All ages (See Examples)

SKILLS LISTS:

NOTE: For students with some sight, sleep shades are a tool of instruction essential for the development of all skills. The specific skills listed here are those which are especially brought out in the Examples given, and/or when discussing the reasons for the shades.

PRIMARY SKILL EMPHASIS:
Attitudes toward blindness
Understanding vision and partial vision
Flexibility and confidence
General travel

ADDITIONAL SKILL EMPHASIS:
Examining things tactually
Obstacles in path
Sound direction and meaning
Detecting step-downs or drop-offs
Posture, grip, gait, and arc

TEACHER PREPARATION: If you are not accustomed to having your students use sleep shades, observe some lessons where they are used regularly. The National Federation of the Blind can direct you to such a lesson or demonstration.

FIGURE(S):

FIGURE 7-1: Sleep Shades for Effective Learning

SEE ALSO (Other Modules):
General Principles
Introducing the Cane
Poor Lighting Conditions
Unexpected Drop-Off or Step-Down
Visually Confusing Appearance
The Blind Travel Instructor

THE USE OF SLEEP SHADES:

Sleep shades are a blindfold sold to the general public for use while sleeping in the daytime. They are an extremely important tool in teaching proper cane travel techniques, Braille, and other alternative techniques used by the blind.

At first glance, it would appear that their use would be counterproductive, that partially-sighted children should be encouraged to use their vision to the fullest in order to be the most able to perform tasks. Actually, most partially-sighted people tend to use their vision to the exclusion of more effective alternatives if not trained to do otherwise with the aid of sleep shades. These partially-sighted people function to some extent like the cartoon character "Mr. Magoo," relying on unreliable vision, making mistakes about what they see, and generally functioning less effectively than they could.

Since blindness is generally viewed as a negative characteristic [although it need not be], the partially-sighted child often feels that it is better to use sighted techniques, even if they are very difficult for him and are less effective than alternative techniques not involving sight. The student may even know his inefficiency, but he is socially conditioned to believe it is better to use sight.

Advantages of Sleep Shades

The use of sleep shades accomplishes two things: (1) it forces the student to practice alternative techniques, and (2) it tends to help the student to accept his own blindness. When a partially-sighted student finds that he *can* function effectively without sight, accepting blindness becomes much easier. It is desirable that a blind person accept the fact so that solutions to the problems it creates can be logically worked out. If blindness is denied, the result is a great expenditure of energy in attempts to hide blindness, and less competence than is possible.

Another advantage of using sleep shades is that many, if not most, children with partial vision will lose more vision as time goes on. Retraining will be minimal or unnecessary for children trained to function without vision. Children with glaucoma, retinitis pigmentosa, optic atrophy, congenital cataracts, macular degeneration, and retinopathy of prematurity are among those who generally can expect to have very little vision by the time they are thirty years old, if not sooner. Of course, there are exceptions, but not many. However, because of the above mentioned tendency to deny blindness, there is an equal tendency to deny that vision will decrease (sometimes supported by the attending ophthalmologist). Since all students with partial vision should wear sleep shades for training purposes for the reasons given above, it may be wiser not to engage in the argument as to whether a child's vision will or will not deteriorate, in establishing the agreement for the student to wear sleep shades. Occasionally, parents or teachers do recognize that training with sleep shades will be useful as the child loses vision.

All of this is not to say that a partially-sighted child should not use the vision he has when this is truly the most efficient way to do something. The use of sleep shades should not be construed as an intent to deny or degrade the sight which exists. We live in a sight-oriented world, and it is unlikely that any partially-sighted child will not use the vision present. Society will encourage and teach him to do so. Sleep shades are merely a vehicle to teach the alternatives in the most efficient way.

Overcoming Resistance

Because of the stigma attached to blindness, the teacher is likely to meet resistance to the use of sleep shades – from the student, the parents, or perhaps other school personnel. For this reason, it is most important that the teacher know the reasons for their use and be able to explain them with conviction. Most resistance can be eliminated by a clear explanation of their purpose, coupled with a firm stand on their use. The teacher who is hesitant or doubtful about their value may encounter problems which will eventually preclude their use altogether. The teacher who handles sleep shades as a matter of course, accompanied with appropriate explanation, will have relatively few problems.

Consistency is essential in minimizing problems with students generally and the same applies to sleep shades. The teacher should *not* allow the student to make decisions regarding when not to wear sleep shades. Extra sleep shades should be available in the event of loss or damage, or the teacher may elect to keep each student's sleep shades between lessons.

Most students will not particularly like wearing sleep shades. A clear explanation of their purpose will often help. However, although it is desirable for a student to use them cheerfully, the resistant student will nevertheless learn much more with them on than off. A student will learn the skills of blindness much better and exercise more caution with sleep shades on.

A Dramatic Example

To illustrate the fact that it is actually safer for a student to wear sleep shades, consider this example. Mel disliked school and was generally regarded as rebellious and careless. With very poor vision, he often could not see well enough to perform a task accurately with vision alone. Mel handled this by bravado, rushing through the task with false confidence. In home economics (not wearing sleep shades) he nearly cut off the tip of his finger by reaching into the blender while the blades were rotating.

"We just can't have Mel in my class," said the industrial arts teacher with panic in his voice. "He'll cut off his whole hand."

The itinerant teacher, however, urged once again that sleep shades be used. "With the shades," she explained, "Mel will realize that he really cannot see things, and will be more motivated to use good techniques."

Realizing that Mel would resist, the principal called him in and made it clear that this was how it would be done. Standard safety goggles were modified to obscure vision. Mel was nervous and resentful at first, but at least he was cautious. Gradually he did learn alternative techniques for the basic power tools, and he also observed the general safety rules much better than he had in home economics. Slowly he gained some genuine confidence based on real competence. He was justly proud of his completed project. And his hands were very much intact.

Mel Was Not Unique

Many students, if not wearing sleep shades, use an unsafe approach much like Mel's former behavior, although it is rarely quite so obvious or spectacular as in Mel's case. Realizing (consciously or unconsciously) that they cannot really see well enough to work accurately by using vision, but believing there is no good alternative, they plunge ahead by guessing and hoping.

Other students, if not wearing sleep shades, react by being overtly fearful. They too gain confidence by wearing sleep shades during all practice sessions. This seems paradoxical and needs to be repeatedly explained, but it *does work*.

"How can this be??" exclaimed Joyce in amazement after several cane travel lessons with sleep shades. "I think I actually get around *better* with my sleep shades on than without them!" As Joyce's teacher explained, she was at last learning techniques which were safer and more reliable than her inadequate vision–techniques which she had never really used during previous lessons without sleep shades. Much later, when she had learned them thoroughly, Joyce would be able to use these techniques all the time, even when not wearing shades.

Wearing sleep shades and using proper techniques is safer, more comfortable, and more efficient.

Evaluating Progress

Since resistance to sleep shades is common, it is not unusual for students to peek under their sleep shades or take them off when they become frustrated. It is possible to look under sleep shades without actually touching or removing them (by moving various facial muscles and disarranging the shades slightly, etc.) Therefore, often the only way the teacher knows about the cheating is to observe how the student is performing the task. Whether the teacher is sighted or blind, this observation of performance is the best way to know if a student is cheating. For instance, if a student veers to avoid objects without contacting them with the cane, or skips down the page without following the line tactilely, it is likely that cheating has occurred. The blind teacher will encounter the objects avoided by the student and can hear the way the hands move in the reading of Braille. Periodic discussions of the value of sleep shades also help reduce the incidence of peeking.

Also note that with younger children, the regular shades are genuinely too large, and the child may be unable to avoid peeking. Adding a small amount of fabric around the nose solves this problem.

Conclusion

Ultimately, whether a child likes wearing sleep shades or not, they are a useful tool like any other. If a child doesn't like to work math problems by hand, for instance, we do not simply omit this from his curriculum.

After a student can travel competently and needs no more training, and after a student has learned to read and write Braille with ease, there is no more need for sleep shades when using those skills. The skills that were learned efficiently by wearing sleep shades will continue to be used.

REMARKS: *Inform Parents and Educators*

When you first describe your proposed instructional plan, include an explanation of sleep shades and their importance. Write them into the IEP. Make it clear that the use of shades is an integral, necessary part of instruction, not an optional idea.

When their child is beginning instruction, it is important for parents to observe a competent traveler. Ask that traveler to wear sleep shades during the demonstration. (Even if he/she is totally blind, this is a good idea. It will prove that he/she really is not relying on even light perception, and it will show that the shades are not uncomfortable.)

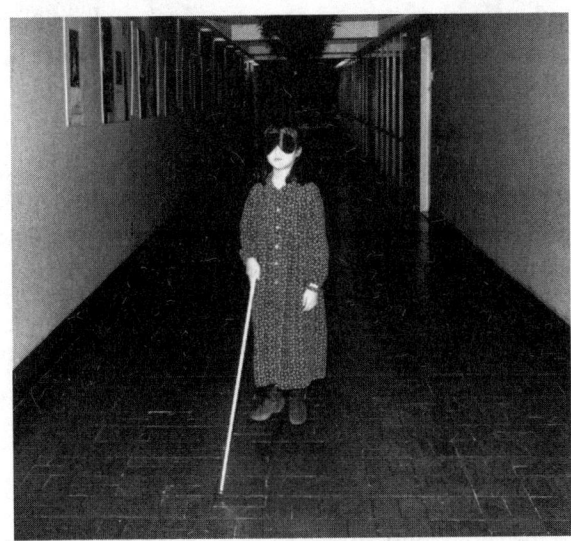

**Figure 7-1
Sleep Shades for Effective Learning**

ACTIVITIES:

EXAMPLE 1: *AGE 12 AND UP*

For a reasonably mature student age 12 and up (and often even somewhat younger), introducing the sleep shades is very much the same as for an adult.

A student of this age should be included in the IEP meeting where instruction is decided upon. Sleep shades should be included in the overall description—as part of the matter-of-fact explanation of methods, not as a tentative afterthought. They should be written into the IEP as a condition. (See Objectives, above).

When starting instruction, encourage the student to examine both cane and sleep shades, and to try on the shades and check for comfort. Review the reasons for use—in a brisk tone that implies information rather than cajoling:

- They shut out vision so that the other senses and the cane must be relied upon. Without this, the new skills will not be learned.
- With shades, it will be abundantly clear that travel is accomplished without vision. Otherwise it would be unclear how much success is due to vision and how much to alternative techniques. Later, with full understanding, a person can combine visual and alternative techniques during travel outside of lessons.
- If more vision is lost in the future, retraining will not be necessary.

At first, provide a very easy setting to promote confidence and a smooth stride. A long hallway is good. Warn of obstacles at first, to avoid beginning with awkward jolts. Continued careful programming—neither too hard nor too easy—encourages continued good technique and confidence.

Anticipate and prevent problems. Occasionally ask whether comfort could be improved. A choice among two or three pairs often provides both practical and psychological improvement in comfort. Be sensitive to concern about messy hair.

The student should put the shades on and take them off himself, but the teacher should decide *when*. Be definite about this—either by direct statement each time or by ongoing convention. ("Put them on each time we go out the door to leave for a route, please; then when we return and get inside the building you may take them off.") Shades should *not* be removed for reasons of conversation, retrieving a dropped object, etc. Actions in the course of the lesson should be accomplished by alternative techniques.

The older the student, the more important it is to include him in planning and to enlist his agreement and support. If a younger student is reluctant, it is usually possible to secure cooperation by making expectations clear and by shaping the situation. But if a teenager is really not in agreement, it may be virtually impossible to make progress; more discussion is necessary with parents, school staff, and the student.

Even with the most cooperative student, take care that many aspects of instruction are clearly pleasant. Arrange increasing privileges and opportunities. Keep a list of accomplishments. Provide reassurance and encouragement when work is difficult.

EXAMPLE 2: *AGE 8*

Shades are introduced to a student of this age in a manner similar to that with an older student, but with allowances for less maturity.

The student may or may not be included in IEP planning sessions. As with many other things for children of this age, the plan for instruction may be presented to the child as an already-decided fact. However, it is important to explain in a positive manner and encourage the child to voice any questions or concerns. (See also the Module, "Introducing the Cane.")

Explain reasons for the shades in the same general way as described above for older students. But use appropriate vocabulary, and be alert to prevent misunderstandings. For example, the student may get the impression that he will soon be required to wear shades literally *all* the time – beyond the lessons and even at home.

Standard-sized shades may be too large to fit well and to occlude all vision. If necessary, sew a little extra fabric around the nose.

The first session should have relatively little actual instruction. Spend most of the time getting acquainted and putting the youngster at ease.

Do not expect the shades to be worn for the full period. Instead, ask the student to wear them for 3-5 minutes twice:

(1) during an enjoyable activity which is easily done without sight – for example, telling riddles or talking about hobbies.

(2) after initial explanation of stance, walking on a flat surface with no obstructions and with some physical assistance.

These two brief experiences assure an easy, successful beginning.

During **the second session,** begin requiring shades during all actual instruction. Note, however, that you can bend the definition of a "lesson." With a young beginner, I may say, "For ten minutes we will have a lesson on walking on the flat, level floor. Then we'll take a break and talk awhile. Next we'll go up and down stairs a few times." I may define the "break" as not being a "lesson," and allow the shades to be removed. Also, when we finish on the stairs, I may state that "the lesson is over," and let the student walk back without the shades (though still using his cane).

In later sessions, I expand the definition of the "lesson," so that that student wears the shades for 20 or 30 minutes at a time, as appropriate for his age.

(Note: This kind of phasing in is not advisable for an older student who should be able to work for an extended period of time in the standard manner. But short sessions, *determined by the teacher,* can be important in helping a young beginner get accustomed to a new experience.)

Continue to have some "pure fun" at the end of the lesson frequently. Examples include: free time to examine interesting things (with or without shades); a chart or booklet of accomplishments; a game or treat at the end of each unit; etc. Less mature children may need an approach more like that suggested for a four-year-old, below.

The "fun" activities should be contingent upon cooperation in the use of shades, as well as other things. Any lack of cooperation should be handled in age-appropriate ways.

EXAMPLE 3: *AGE 4*

Lesson 1: Get Acquainted

For a young child, it is very important to spend time establishing rapport before beginning actual instruction. The first session should be a pleasant "play" session in a familiar location, with familiar activities and materials. The parent or preschool teacher may remain nearby or even join in.

Ask parents or preschool teachers what the child especially enjoys. Ask them to introduce you, and to help you plan initial sessions which are enjoyable and familiar. Examples include:

- The child shows and demonstrates favorite toys.
- Student and teacher play with clay, construction sets, etc.
- The child goes about his usual activities, while the new teacher goes along and makes friendly remarks.

Lesson 2: Introduction

Begin with a brief "fun" activity, such as examining two favorite toys.

Then show the child the cane, and encourage interested discussion. Consider showing several canes of various lengths (certainly including your own cane, if you yourself are blind). Show how the length is determined in comparison to a person's height.

Teach vocabulary: cane, tip, handle, etc. The child may enjoy answering questions as you (for example) place the tip in his hand and ask, "What is this part called?" Look at a separate cane tip, as well as the tip on the cane.

Do not hurry this discussion. It is an age-appropriate activity which sets the stage for instruction. Encourage the child to examine the cane(s) thoroughly and ask questions himself. Begin to show how the cane is held and moved.

Show the child the sleep shades. Ask him to repeat the name. Explain that the name comes from the fact that some people use them to help them sleep in the daytime; encourage amusement.

Continue, "I'm going to show you how these shades fit on your eyes. I will put them there for just a minute so you can find out what they feel like. When they're on, you won't see things with your eyes, but you can hear with your ears. I will make some animal noises, and you tell me what they are. OK, hold still, now....There! Meeoww....."

If the child is especially immature, introduce the shades by simply holding them over his eyes momentarily, rather than putting the elastic band around his head the first time.

After taking off the shades, spend a few more minutes with a general get-acquainted activity, as in Lesson 1.

Lesson 3: Seated Activity With the Shades

Examine the cane and shades again. Review vocabulary and explanation. Compliment the child for what he remembers.

Introduce a "fun" activity which can very easily be done without sight and does not involve going anywhere. Good examples are:

- Examining interesting textures and objects by touch, as the teacher hands them to the student.
- Eating a very simple snack, such as a cookie or cracker
- Drinking juice
- Singing, talking, telling jokes, etc.
- Listening to music

Explain, "You remember that these are called sleep shades – or shades, for short. Last time I put them on your eyes for just a minute.

"Today you will wear them for a little bit longer – long enough for us to do something extra fun. With the shades on, you won't see things with your eyes. But you can hear, and taste, and smell, and feel. The shades will help you notice hearing and feeling and so on. Here they are; I'm going to put them on you. I will take them off pretty soon; don't touch them, please... OK, ready for the fun. First, here's a really, really fuzzy toy dog...."

Three to five minutes is a good length for this first experience. Short experiences are important in establishing that (a) wearing the shades is not uncomfortable or frightening; and (b) the teacher controls when they will be worn. A child of this age might genuinely have great difficulty tolerating a new experience for a longer time at the very beginning.

With a very young student, it is usually best not to allow him to touch the shades at all, at least at first. The easiest way to prevent his trying to remove them is to insist that only the teacher touches them. ("If they don't feel right, tell me about it. *I* will take hold of them and fix them.") If after a few sessions the student seems reliable, you may decide to allow him to put them on and take them off–provided that he follows your directions.

Lesson 4: Walking While Wearing Shades
Select a location suitable for the first actual cane instruction: a flat surface with considerable space free of obstacles. Go there with the child (without using shades).

Show the child how to hold the cane.

Continue, "You remember the sleep shades – here they are. I'll put them on over your eyes... there. Now, the shades will help you learn what your new cane can do. It can do a lot of things! Some people even like to say the cane can talk! Now, there's nothing in the way here, and the cane and I are going to show you some new and fun things...."

Physically assist the child to tap the cane and walk ahead. Then announce that a wall will soon be found; help him find it with the cane (striking it more than once for emphasis). Turn around and proceed to the opposite wall or another suitable object, etc.

Again, 3-5 minutes is a good length of time for this initial experience. Remove the shades and follow with a short play session.

Further lessons
For most children at age 4, after about four sessions as above, it is reasonable to expect the shades to be worn for the duration of an age-appropriate practice session. (The Module, "Introducing the Cane," discusses the length and nature of age-appropriate sessions. Also, in the *Handbook,* see the chapter, "Cane Curriculum (Under 8 and Special Problems)."

If the child is especially immature, it may be wise to keep devoting much of each session to "play"–contingent upon completion of a short activity with the cane as you direct. Even for a mature child of this age, a short "fun" activity at the end is desirable.

Sometimes the fun can occur naturally with the lesson. If the child is learning his way around the playground, he can climb on equipment for awhile afterward. Otherwise, a short period (5 minutes or so) of unrelated "fun" is desirable

and appropriate for this age.

Save the greatest "fun" for last, as added motivation. If there is much fussing about the shades, or the lesson is otherwise very unsatisfactory, the "fun" may be conspicuously omitted. ("I'm sorry, but we won't have time to do any playing today. We used up all our time talking about being quiet in the hall. But next time I will plan some playtime, and I'm sure you'll do your work fine.")

Below Age 4

Many instructors prefer to wait until age 4 before using sleep shades in instruction. Little research has been done on their use below that age.

EXAMPLE 4: *A STUDENT ACCUSTOMED TO OTHER METHODS*

What if a student has had instruction elsewhere and did not wear shades?

It is usually unwise to attack the methods used by the previous teacher, since the student and his family may have been fond of him or her. Instead, explain your reasons for using the shades. Emphasize that this is the method used in your program; compare it to differences in math or other subjects.

The younger the student, the less he/she will be surprised by the idea of shades. Everything seems new and different to a young child. His/her parents may feel uncertain at first, however. All parents, as well as older students, should receive careful explanation and demonstration, as discussed above for initial planning.

Sometimes a student has been wearing sleep shades for Braille instruction and some daily living skills work, but not for travel instruction. If shades have been introduced in one of those settings first, minimal explanation and adjustment should be needed for using them in travel. Note, however, that in another setting the student may have been allowed to remove the shades when moving around.

EXAMPLE 5: *A LOWER-FUNCTIONING OLDER STUDENT*

When an older student has a mental disability, instruction should be approached as for a younger student, but in an age-appropriate manner.

Rob is 15 years old and attends a special class. He seems much like a five-year-old. He does not read.

For Rob, an approach much like that described for a four-year-old is called for – but in an age-appropriate manner.

While getting acquainted, ask Rob to show you things he particularly enjoys – games, for example. Play a game with him.

When first introducing the shades briefly, tell riddles rather than using childish animal sounds.

Age-appropriate "fun" activities at the end of a session might include touring an interesting area at leisure; playing checkers; making a booklet or chart.

Ask classroom teachers about how much to expect how soon; activities the student especially enjoys; and behavior control.

EXCEPTIONS AND SPECIAL CIRCUMSTANCES:

There are a few medical conditions which really may cause delay or changes in the use of sleep shades.

Injury: If the student has had a major injury to the head or face, check with a nurse or doctor about possible precautions.

Hearing Impairment: If a student has usable vision and a substantial hearing loss, it may not be wise for him to wear sleep shades when traffic is involved. Following are suggestions:

- The student wears shades while walking with the teacher (not independently), and while standing near traffic. This enables him to learn as much as he can about traffic sounds, in a very safe manner.
- Advice is provided by an instructor experienced with students who have impairment of both hearing and vision.
- The student wears shades for practice sessions which do not involve traffic, but does not wear them when practicing independence around traffic.

Emotional Problems: Fear and emotion are often given as a reason to avoid or delay the use of sleep shades – usually without real basis. Ordinarily, any fear or concern is a natural part of learning a new skill; it is overcome with reassurance, practice, and gaining confidence. Especially with a younger child, it is usually the *adults* who may be concerned. The student usually accepts the shades if others do. In time, the shades prove themselves as a valuable tool; the student learns to depend on alternative techniques instead of trying to depend on inadequate sight.

Occasionally, however, you may have a student who truly has major emotional problems. Consult with other staff and obtain medical information. Ask, by comparison, what would be done if the student needed to learn some other new physical skill – swimming, for example.

The IEP team should decide whether emotional difficulties really do warrant a delay or modification in instruction. Sleep shades should not be singled out, however. If the student is not ready to begin regular cane travel instruction, he is not ready. When he is ready, he should be able to use sleep shades along with the cane (though perhaps with extra reassurance and other modifications in the overall instruction).

Light Sensitivity: It is a good idea to warn every student: "When you take the shades off, it will be like coming from a very dark movie into a bright light. You may want to close your eyes when you take the shades off, and open them slowly."

Some eye conditions cause extreme sensitivity to light. This can result in extreme discomfort after removing the shades. Help the student find ideas to minimize discomfort. Should sunglasses be available immediately? Might he hold his hand above his eyes, shielding them for a short time? Should he take off the shades only indoors?

CAUTION: Always be informed about *any* medical conditions which affect a student.

Avoid letting sleep shades be passed around, lest eye infections also be passed around. When a student leaves the program, discard the shades that he has used.

COMBINING VISION WITH ALTERNATIVE TECHNIQUES:

An adult who has traveled under sleep shades will figure out an appropriate personal combination of techniques to be used outside of lessons, some using sight and some not. For example, a person may see the outlines of buildings visually, but rely on the cane to find steps and doorways. Children, however, may not do this on their own. Instead they may travel increasingly well under sleep shades but immediately revert to the old hesitations when the sleep shades are off.

Ted was terrified of crossing streets, since he did not really have enough vision to judge traffic movements. Using sleep shades, he learned to listen carefully and cross confidently. But one day after the lesson, when Ted had his cane but was not wearing sleep shades, he was asked to cross a street—and he froze! The teacher, seeing no cars coming from any direction, asked in bewilderment what was wrong. "I'm waiting for those," replied Ted as he pointed to two *parked* cars. He was relying on his eyes instead of applying what he had been taught.

It may be desirable for the travel teacher occasionally to help the child use alternative techniques when the eyes are not covered. Explain that partial sight sometimes gives such inaccurate or incomplete information that it should be disregarded. ("Never mind what you see with your eyes. That won't help. Listen with your ears, and pay attention to your cane.")

Make a clear separation between this kind of practice and the regular lessons in which sleep shades are always used. You might label the combination work as "extra practice," and possibly carry it out in a different location.

RELATED PRACTICE:
Have the student visit lessons or demonstrations where others are wearing sleep shades.

Wear shades yourself some of the time. You may want to do this even if you are totally blind. It will demonstrate that you do not find them uncomfortable, and will help to prove that you really are using alternative techniques.

A good discussion question is: "Why do you suppose some students have started calling them 'Freedom Shades'?" [Wearing the shades helps the students learn ways to travel more freely and easily. This frees them from being slow and limited. Also, the shades help to free them from unwise dependence on sight in situations where that is inefficient.]

REFERENCE(S):

PUBLICATIONS:

Willoughby and Duffy. *Handbook for Itinerant and Resource Teachers of Blind and Visually Impaired Students,* pp. 55-72, 175-198, 385-392.

Future Reflections magazine.

AGENCIES AND ORGANIZATIONS:

BLIND, Inc.

Colorado Center for the Blind

Louisiana Center for the Blind

National Federation of the Blind

Nebraska Services for the Blind

MODULE 8
POOR LIGHTING CONDITIONS:
Independence at Night
In Dim Light
and
With Glare

OBJECTIVE: The student's independence will be consistent regardless of lighting conditions – including glare, inconsistent lighting, dim lighting, and day vs. night.

AGE OF STUDENT: All ages
(NOTE: Ages are mentioned in relation to circumstances given in a particular Example – e.g., recess in an elementary school. Concepts and techniques apply to all ages. Manner of presentation would be altered according to the student's maturity.)

PRIMARY SKILL EMPHASIS:
Attitudes toward blindness
Understanding vision and partial vision
Detecting step-downs or drop-offs
Flexibility and confidence
General travel

ADDITIONAL SKILL EMPHASIS:
Finding a person
In a crowd or a line
Finding a seat
Responsibility and citizenship
Weather and temperature

SEE ALSO (Other Modules):
  Inclement Weather
  Visually Confusing Appearance
  Sleep Shades
  Walking Independently While Following Someone
  Unexpected Drop-Off or Step-Down
  Auditorium or Theater

TEACHER PREPARATION: Inquire about present level of independence in dim light and in extreme glare. Look for situations and times when the student could encounter these conditions during lessons.

FIGURE(S):
FIGURE 8-1: Safe Travel at Night

REMARKS: Many persons with partial sight travel fairly well in normal daylight, but have significant difficulty at night or under glare conditions. A person may *use* a cane at all times, yet continue to *rely* mainly on the eyes for certain things – e.g., finding doorways or watching for traffic. Or, he may decline to use a cane in daylight at all, believing he "doesn't need the cane unless the light is bad."

The remedy is *consistent* reliance on good cane technique.

First, the student must learn techniques thoroughly while wearing sleep shades, not using sight at all. Outside of lesson time, he may supplement the cane with the use of sight when it is convenient. However, the cane remains in use at all times, and alternative techniques are relied upon whenever sight may be unreliable or inconvenient. (See *Handbook*, pp. 182-185.)

ACTIVITIES:

EXAMPLE 1: *SUDDEN CHANGE OF LIGHTING CONDITIONS*
(*Primary grades*)
"Mrs. Brown tells me that coming in from recess has been hard for you. People have been helping you find your coat hook and find your seat. Would you tell me about that?....

"Thank you for explaining. So, it's very bright on the playground, and then the hallway seems awfully dark. It takes awhile for your eyes to get used to the change....

"Mrs. Brown tells me that you have your cane with you when you're coming in, and we're glad you're remembering. I'm going to help you get the cane to work even more while you're coming in, so that you won't need extra help."
*****

Proceed with the following practice:

   a. Have the student wear sleep shades and practice "coming in from recess" during a travel lesson. Have him go in and out of the rest room; find his coat hook; find the door to his classroom; etc.
   b. Simulate coming in from recess (again, with sleep shades) while you follow with a stopwatch. Everything must be completed in the five minutes normally allowed.
   c. In a special extra lesson, do the same things without using sleep shades. Emphasize relying on the cane regardless of what is seen (or not seen) visually. Again, have the student simulate coming in from recess while you follow with a stopwatch. If he hesitates, trying to focus his eyes, prompt him: "Use your cane! Three more minutes!"
   d. Observe the end of an actual recess, and note that the student arrives at his seat without extra help.
   e. Ask classroom and playground teachers to help you spot-check maintenance of good habits.

EXAMPLE 2: *LIGHTING IS DIM OR UNRELIABLE*
(*Middle School or High School*)

Problem: The student travels well under sleep shades in various environments. At school, however, even though he has his cane with him, he tends to run into people in the west stairway and the north hallway. He has great difficulty finding a seat in a classroom if the lights are off for a film.
*****

You note that the north hall and the west stairwell are rather unevenly lighted. You say,

"I'd like to tell you about an unfortunate high school student I once knew. Although he didn't see well at all, he refused to use a cane at school. One stairway, especially, was rather dimly lighted. One day he was going down in a hurry, and ran into another student – hard.

"The other student thought he had done it on purpose, and slugged him. The blind student hit back, and they both found themselves in the principal's office. As an added complication, one of the young men was White and one was African-American; each thought the other was racially motivated.

"They were both suspended for three days.

"Now, I am pleased to point out that you are *not* making that other student's biggest mistake – not having a cane at all. If he had had a cane, it's very likely that the other student would have given him space, or at least would not have thought he ran into him on purpose. There probably would not have been a fight. Just having a cane with you provides identification and prevents a lot of problems, as we have said before.

"But I think maybe you sometimes have part of the same problem: you may not be *using* your cane consistently here at school. I think sometimes you rely on your eyes and your memory, and just sort of carry the cane. Then when the light is poor, you run into people or can't find your way. What do you think?....

"It's been quite awhile since we've had an actual lesson here at school, since you're doing so well downtown. I think we've been neglecting certain points, and I'd like to do some work here...."
*****

Proceed with the following practice:

   a. The student, wearing sleep shades, practices walking up and down the west stairway; going to an unfamiliar room in the north hallway; finding a seat in a darkened classroom (with pre-arrangement, in a room which is vacant at the time); etc.
   b. If desired, the above is repeated as a special extra lesson without sleep

shades.

c. Explain that you will occasionally observe while the student is going from class to class. You will not say anything at the time (you will just walk along casually nearby, and not make it obvious that you are observing), but will discuss it later.

EXAMPLE 3: *AT NIGHT*
(*Middle school or high school*)

Problem: the student never walks independently at night. In fact, he dislikes going anywhere at all at night. He travels quite well in the daytime, and while wearing shades during lessons; however, at night he hangs onto someone else.

*****

Talk about daytime travel vs. evening travel. Emphasize that travel under sleep shades trains a person to use techniques not requiring any sight. Even if a person uses partial vision to some extent in daylight, he should easily be able to change emphasis at night and place more reliance on the alternatives.

"Imagine you are wearing sleep shades," you might say. "You get along fine when you are really wearing them. Try imagining that you do have them on."

Depending on circumstances and the student's abilities, arrange experiences such as the following:

a. Practice in poorly-lighted areas of the school, as in the Example above.

b. On a very bright day, ask the student to walk around outside and then come inside to complete specific tasks immediately (as in Example 1, above.)

c. Practice outdoors when weather causes extreme glare or other adverse visual conditions.

d. Arrange a session after nightfall. This might be in conjunction with an evening conference; after the early sunset in winter; or by some other scheduling arrangement.

First, practice as usual with sleep shades in situations which particularly bring out the value of the cane: crossing streets, meeting unexpected step-downs, etc. Then continue with comparable practice as a special extra lesson without sleep shades. Urge the student to "imagine the shades are still on" and rely mainly on alternative techniques. *Disregarding* visual input is wise when it is unreliable or so incomplete as to be confusing.

e. The above practice (first wearing shades, and then immediately practicing in a similar way without shades in poor light) may be done without the travel teacher being actually present. A mature student may practice alone. Parents or others may assist. But the helper must really understand that alternative techniques are superior to the attempt to rely on inadequate vision.

In time, the student will learn to integrate the use of his vision with alternative techniques in the way most advantageous for him individually. But, especially at first, it is often good advice to say, "Never mind what you see with your eyes."

It may be helpful to time activities with a stopwatch, record the number of hesitations, etc., both with sleep shades and without.

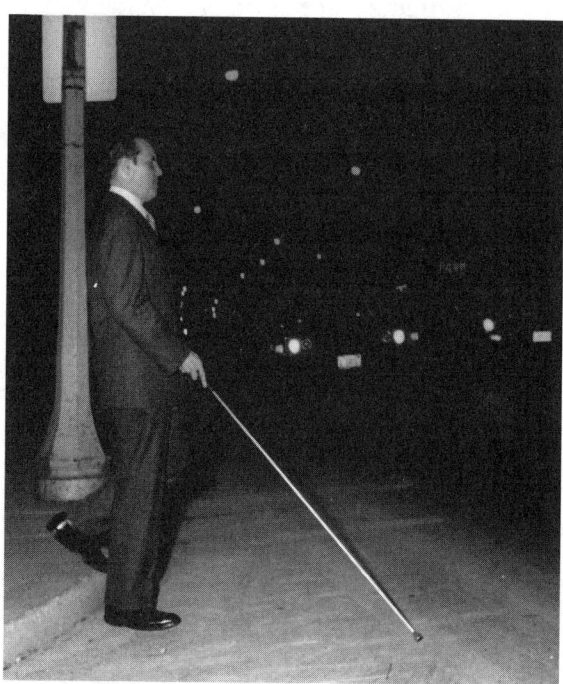

**Figure 8-1
Safe Travel at Night**

REMARKS: A student may comment, "I get along fine in good light, even if I'm not really using my cane. Why can't I just leave it – or use a folding cane and keep it folded – in the daytime? I only need it at night!"

The *Handbook* discusses this question in detail. Essentially, these are the main points:

- We never can be sure what lighting conditions will exist from one minute to the next. A light bulb may burn out; the weather may change; lighting may vary for any number of reasons.
- If a person uses a cane only part of the time, techniques will never become automatic, polished, and reliable. Techniques will not be fully effective even when they are used.
- If a person really cannot travel well under poor lighting conditions, then his eye condition is such that he actually would benefit from using the cane at other times, even though the need may not be so obvious.
- The main reason for avoidance of a cane is the lack of acceptance of blindness as a respectable characteristic. When positive attitudes are attained, the subject is viewed objectively.

REFERENCE(S):

Willoughby and Duffy, *Handbook for Itinerant and Resource Teachers of Blind and Visually Impaired Students,* pp. 157-198.

Richard Mettler. *Cognitive Learning Theory and Cane Travel Instruction: A New Paradigm,* pp. 66-106.

MODULE 9
RIGHT AND LEFT

OBJECTIVE: (*Preschool and Kindergarten*) The student will correctly name left and right in regard to parts of his/her own body.

OBJECTIVE: (*Elementary grades and up*) The student will correctly name left and right, both in regard to him/herself and in regard to another person's frame of reference.

OBJECTIVE: (*Elementary grades and up*) The student will turn left or right according to verbal directions.

AGE OF STUDENT: Preschool and up (See Examples)

TEACHER PREPARATION: Be familiar with the typical level of understanding for each age group.

PRIMARY SKILL EMPHASIS:
Right and left
Corners, turns, and angles

ADDITIONAL SKILL EMPHASIS:
General travel
Compass directions
Communication and instructions
Landmarks
Orientation overall

SEE ALSO (Other Modules):
Home—Contents of Room
Walking Across Open Space
Street Crossing With Little Traffic
Compass Directions

REMARKS: Learning the concept of left and right is a developmental process for young children.

At the preschool level, children are still learning even more basic relationships such as "behind," "in front of," and "beside;" however, they can also proceed with understanding "left" and "right."

By age 5 or 6, most children can name left and right in relation to their own bodies. Many children learn even faster than this, either by natural ability or because of extra emphasis. Since this skill is very important for blind children, we should strive for early learning.

When a young child cannot yet reliably name left and right, it is important that she frequently hear other people naming them for her. This provides important readiness background.

REMARKS: A vocabulary problem occurs with the many meanings of "right." It can mean the opposite of "left," the opposite of "wrong," and even "a 90-degree angle." To prevent confusion and endless puns, I tend to say "Correct," or "Yes, that's it."

ACTIVITIES:

EXAMPLE 1: *INTRODUCTION*
(*Preschool/kindergarten*)
Wearing something on one arm or hand is very helpful at first. This may be a toy watch, ring, bracelet, etc., or just a rubber band.

Work with classroom teachers, parents, and others to encourage strong emphasis on left/right. Many games and songs, such as "Looby Loo," include this already. Others, such as "Simon Says," easily incorporate it. As the travel teacher for a young child, you can sometimes include such games and songs in your lessons. Besides teaching directionality in an appropriate way, they add variety and fun.

Following are examples of games and activities:
- Use singing games which incorporate left/right
- Briskly direct several amusing motions such as:
   *Touch your right ear
   *Put your left hand on your nose
   *Hop on your right foot

*Touch the wall with your right hand
*Wave with your left hand
- Direct the child to walk a short distance to find something, as:
    *Turn to your right and find the wall.
    *Go to your left and find a desk.
    *Go to your right and sit down in a chair.
- Ask questions in which the answer involves left/right. For example, in a familiar classroom ask, "Think about where we are. Point toward the toy shelf. To get there, will you be going left or right?"
- Seat the child at a desk or table. Say, "I will place a toy car on the left side of your desk. See how fast you can find it." (Tap *both* sides of the desk as you set the car down.)

EXAMPLE 2: *REVERSING DIRECTION IN RELATION TO SURROUNDINGS*
(*Preschool/kindergarten*)

A child of preschool age begins to learn that when she herself turns around, her own left/right is reversed in relation to the outside world. Emphasize and discuss this as the child matures.

For example, ask the student to walk along the hallway, noting that the water fountain is on her right. Then have her turn around and come back past the fountain again; it will be on her left.

This kind of exercise should be done frequently. It is particularly effective with a distinctive sound feature – a humming fountain, the music class, etc. However, it is also important to discuss this when there is no distinctive sound. For example:

"Stop here, please. Tell me again what we will find at the end of the hall.... the gym, yes, that's correct. Now, as we go toward the gym, can you tell me whether the library is on our right or our left?... OK, I'm not going to tell you whether you are correct in saying it is on the left. Go ahead, please, and walk along the left side of the hall. Look for the big library doors....Are they there?"

EXAMPLE 3: *ANOTHER PERSON FACING THE SAME WAY*
(*Preschool/primary grades*)

It is one thing for a child to learn left and right in relation to her own body. It is quite another for her to transpose this concept into someone else's frame of reference.

When a young child is still uncertain about left/right in relation to herself, do not place emphasis on understanding different points of view. Instead, for variety and added understanding, help the child examine left/right on someone else who is *facing the same way* – as, with his back to the child. The other person's left arm will then be on the same side as the child's left arm. Consider having this other person wear (at least temporarily) a duplicate of any "marker" the child may be using – e.g., a watch on the left arm. (A rubber band will do if an actual equivalent is not readily available.)

The "other person" may not be an actual person – it may be a doll or a teddy bear.

During this stage, the child will begin to grasp a part of the idea of a "different frame of reference." She will realize that other beings have left and right sides also. She will hear you say, "Now the teddy bear is facing the same way you are," and begin to realize that something is different if the teddy bear is *not* facing the same way.

EXAMPLE 4: *A PERSON FACING THE OPPOSITE WAY*
(*Kindergarten through elementary grades*)

Help the child learn that turning around results in reversal. For example, with a kindergartner, stand with your back to the child as she finds the rubber band to verify your left wrist. Ask her to stand still while you turn around and face her. Compare arms again.

As the youngster matures, include more advanced work. Explain, "When you are thinking about which is someone else's right or left side, first you need to think of that person facing the same way you are. You may need to turn that person around – either for real, or in your head – so that he's facing the same way you are.

Then, keep track of one side as you think about how he can move into another position."

Stand *facing* the child. Ask *her* to arrange things so that you both face the same way. (She is permitted to move herself and/or you.) Then verify that both of you are facing the same way, and note a particular part of your body (e.g., left arm with watch). Turn around again, with the child examining your motion as much as possible; note that the arm is now on the "other side" in relation to the child, but still "on the left" to you.

Repeat this with a teddy bear or doll. This may be even clearer to the child, as she can easily hold onto the teddy bear's left arm while the bear is moved around.

EXAMPLE 5: *CONTINUED PRACTICE*

Include directional names continually in travel lessons, as well as other activities. Following are a few examples:

Preschool/primary grades:
- As the student walks along, give directions for practice:
    * Turn right and touch the wall.
    * Turn right, find a seat, and sit down.
    * Turn left and step onto the grass.
    * Find a pole on your left.
- As you walk around the school with the student, ask questions such as, "Look on your right. What do you find?".... The desired answer may be in general terms ("the wall") or specific ("the door to Mr. North's office").
- Beforehand, place (or plan) a few "fun" items in specific places. As the student walks along, give directions:
    * Turn right and touch the wall. Down by your feet you'll find a box, and you may look inside.
    * Turn right, find a seat, and sit down. Then I will tell you a riddle.
    * Turn left and step onto the grass. Keep going and find a tree with nice-smelling blossoms.
    * Find a pole on your left. Look at the funny balloon tied to it.
- Have a treasure hunt with Braille clues which emphasize directionality, as, "Go to the left side of the sink."

All ages:
Integrate left/right directions into any and all practice. For a young child still working on the concept, adults should often say, "Now we are turning right," even if the child cannot yet state this independently. As the student gains in understanding, incorporate left/right into explanations continually.

- "The first door on the left..."
- "Turn left at the first hallway."
- "The counter is on your right as you enter."
- "When you're coming back from ___, will you hear the traffic on your left or your right?"

Left/right directionality is the main characteristic used in distinguishing some items such as switches or buttons.

- The switch on the left is the kitchen light.
- With water faucets, the one on the left is hot and the one on the right is cold.
- On this tape machine, the second button from the left is *play*.
- In Home Economics, each even-numbered area has the stove on the right; each odd-numbered area has the stove on the left.

EXAMPLE 6: *VARIOUS FRAMES OF REFERENCE*
(*Elementary grades and up*)

Some children, even at quite a young age, are intrigued by directional concepts and enjoy a sophisticated discussion. Others find it confusing to discuss more than one idea at a time. However, by the upper elementary grades a student should be introduced to interrelationships. For example:

- Your own left/right is in relation to your own body. Left/right in regard to someone else is in relation to that person's body. This can also apply to an animal, a toy, a vehicle, etc.
- Other completely different frames of reference, such as up/down, may be

discussed by comparison.

– If we speak of the left or right side of a particular room, it tends to be in relation to our own bodies as we face the front of the room. In a theater, we usually discuss direction in terms of the audience, but the actors have a reversed frame of reference.

– Walk past a humming refrigerator on your right; turn around; walk back past the same refrigerator, which is now on your left. The refrigerator has not moved. You have moved, and you have changed your frame of reference in relation to the refrigerator and its surroundings.

– Compass directions (NSEW) are not in relation to anyone's body. They are in relation to the poles of the Earth. One person may extend her left hand toward the north, while someone else (perhaps facing her) is extending her right hand toward the north.

– Although "north, south, east, west" is a different frame of reference than "left, right," the two interrelate in a consistent way. For example, if you are facing *north*, your *right* side will always be to the *east*. Analyze this for the various compass points.

– Some students will enjoy learning orientation terminology for space ships, where the ship and people move freely in every direction.

– When a member of the public gives a blind person directions, he/she may misspeak in terms of "your right" or "your left." Many sighted people do poorly in this regard.

REMARKS: Carefully consider how much discussion of various frames of reference is appropriate for a student at a given time. A young child may be easily confused. On the other hand, it is important for the maturing student to understand interrelationships.

EXAMPLE 7: *OLDER STUDENTS HAVING DIFFICULTY*

By age 5 or 6, most children can name left and right correctly, at least in relation to themselves.

If a person is ambidextrous (using both hands with relatively equal facility), she may have more than average difficulty with naming left and right. The same may be true of left-handed persons, perhaps because they are often forced to do things right-handed to accommodate society. Talk with classroom teachers about helping a young child settle on a hand preference without unwise coercion.

Handwriting is a task that requires young sighted children to settle on hand preference; make sure that Braille students also have tasks with one hand clearly dominant.

If an older student continues to have trouble with left and right, continue the practice described for younger children, but in an age-appropriate way. For example, instead of using a teddy bear for naming sides of the body, an adult-type costumed doll from South America might be used.

EXAMPLE 8: *TURNING 90 DEGREES*

Most commonly, "turn left" or "turn right" means approximately a 90-degree turn. Beginners should be taught to approximate this, and advanced students should realize that this is what usually is meant.

It is *not* realistic to expect to make a perfect 90-degree turn to the left (or right), proceed in a perfect straight line, and unerringly locate a small item. (See the Module, "Walking Across Open Space.") It *is* realistic to expect the student to turn approximately 90 degrees on the correct side and proceed essentially straight. Depending on the distance involved, some correction or exploration should be assumed at the destination.

For example, suppose the student is at a table in the middle of the lunchroom. The dirty-dish window is on her right, 20 feet away. The student will probably need to look around a bit when she reaches the wall with the window, rather than expecting always to arrive "straight as an arrow." Of course, she may also be aided by finding a noisy line of students.

A beginner: When a beginner is learning to "turn left" or "go to your left," it is helpful to direct her toward a large, easily-found item which is within a very few steps – the wall, a large piece of furniture, etc.

It is also helpful to practice turning while remaining close to a wall. The child can reach out her hand to touch the wall as she faces it; after turning 90 degrees to the left; after she has turned 180 degrees and is facing away from the wall; etc.

Teach the child to point in a given direction upon request. (Help her use the conventional gesture in a natural way.) Sometimes, tell her to point in the correct direction (e.g., to the right), and then direct, "follow your hand."

Building understanding: As the student matures, expose her to various additional names for a "normal" turn – e.g.,

- 90 degrees
- Sharp left/right
- Right-angle turn (note the pun in "turn left, at a right angle")

Emphasize that this kind of turn is ordinarily meant when someone says "on the left" or "turn left."

Tactual diagrams are useful in illustrating a 90-degree angle. They also help in discussing turns which are not 90 degrees – a situation which tends to be vague and confusing in daily life. Consider these remarks:

> "The street kind of meanders to the left."
> "It's a 'Y,' and you need to keep right."
> "Angle to the right – but not sharp right."
> "Go to your left, and then double back a bit."

A mature student should learn to describe angles in terms of degrees. But common expressions should be discussed also.

Remind the student that in getting directions from someone else, it is often helpful to point in the direction she thinks is meant; the other person will correct her in case of misunderstanding. A member of the public is likely to misspeak and say "on your right" when he means "on my right."

Avoid overemphasizing a precise angle. The approximately correct angle of approach should be supplemented with other clues and landmarks.

MODULE 10
COMPASS DIRECTIONS

OBJECTIVE: (*Lower elementary grades*): The student will state the four cardinal directions (NSEW). When north is known, he/she will indicate any of the four directions on request.

OBJECTIVE: (*Fourth grade and up*): The student will state the four cardinal directions and the four intermediate directions (NW, NE, SW, SE). When north is known, he/she will indicate any cardinal or intermediate direction. He/she will convert information about "left and right" into information about compass directions, and vice versa.

AGE OF STUDENT: Preschool and up (See Objectives and Examples.)

PRIMARY SKILL EMPHASIS:
Compass directions
Maps

ADDITIONAL SKILL EMPHASIS:
Right and left
Communication and instructions
Corners, turns, and angles
Landmarks
Orientation overall
General travel

SEE ALSO (Other Modules):
Right and Left
Around the Block
Asking Directions And Figuring It Out
Rural Environment

TEACHER PREPARATION: Be familiar with the typical level of understanding for each age group.

ACTIVITIES:

EXAMPLE 1: *VOCABULARY AND BASIC CONCEPTS*
The following approximate *sequence* of basic understanding begins in the preschool years and should be well along by about age 9:

(1) The student recognizes that the words "north, south, east, west" refer to directions in the environment.

(2) The student can recite the four cardinal directions. In at least one familiar place, she can face north upon request, and then can point out the other three directions while facing north.

(3) If one direction is known, the student can face in any direction and point out each of the four cardinal directions.

(4) If one direction is known, the student can point out any cardinal direction or any intermediate direction (NW, etc.)

(5) The student can convert information about left and right into information about compass directions, and vice versa. (This ability is gradually developed while the above skills are being developed in sequence.)

The instructor needs to understand this sequence of development. If a student has trouble with a higher level of skill, there may need to be reteaching at a lower level.

The student can understand directions as they relate to herself, facing in one particular direction, before she can grasp varying viewpoints. The Module, "Right and Left," has detailed suggestions for working with various viewpoints.

Especially for a beginner, it is important to have one familiar location where directions are clear-cut and often recited. A school hallway is especially good. Stand with the student (both of you facing north) and discuss: "North is toward the office...west is toward the fifth grades...south is behind us, toward the gym...and east is out the front door."

One of the best exercises is to go around a city block. The Module, "Around the Block" gives detailed suggestions.

EXAMPLE 2: *DIFFERENT FRAMES OF REFERENCE*

The Module, "Right and Left," discusses the relationship of various frames of reference:

- Left and right in relation to one's own body
- Left and right in relation to someone else's body
- Left and right in a room, auditorium, or vehicle
- Compass directions (in relation to the Earth)

Even a child under 8 can begin to discuss how these frames of references, and others, relate to one another. As the student matures, she should discuss this in detail.

When a student is turning (for example) east, ask her whether she is turning left or right, and analyze the relationship. Explain that in the future, you may not give "left and right" directions, but only compass directions, in assigning a route. Giving only compass directions—and noting how well the student can convert this information into actually walking the desired route—is valuable practice.

The concept of left and right should receive the major emphasis until it is mastered, since it is the more basic.

See the Module, "Right and Left," for detailed discussion of integration of concepts.

EXAMPLE 3: *CONCEPT INTEGRATION*

With a child of 10 or younger, avoid discussing too many aspects of compass directions at once. If the student is still learning such concepts, she may be confused by discussing all of these on the same day:

- Northeast corner of the block
- Walking west
- Turning left
- Walking on the south side of Elm Street
- North side of the block
- Traffic moving east on Elm
- The street is to our right; buildings are on our left

To avoid confusion for a young child, select one (or a few) of these concepts to be discussed at a particular time. Gradually help the maturing student to integrate them so that she can discuss all of them at the same time.

A beginner over age 10 should be able to discuss and relate several concepts together immediately. However, watch for possible need for simplification at first.

EXAMPLE 4: *CONTINUED PRACTICE*

Almost any practice session can easily include compass directions.

For a young child still working on the concept, the teacher can often say, "Now we are going east," or "We are on the north side of the building," even if the child could not yet state this independently.

Continual reinforcement is essential. Gradually expect more and more independence; do less and less re-explanation and simplification. Students must be exposed to cardinal directions *repeatedly* to acquire the habit of thinking in these terms as they travel about. Many lessons should focus on this in the ordinary course of acquiring skills.

Help the student internalize concepts of rotation—e.g., when you face east, north is on your left; when you face south, north is behind you.

Some find it helpful to relate compass directions to a clock face.

Relate directions to locations or features the student understands. For example:

- Often there is a conspicuous local landmark. In Boulder, Colorado, directions are clarified by the mountain range to the west. Other examples would be a river, a main highway, the ocean, etc.
- The student should know that the sun rises in the east and sets in the west. She can feel the sun's warmth and directionality in early morning and late evening.
- As elementary geography is learned, travel can be related to a map (in

actuality or in imagination). You may say, with varying degrees of humor, "We need to go toward New York," "This route goes south, toward Ames," or, "You don't want to go to Canada today."

The purpose of learning cardinal directions is to build a mental picture of the relationship of things to one another. When this occurs, the student understands that if she is in the northeast corner, there may be several routes to get to the southwest corner. But if cardinal directions are not used, pure memorization of fixed routes will be the result.

When the student really understands where she is in relationship to where she wants to go, she can get there without a specific route being assigned. It is desirable occasionally to let a student choose her own route from one place to another, to test whether she is doing good mental mapping or not. For example, if she is directed to proceed from the school to the bank along a specific route, she could be invited to choose a different route for return. Students who can devise an alternate route are demonstrating good mental mapping. Those who (in returning to the place where they started) must reverse their path without variation, either aren't at all adventurous or don't know how to use mental mapping skills.

MODULE 11
ROUGH TERRAIN

OBJECTIVE: The student will walk on varied surfaces – including sand, grass, and pebbles – at a speed appropriate for the situation.

AGE OF STUDENT: These examples are presented as for preschool or kindergarten. An older student will not ordinarily need much help and explanation, but merely experience in walking on various surfaces.

PRIMARY SKILL EMPHASIS:
Varied terrain
Flexibility and confidence
General travel (outdoors)
Detecting step-downs or drop-offs

ADDITIONAL SKILL EMPHASIS:
Examining things tactually
Climbing, clambering, crawling, etc.
Open space
Weather and temperature
Barefoot walking
Hills and inclines

TEACHER PREPARATION: Look for places where a surface consists of pebbles, gravel, sand, wood chips, etc. Consider arranging to walk where students are not ordinarily allowed, such as in a garden.

Note the child's maturity and previous experiences with such surfaces. Introduce a young child to such experiences carefully – very gradually, if necessary. Do not expect independence at first. Be firm, however, in expecting her to learn.

FIGURE(S):
FIGURE 11-1: At the Beach

SEE ALSO (Other Modules):
Inclement Weather (Including Ice Underfoot)
Back Yard Boundaries
Back Yard (Overall)
More Ideas for Lessons at Home Outdoors
What's Out There? (On the School Grounds)
Sidewalk Flawed or Obstructed
Walking Independently While Following Someone
The Great Outdoors
Rural Environment
Swimming Pool or Beach
Posture, Gait, and Arc
Description of Basic Techniques

ACTIVITIES:

EXAMPLE 1: *GRASS*

Walking on a grassy surface should be very natural and easy. Lack of experience, however, can lead to fear or avoidance. See that your student walks on grass often.

With a young child, a good exercise is to walk back and forth in such a way that she keeps crossing one or more sidewalks. Ask her to announce "Grass!" or "Sidewalk!" each time the terrain changes. This is an enjoyable way to call attention to the contrast.

(NOTE: With a child of kindergarten age or younger, be especially careful of vocabulary. If you call a surface "cement," but the child's family calls it the "sidewalk," she may genuinely not realize that it is the same thing.)

If an appropriate and safe situation is available, provide the experience of walking barefoot.

The beginner may complain that the cane tip continually catches; but with practice this need not be a substantial problem. The cane should tap at each end of the arc and *not* be slid along the surface. The Module, "The Great Outdoors," Example 1, describes a loose grip which is helpful on very uneven terrain. Help the student learn to bounce the tip deftly so that it rarely catches.

EXAMPLE 2: *PEBBLES*

"Now we're going to practice walking together while you hold my hand, and while you keep using your cane well. What are we walking on now?...Yes, this is grass.

"Your cane helps you know what is in front of us. Pretty soon your cane will find something different on the ground. Tell me when you find it...Yes, your cane makes a scratchy sound now. We'll walk together a little farther and then you tell me what this is...OK, yes, it's kind of like sand, isn't it? Reach down and touch it with your hands...It's kind of like sand, but the pieces are bigger. They're little, tiny rocks. We call them *pebbles* or *gravel*. Let's sit down and look at them for a minute....

"Now stand up, and we'll walk together a little farther. Your cane goes scratch, scratch!...Now we'll turn around. I'll let go of your hand, and you walk on in front of me....Good! It's interesting to walk on little pebbles."

See also the Module, "The Great Outdoors," Example 1.

EXAMPLE 3: *SNOW AND ICE*

Snow and ice provide an irregular terrain which is constantly changing. See the Modules, "Inclement Weather" and "The Great Outdoors" (Example 1), for detailed suggestions.

REMARKS: Sliding the cane from side to side, rather than tapping it, may be desirable on some surfaces. Holes, puddles, and other irregularities are often found more easily with this technique.

RELATED PRACTICE: Sometimes "solid" ground provides comparable experience. Mud may harden into a rutted, irregular surface. A flagstone patio or an old sidewalk may be rough and inconsistent.

Avoid having consistent terrain continually. Help your student be alert for unexpected changes and irregularities underfoot.

FOLLOW-UP: Frequently provide experience in walking on different surfaces. If the student hardly ever does this, she is likely to be needlessly nervous. Look for various surfaces. Following is a partial list:

    Wood chips or mulch
    Pebbles of various sizes
    Closely mowed grass vs. deep grass
    High weeds or underbrush
    Sand of various consistency
    Various sidewalk and road surfaces
    Fallen leaves
    Dirt road or path (smooth or rutted)
    Broken sidewalk
    Wet surfaces, including mud
    Snow
    Ice
    Wading in a stream
    Mountains, caves, etc.
    In a rock garden
    Between the rows in a cultivated field
    At the edge of a road that has no curb

CAUTION: Always consider possible hazards. General ones include ticks, poison ivy, nettles, etc. A given student may have allergies. Especially if you are new to the area, be sure you are familiar with necessary precautions when accompanying a student in a natural environment.

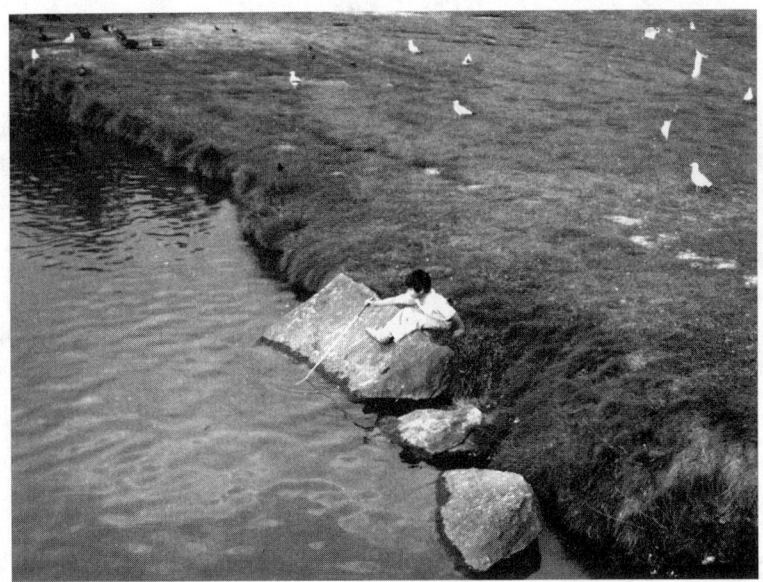

**Figure 11-1
At the Beach**

MODULE 12
CARRYING THINGS

OBJECTIVE: The student will carry objects in age-appropriate situations, with appropriate overall gait and posture. Regardless of whether an object is being carried, the student will not use the free hand for exploration which should be done with the cane.

(NOTE: Objectives for daily living skills may also apply.)

AGE OF STUDENT: All ages

PRIMARY SKILL EMPHASIS:
Carrying things
Stairs
Daily living skills
Flexibility and confidence
Stowing cane
Walking in company with others

ADDITIONAL SKILL EMPHASIS:
Doors and doorways
Detecting step-downs or drop-offs
Human guide
Posture, grip, gait, and arc
Purchase or transaction
Right and left
Responsibility and citizenship

FIGURE(S):
FIGURE 12-1: On the Stairs

SEE ALSO (Other Modules):
    Utilities and Trash
    Doors and Doorways
    Lunchtime
    Errands
    PUBLIC BUILDINGS Modules
    Inclement Weather
    Posture, Gait, and Arc
    Description of Basic Techniques

REMARKS: During the very first lesson(s), when the student is first learning how to hold and use the cane, it may be counterproductive to carry anything. Soon, however, the student should carry an object part of the time. Otherwise he will build habits of relying on the free hand as a travel aid, and will believe that he must *always* hold the handrail on stairs. The student may come to feel that carrying something is very difficult.

ACTIVITIES:

EXAMPLE 1: *COMFORTABLE AND NATURAL*
As soon as the student has had some experience in basic cane usage, ask him to carry something. If possible, there should be a real purpose. Most students need to carry books and supplies from place to place. A box may be delivered to a classroom or office. Chairs need to be moved around.

Help the student carry the item in a natural and comfortable way, avoiding awkward positions or habits.

Many students need little or no instruction in this respect, but simply carry things naturally from the beginning. Nevertheless, the teacher should check this from time to time.

EXAMPLE 2: *TOTE BAG OR BRIEFCASE*
In the primary grades, often the child has most classes in one location, with only intermittent need to carry things. From the intermediate grades upward, however, students usually move from one classroom to another, taking along books and personal possessions. This should be practiced before the need arises.

The student should have a backpack, tote bag, or briefcase, to avoid fussing with loose objects. Guide the student and family, if necessary, in getting a suitable carrier. Help boys avoid the kind of totes which seem feminine. If the family cannot provide a suitable carrier, the school may need to get one and lend it to the student.

Help the student organize his belongings and plan where to keep things, so that no more weight is carried than necessary.

EXAMPLE 3: *FINDING DOORWAYS WITH THE CANE, NOT THE FREE HAND*

An important reason for carrying things during cane lessons is to prevent the habit of feeling around with the free hand. The student should frequently practice finding doorways (and other things) along the wall on each side, particularly the side where the hand is not holding the cane. With proper usage, the cane tip easily detects the different sound and feel of the door – it is less solid than the wall, and probably made of a different material. Often the door is slightly set back.

EXAMPLE 4: *ON STAIRS*

The need to carry things is one reason why students should quickly learn to use stairs without necessarily holding the railing. (See Figure 12-1) As soon as the student learns stairway techniques, have him carry something at least occasionally. Sometimes insist that he not touch the rail or wall – not even lean on it. Provide practice on steps that have no railing.

The blind person who believes that he must always hold a rail is unnecessarily handicapped. If your student really does have additional physical problems such as cerebral palsy, consult a therapist regarding how much to expect on the stairs.

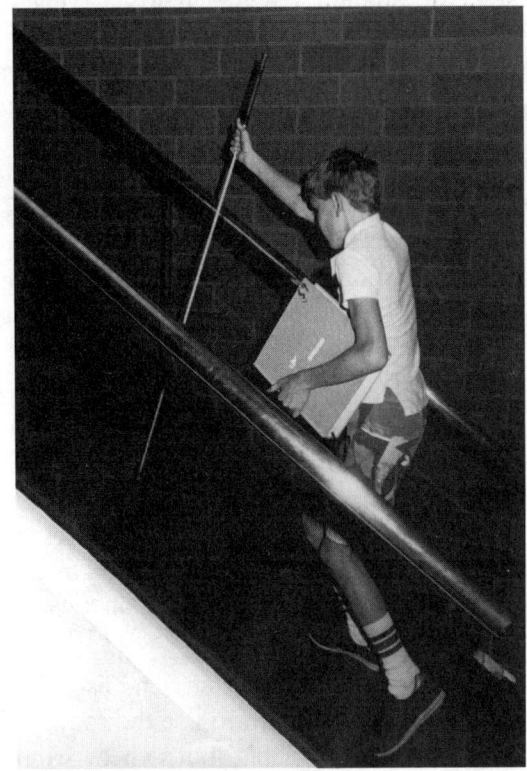

Figure 12-1
On the Stairs

EXAMPLE 5: *LUNCH TRAY*

Many competent blind adults prefer assistance for carrying a loaded tray at a cafeteria, especially with soup. However, every student should be able to carry a tray of food for at least a short distance. The question comes up continually in school and in college, and from time to time elsewhere. Obtaining help may be difficult and tends to set the person apart.

Examine the layout of the school lunchroom, and think about what should be expected of your student at this time. At the least, he should learn to help himself to accessible items such as silverware; make his own choices of foods, as appropriate; and carry a tray a short distance.

Experiment with various ways of holding the tray. The tray may be more stable if held against the chest, with the arm underneath; however, this may increase the chance of food being spilled onto clothing.

Consider making two trips.

Even if the student receives help carrying the tray to his seat, he should carry it himself afterward to the garbage area. He can throw away paper trash, scrape garbage, and place the tray and utensils in the designated spot.

EXAMPLE 6: *ITEMS NOT EASILY CARRIED IN ONE HAND*

Provide experience in carrying things that are not easily held in one hand, but are not too heavy for one person.

One aspect is the matter of carrying several things at once. Some students do not realize that a suitably-shaped object (such as a book) can be carried under the arm. See that the student practices this, and that he sometimes carries one object under his arm and something else in his hand. Note other miscellaneous ways of carrying odd items.

A very bulky object may require the use of two hands. Some people learn to use the cane fairly normally while doing this, but others cannot. Discuss safety concerns about carrying an object which prevents normal cane usage.

Consider options: (1) If the area is familiar, with a certainty of no unknown step-downs, etc., it may be safe to proceed carefully without normal cane usage. A large object may act as a "bumper;" however, there would be no good way to detect unexpected step-downs. (2) Another person might provide verbal or physical guidance. (3) In some cases, making two or more trips may prevent the need for carrying a large load. (4) If a load cannot be carried safely, one should seek the help of another person or use a cart.

Sometimes the question should be, "Does all of this really need to be carried now?" In school, perhaps the student is carrying too much around due to poor planning or inappropriate techniques. When shopping, consider leaving a large purchase somewhere and returning later – at the store where it was bought, or in a coin-operated locker.

If an object is carried without normal cane usage, the cane should not be forgotten. In a small, contained area, the student may set the cane down and return to get it. Often, however, the cane should come along – carried under the arm or in the hand. In some circumstances it is easiest for someone else to bring the cane along – rather like the comparable example, "I'll carry this box if you'll bring my coat."

EXAMPLE 7: *USING A CART*

Provide experience with various kinds of carts:

- Grocery carts of various kinds
- Low, flat "dollies"
- Hand carts with two wheels
- Media carts commonly used in schools to transport projectors, boxes, etc.
- Strollers and baby carriages

If a blind person pushes a cart in front, the cane cannot be used effectively. In a very familiar, controlled setting this may be acceptable – for example, when moving supplies around in the storeroom. Also, the cart can act as a "bumper." However, there is no way to find step-downs efficiently and safely; things may be broken or scratched; and the feedback from the terrain is vague at best.

Often the best solution is a very simple adaptation, but one which is often forgotten: *pull* the cart instead of pushing it. The cane can be used normally, and walking is safe and comfortable. If the cart is wide, the cane's arc should be widened.

With some carts it is necessary to be sure the easily-steered end is toward the front. A few things (such as children's strollers) may be designed so that the handle comes out if pulled; a slight alteration may be needed.

A cart is *not* appropriate for routine passing from class to class. If heavy items must continually be moved around, there is a need for better planning and/or more appropriate techniques (e.g., Braille rather than reliance on a CCTV). See the chapter, "General Classroom Arrangements and Study Skills" in the *Handbook*.

EXAMPLE 8: *TWO PEOPLE WORKING TOGETHER*

Discuss safety from several viewpoints. Muscle strain can occur from trying to lift a too-heavy object, or from bending and lifting with the back muscles instead of leg muscles. As above, if a large object keeps one from learning what is ahead, accidents may result.

Independence should not mean foolhardiness. Everyone should seek help at times. If an object is too heavy or unwieldy, seek help. The student should practice carrying a large object with one or more other people. The blind person may lead, using his cane and supporting the object behind him. The blind person may walk backward, with verbal and physical guidance from the other person (not unlike a sighted person in the same position). The blind person may be behind the object while the other person leads. Similar options exist when two people move a cart.

Again, the cane should not be forgotten if it is not actually used in a given situation. In a small, contained area, the student may set the cane down and then return to get it. Often the cane should come along – carried under the arm, in the hand, or on the cart.

EXAMPLE 9: *WHEN NOTHING IS CARRIED*

See that the student keeps his free hand down in a natural position when he is not carrying anything. Some students tend to hold that hand in an awkward position which may look effeminate for a boy and look peculiar for anyone. If this is a problem, ask the student to carry something and pay attention to the hand position. Then ask him to proceed without carrying anything, but to keep the hand and arm in roughly the same position.

Insist that the student *not* use the free hand to look for doorways or other features which should be found with the cane.

It may or may not be wise to discuss the natural swinging movement of the arm during walking. Usually this comes about naturally when the student walks quickly and normally. Discussion may lead to attempts to swing the arm artificially, with unnatural motions. At the same time, some students may incorrectly believe that the arm should be held still. Observe the student's overall posture and make suggestions if needed.

REFERENCE(S):
Willoughby and Duffy. *Handbook for Itinerant and Resource Teachers of Blind and Visually Impaired Students,* pp. 197, 225-238.

MODULE 13
IN A CROWD

OBJECTIVE: In a setting crowded with many people, the student will use appropriate cane techniques (including the "pencil grip"), and move at an appropriate speed.

AGE OF STUDENT: Elementary grades and up

PRIMARY SKILL EMPHASIS:
In a crowd or a line
Human guide
Walking in company with others
Obstacles in path
Posture, grip, gait, and arc

ADDITIONAL SKILL EMPHASIS:
Flexibility and confidence
Finding a person
Purchase or transaction
Meeting the public
Moving straight ahead

SEE ALSO (Other Modules):
   Human Guide
   Description of Basic Techniques
   Posture, Gait, and Arc
   Lunchtime
   Walking in a Line of People
   School Bus
   Walking Independently While Following
      Someone
   PUBLIC BUILDINGS Modules
   PUBLIC TRANSPORTATION Modules

STUDENT BACKGROUND: The student should first become familiar with the regular position for holding and arcing the cane. If a young student (primary grades or below) is taught the "pencil grip" position before she has had considerable practice with the regular position, she may become confused. At the same time, the relatively short cane used by a small child makes the alternate position less necessary.

An older student, however, should be able to learn and understand both positions almost immediately.

FIGURE(S):
FIGURE 13-1: Pencil Grip
FIGURE 13-2: In a Crowd

ACTIVITIES:

EXAMPLE 1: *INTRODUCTION*
Review the regular position, with cane extended and tapped in a generous arc. In a large crowd of people, this takes up more space than is readily available. It may cause inconvenience to oneself or others. Also, in such a crowd it is usually not possible to walk fast.

The student learns and practices the "pencil grip" position (also called "pulled up," "near vertical," etc.) (See Figure 13-1.) The tip of the cane is only about one step in front. The grip may be modified, and may be below the handle. The arc is not generous, though it should still "cover" both feet.

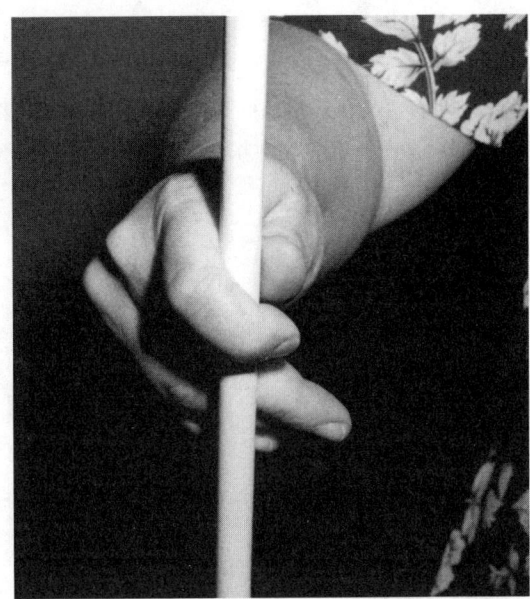

**Figure 13-1
Pencil Grip**

If a crowded hallway is readily available, practice there. Otherwise, simulate a crowd yourself (possibly helped by one or more others). Brush against the student from various directions, stay close in front of her, etc. Also, the student can simply be asked to imagine a crowd at certain times.

EXAMPLE 2: *AT SCHOOL*

Call attention to crowded situations at school, and see that appropriate techniques are used. Make sure the cane is not moved so forcefully as to "whack" classmates' ankles hard.

If next year the student will attend a school with much more crowded halls, she should go there this year and practice while classes are passing.

She should avoid turning a corner too quickly and extending the cane suddenly in front of people coming around the opposite way. Such a sudden appearance may trip people.

EXAMPLE 3: *PUBLIC PLACES*

Go to a mall or other public place where crowds are present. Part of the time, the student should walk independently to a given destination. At other times, she may take the arm of the teacher for convenience in staying together. Review the concept that the cane should be used even when a human guide is available.

Include variations in terrain underfoot. Help the student learn to react quickly to step-downs as well as obstacles, while using the pencil grip and walking slowly in a crowd.

The traveler should not walk fast with this position, because the cane does not extend very far in front; however, one does not normally walk fast in a crowd.

Help your student to relax and hold the cane loosely. If someone trips on it, the traveler should drop the cane immediately. This saves the other person from falling, and it keeps the blind person from suffering a wrenched hand and/or a broken cane. Also, a relaxed and steady motion of the hand helps to keep the cane from being caught on things.

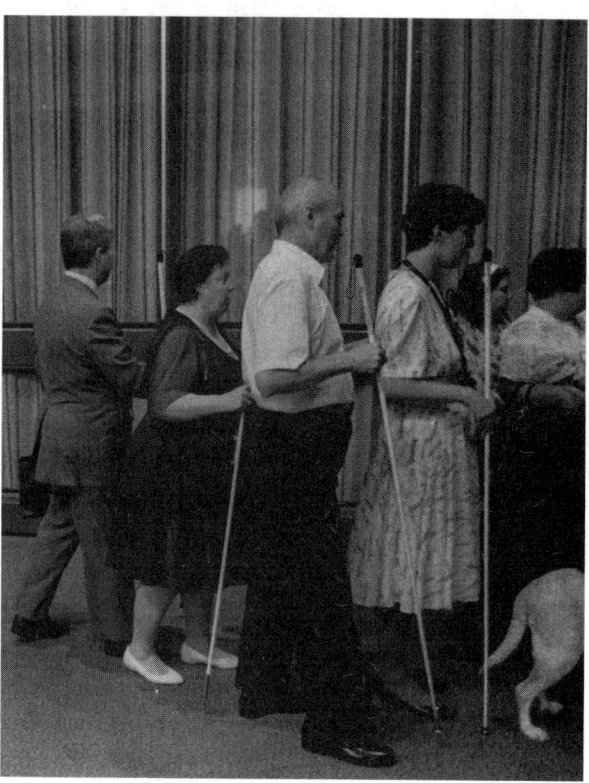

Figure 13-2
In a Crowd

CAUTION: When away from the school with a young or inexperienced student, carefully avoid getting separated in a crowd. If the student would easily become lost or frightened, it may be best for the student to take the arm of an adult while practicing the shortened-up grip in a crowded public place. Later, with more maturity, she will walk in a crowd in public without taking someone's arm.

REFERENCE(S):
Richard Mettler. *Cognitive Learning Theory and Cane Travel Instruction: A New Paradigm*, pp. 119-20.

AT HOME
INDOORS

MODULE 14
HOME – CONTENTS OF ROOM

OBJECTIVE: In his or her home, the student will locate and name three features in each major room.

AGE OF STUDENT: Preschool

PRIMARY SKILL EMPHASIS:
General travel (indoors)
Orientation within a room
Right and left
Corners, turns, and angles
Floor plans
Communication and instructions

ADDITIONAL SKILL EMPHASIS:
Stairs
Doors and doorways
Examining things tactually
Stowing cane
Compass directions

SEE ALSO (Other Modules):
What Is a "Room"?
Doors and Doorways
Right and Left
Compass Directions
Orientation Inside New Classroom

REMARKS: These descriptions assume the student is four years old. A child who is even younger may not yet be ready for these activities as written. If necessary, work on a small part only – e.g., finding the refrigerator. Build toward the more complex activities described.

ACTIVITIES: *Note:* Ordinarily, a person does not use a cane within his own home. Therefore, it may be decided that the cane will not be used during the first Example. However, having the child use the cane at this time should be carefully considered, since reasons such as the following may apply:

– The child does not yet find his way around confidently in his own home.
– The child is still working on very basic technique, and any opportunity for practice with the cane should be used.
– Comparison of the child's home with the other home would be made easier by using the same mode of travel in both places.
– The teacher is establishing the fact that the cane will be used at all times during "lessons"; it is hard for the young child to understand exceptions.

EXAMPLE 1: *A ROOM IN THE CHILD'S OWN HOME*

In his own home, the child goes independently to the kitchen. He finds and names each major feature: refrigerator, sink, stove, microwave oven, table, dishwasher, etc. This is done twice, as follows:

(a) The student walks all around the kitchen in a logical sequence and names each fixture as he comes to it.
(b) The teacher names each fixture (not in sequential order) and asks the child to find it. Each door or entrance is also named and found.

Other rooms may be examined in a similar way. However, for a very young child it is best to deal with only one room at a time when comparing two different homes.

Compass directions can easily be included as part of the lesson. However, the concepts of left and right should receive the greatest emphasis until they are learned.

EXAMPLE 2: *THE SAME ROOM IN ANOTHER HOME*

After reviewing his own kitchen, the student goes outside with his cane. He walks independently to the neighbor's house (or to the car). Arriving at the other home, he walks to the door and rings the bell.

Assist the child as needed. In giving directions, tell him as much at a time as his maturity allows. In the example below, at each ellipsis the teacher might pause for the child to carry out another part of the directions:

"The Allens' is the fourth house south of yours. Walk out your front door, and turn left at the big sidewalk....Now count four driveways....Yes, this is the fourth driveway.

"Turn left and walk up the driveway. Look with your cane for a little sidewalk going to the right.....It will curve some, and just keep following this little sidewalk....Go on up to the door – your cane will tell you if there are any steps. The front door is easy to find.... Ring the doorbell. Remember, if you can't find the doorbell button, or if you try it and nobody comes – then knock."

Inside the other house, unless it is very familiar, the child continues to use his cane. After greetings, an example of directions would be: "This is a *split level* house. We came in the door, and we're on kind of a landing in the middle of the stairway now. Look with your cane – you'll find stairs going up and stairs going down. Find them and go *up*.... Turn left. Now check the wall on the right with your cane.... When you can turn right, you'll find the kitchen."

In the kitchen, the child is given a tour by the neighbor. (Help the child set the cane down appropriately if necessary while examining things by touch.) He examines each item by touch. Depending on his experience, he may open each thing to understand what it is (e.g., feel the cold inside the refrigerator).

Compass directions can easily be included as part of the lesson, according to the child's maturity.

Compare this kitchen with the child's own, as:

- "What things does your kitchen have that aren't here?"
- "What does this kitchen have that yours does not?"
- "Both kitchens have refrigerators. But how is this one different from your own?"
- "We're standing at the sink, and the stove is on our right. If you stand at the sink at home, what's on the right?"
- "We've found a lot of things that are at the wall. Is there anything out in the middle of the room, not against a wall?"
- "Get your cane now, and come over here to this door. Open the door and walk through it. Then tell me what is on the other side." (The child finds that it leads outdoors.) "Can you go straight outside from your own kitchen?"
- "With your cane, let's find the doorway where we came into the kitchen... When we go through it, what room are we in?" (The child finds a large table and recognizes the dining room.)

Discuss the overall room size and floor plan, according to the child's ability to understand.

The child walks (with his cane) back to the front door. If able, he retraces his steps without being given directions.

The child thanks the host or hostess, and walks back to his own home (or to the car).

MODULE 15
WHAT IS A "ROOM"?

OBJECTIVE:
(1) The student will name and locate the structural elements of a typical room: walls, floor, ceiling, doors, and windows.
(2) In his/her home, the student will locate and name three features in each major room.
(3) In the classroom, the student will locate and name his/her own seat, the doorway, and four other significant features. He/she will walk between any two of these upon request.

AGE OF STUDENT: Preschool through primary grades (See Examples)

PRIMARY SKILL EMPHASIS:
Corners, turns, and angles
Structure of buildings
Floor plans
Orientation within a room
General travel (indoors)

ADDITIONAL SKILL EMPHASIS:
Doors and doorways
Right and left
Landmarks
Stowing cane
Examining things tactually

SEE ALSO (Other Modules):

> Home – Contents of Room
> Outside and Inside the House
> Outside and Inside the School
> Orientation Inside New Classroom
> Unfinished Basement, "Crawl Space," or Attic
> Porch or Deck
> Doors and Doorways
> General Overview – Buildings

REMARKS: Lessons like this are *not* the beginning of the child's understanding of room structure. All young children (with reasonable opportunity) gradually build understanding of the parts of a room and of the general whole.

Most of this Module is unnecessary for many students, even at a young age.

Nevertheless, some organized practice is helpful from time to time. A student may understand a concept well in most respects, yet lack the vocabulary to follow verbal directions easily. She may harbor incorrect assumptions or overly-rigid generalizations.

Also, reviewing concepts can be a pleasant way of practicing physical skills. For example, a student may understand what a corner is, and walk around one while feeling the wall with her hand, yet need practice in turning smoothly while using the cane. Discussing room structure can be a pleasant way to provide needed practice.

TEACHER PREPARATION: Analyze the student's current level of understanding, as above.

Select a room which gives the best opportunity to demonstrate concepts and characteristics. Ideally it would be a room with four square walls and four square corners, where any furniture can easily be moved away from the walls, and where the ceiling is not extremely high. Select the room closest to this ideal, and compensate where necessary. For example, if there is a built-in cupboard, explain that the wall continues behind. If the ceiling is very high, mention that it is there, and go to another room to actually touch a ceiling.

According to the student's ability, select rooms with variations.

ACTIVITIES:

EXAMPLE 1: *A YOUNG CHILD IN HER OWN HOME*
(*Preschool*)

Examining walls, without the cane
Select a corner in which to start. Discuss the concept of *corner*, and place a distinctive object in this corner. (Since the concept of four walls is

to be brought out, it is important to start at a corner. There may already be a distinctive item there, such as a recliner. Regardless, it is pleasant and helpful to place a "marker" so that the starting corner can easily be recognized when you return. A stuffed toy is good.

The child walks along each wall, touching it continually with her hand. Announce that this is "Wall #1." Discuss the surface–painted plaster, wallpaper, etc. Note any structural features such as windows and doors.

When arriving at the next corner, announce "corner," and name "Wall #2." Continue in the same manner.

On the first trip around, disregard furniture as much as possible. Try to walk directly along the wall. When the starting corner is found again, greet the stuffed animal. Summarize: four corners and four walls.

Noting furniture along each wall (*without the cane*)

Walk around the outside of the room again. This time, however, pay attention to any furniture that is normally near the wall. The child examines each briefly by touch and names it. Note such things as: the piano is in Corner #2; the couch is in the middle of Wall #3.

Four walls and four corners (*using the cane*)

Walk around the room again, with the cane. How does the tip sound when it strikes each particular piece of furniture? When it strikes the wall? The door?

(NOTE: A young beginner, especially in a large house, may benefit by using her cane in the home regularly. If the child does not ordinarily use her cane inside her own home, explain that for this lesson the cane will be used, to help in practicing for use elsewhere.)

The floor

"We've looked at the four walls, with the four corners. We also saw windows and doors. The walls are all *beside* us. Now let's notice another part of the room. What part of the room is *under* us?"

With the cane, walk back and forth across the room, thinking about the floor and how the cane tip sounds. If the floor has more than one kind of surface, such as rugs and bare wood, listen to the change of sound and feel.

Also note any objects that are out in the middle of the room and not close to any wall.

The ceiling

"Now, there is one more part of the room. Most of the time we don't touch it–and children, especially, can't touch it very easily. But I'm going to help you touch it today. What part of the room is *over* us?....Yes, the *ceiling*."

Provide a way for the student to touch the ceiling. She may be lifted up, or held on the shoulders. She might stand on something or climb a ladder. Feel the surface and discuss it. Talk about other times she has touched a ceiling. Do all rooms have ceilings?

"When we touch the ceiling like this, we are *inside*. If we went outside and climbed up on top of the house, we would say we were on the *roof*. The *roof* is what we call the top of the house *outside*, and we call it the *ceiling* when we look at it from *inside*." (If the student can understand, explain that usually there is an attic or space between the outer roof and the inner ceiling, and that the roof is made of weatherproof materials.)

VARIATION(S):

- Repeat with other rooms in the home. Compare.
- Repeat with rooms in other homes or other buildings. Note overall differences–e.g., Grandma's house has wallpaper instead of paint.
- Describe the walls by compass directions, and the corners by intermediate directions (NW, SW, etc.).
- If practical, arrange for the child to go up a ladder and touch the roof, or even climb onto it. It may be better for the parents to do this, rather than the teacher.

EXAMPLE 2: *A ROOM AT SCHOOL*
(*Preschool or kindergarten*)

(NOTE: if the student is just beginning to learn cane usage, or has particular difficulty with the concepts presented here, the walls may be examined first without using the cane. Usually, however, the student at school should use the cane for this Module. When she does examine something with her hands, she may set the cane down beside her, or let it stand loosely inside her arms.)

A simple, "ideal" room: Go to a room where there is minimum furniture along the walls. (The gym may be a good choice.) Select a corner for starting; note a distinctive landmark there, or place an object as a marker.

Walk along each wall, tapping the cane along the wall continually. Feel the wall from time to time and discuss its surface. Name each compass direction (e.g., "Now we are walking along the north wall.") The student announces each corner, and names (with help, if needed) the compass direction for the next wall. Note structural features such as windows and doors as you pass them. The cane should find the doors.

Repeat, this time naming each corner with the intermediate compass direction. If the student has not been introduced to this concept, the teacher gives the corner names as a readiness activity.

Verify that there are four walls. Is the room *square* (with four equal walls) or is it a *rectangle*, with two walls longer than the others?

Walk across the middle of the room, noting the surface texture(s) of the floor.

Discuss the ceiling. Touch it if practical. If it cannot be reached with the hand, consider lifting up a pole or yardstick (it is better *not* to lift up the cane, lest bad habits be encouraged). Perhaps toss a ball or another small object, and hear it hit the ceiling.

EXAMPLE 3: *THE CLASSROOM*
(*Preschool or kindergarten*)

Walk around the perimeter of the student's classroom. Probably there are various shelves or other features against the walls. Touch the wall wherever it is practical, and realize that the wall continues behind various things. Name the four walls and corners as above.

Enjoy a quiz or game to practice naming what is along each wall. Suggest that the child try to answer from memory and then verify by examination. Examples include:

- Name everything along the north wall.
- Name everything along the east wall, in sequence, starting from the door.
- The paint easel is in which corner?
- If you start at the paint easel and walk along the south wall, whose desk will you come to first?
- If you come in the door from the hallway and walk straight ahead, what wall do you come to?
- Which walls have windows?

Note the floor surface.

Discuss the ceiling, touching it if possible.

Repeat the above with other rooms which have a square or rectangular shape.

EXAMPLE 4: *THE HALLWAY*
(*Kindergarten and above*)

With a young child, select a hallway that is relatively short and well-defined. Explain that a "hall" is much like a "room," but is long and narrow, and is used mainly to go somewhere else. Walk around the equivalent of "four walls." Note that at the side there are long, normal walls (probably with doorways in them); at each end there may be a connection to another hall.

Examine the floor and discuss the ceiling. Emphasize the concept of walking *beside* a given wall, as compared to walking *toward* it.

A tactual diagram may be helpful. It may show one particular hallway, or the relationship of several halls which define the overall floor plan.

With an older student, more sophisticated analysis is appropriate. The definition of a "hall" is actually somewhat arbitrary. There may be in-between situations, such as a wide hallway or lobby which has furniture groupings.

Compare various hallways. Note characteristics such as:

- Width
- Length
- Doorways on each side
- Connections at the ends
- Other hallways branching off from the middle

EXAMPLE 5: *ROOMS WITH UNUSUAL SHAPES*
(*Kindergarten and above*)

Locate and examine rooms (or areas similar to rooms) that are not simple squares or rectangles. For example:

- A triangular corner room
- A room that has a complex shape, with "jogs" in the walls
- A room with one or more diagonal walls or curved walls
- An enclosed patio or porch which seems like a room but has no ceiling. How can you tell that there is no ceiling?
- A niche or alcove, set back into a wall but not completely enclosed
- Movable, folding walls
- Room dividers which go only part way to the ceiling
- Closets. (Look at a small one and then at a large "walk-in" closet. What determines whether or not we call it a "closet"?)

MODULE 16
APARTMENT HOUSE OR CONDOMINIUM

OBJECTIVE:
(1) [For a student who lives in an apartment or condominium] The student will go independently to all areas of the apartment complex where children of similar age ordinarily go alone.

(2) [For a student who lives in a single-family home] The student will tour an apartment or condominium complex and discuss the concept of multi-family housing.

(NOTE: Objectives for Tasks of Daily Living may also apply.)

AGE OF STUDENT: All ages

PRIMARY SKILL EMPHASIS:
General travel
Doors and doorways
Stairs
Orientation overall
Floor plans

ADDITIONAL SKILL EMPHASIS:
Structure of buildings
Air currents and echoes
Landmarks
Elevators
Carrying things
Right and left
Compass directions
Sound direction and meaning
Traffic movement
Addresses
Boundaries
Corners, turns, and angles
Emergency procedures

SEE ALSO (Other Modules):
Elevators
What's Out There? (On the School Grounds)
Back Yard Boundaries
Back Yard (Overall)
Home – Contents of Room
Home Address
Utilities and Trash
Swimming Pool or Beach
Alternate Routes Within a Building
Outside and Inside the School
General Overview – Buildings

FIGURE(S):
FIGURE 16-1: Front Entrances and Bus Stop
FIGURE 16-2: To the Garage

ACTIVITIES:

WHEN THE STUDENT LIVES IN AN APARTMENT OR CONDOMINIUM:

TEACHER PREPARATION:
Ask the student's parent to show you areas where tenants ordinarily go. Discuss where the student should learn to go alone at this time.

This requires a frank yet tactful discussion. Parents may find it hard to admit how little the blind child has learned. They may not consciously realize that if someone else always goes along, the child really doesn't know how to get about independently. The best yardstick is comparison with other children of similar age in the same apartment complex.

CAUTION: Recognize security regulations, and be prepared to identify yourself. Ask the parent to introduce you to the manager and/or security personnel. If some doors are locked, determine how entry will be arranged. Carry identification to prove you are a teacher; consider asking the parent to write a note which you can carry with you.

REMARKS: This description assumes the family has just moved to this apartment building. It is assumed that the parents will do at least part of the teaching. If the student has already lived here for some time, the teacher should check and review what is already known, and add skills as necessary.

EXAMPLE 1: *BASIC LIVING AREAS*

Enter building and proceed to apartment: After approaching on the sidewalk, walk up the few steps to the front entrance. Go through the outer door, and use the key to open the inner door. Walk forward down the hallway, with good arcing of the cane. Cane the right-hand wall often enough to note stairwells. At the second stairwell, go upstairs with good cane usage. Turn right. Use cane to count doors (while continuing full arc). Enter with key at third door.

(Note: To reduce the need for carefully counting doors, the family may wish to place a welcome mat which is easy to recognize.)

Recite and analyze the student's complete address—e.g., 7845 Hubbell Avenue, Apartment 209, Arvada, Colorado 80005.

Go to the bus stop or another logical location outside. Then return to the building. Find the correct front entrance (e.g., take the second left turn as you walk north from the bus stop). (See Figure 16-1)

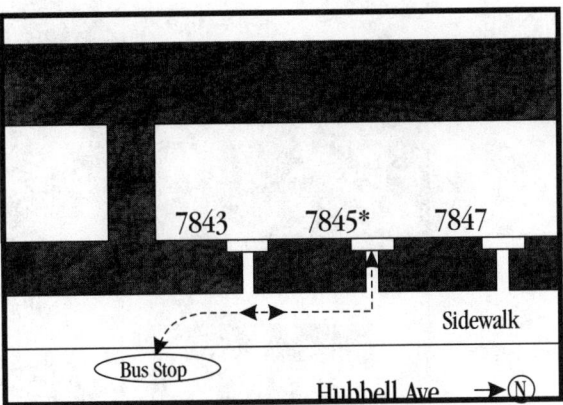

Figure 16-1
Front Entrances and Bus Stop

Practice entering and leaving, between bus stop and apartment. Become accustomed to minor obstacles or changes—people coming and going, boxes in hallway, etc.

Emergency exit: Go to an alternate or emergency exit. The student should be aware of at least one alternate exit, and should practice using it if practical. Is it for regular use, or only for emergencies? Will the same key work?

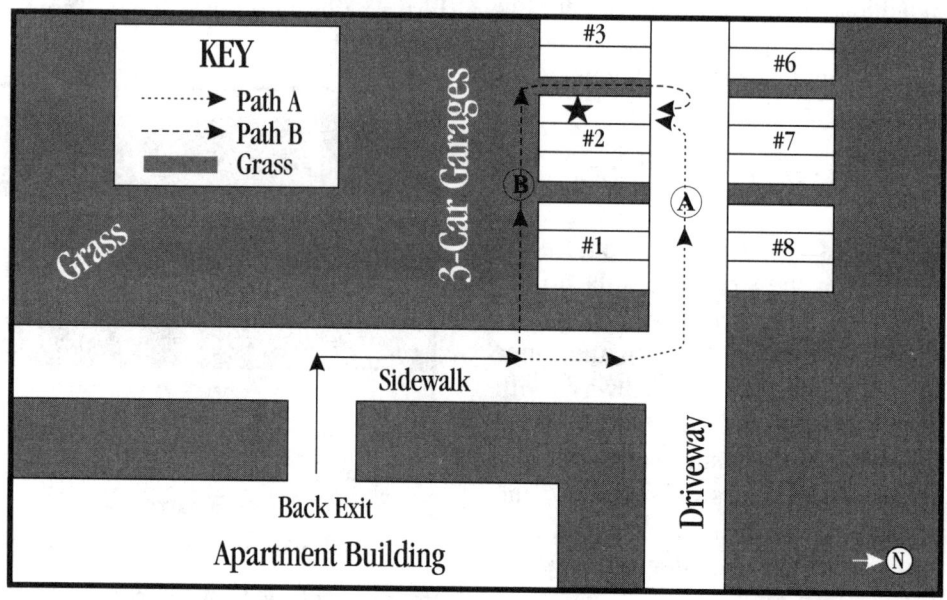

**Figure 16-2
To the Garage**

Garage: (See Figure 16-2) This example assumes that the driveway is to the right (north) of the back door of the apartment house. Garages face the driveway from both sides. The family's garage is on the south side of the drive (facing north), in the second garage from the apartment building.

A person could walk to the driveway and turn left (Path A in Figure 16-2), past the three stalls in Garage #1 and on to the third stall in Garage #2. However, this route requires walking in front of many stalls where cars may pull out suddenly with a poor view.

An alternate route is shown by Path B in Figure 16-2: Go out the back door and turn right (north) at the sidewalk that leads to the driveway, but do not go all the way to the driveway immediately. Instead, on the grass to the left of the sidewalk, look with your cane on your left for Garage #1. Turn west to go *behind* Garage #1 (south of it), still on the grass. Notice, by air currents and/or caning the wall, when you have passed Garage #1. Keep going past the back wall of Garage #2. Turn and walk along the far side of Garage #2, to the front of the garage. Since your family's space is at the far (west) end of this garage, you have now arrived. Use your keys and get the package which your sister forgot to bring in.

CAUTION: As explained above, often an alternative path will avoid the need to walk among cars which may move suddenly and unexpectedly. However, a very young or inexperienced student may not be permitted to go near the drive at all. On the other hand, an experienced older student (certainly by age 12) should be able to walk cautiously in the driveway while listening carefully for doors opening and cars starting.

Visiting another apartment: The student learns to find at least one other apartment. Include the apartment of a friend who would help in case of problems or emergency. Go into the friend's apartment and compare it. Also include the apartment or office of the manager or superintendent.

Laundry room: Locate washers, dryers, and other fixtures. Carry laundry.

A younger child can assist with the laundry. A teenager should take turns at full responsibility. Discuss security precautions as appropriate (e.g., avoid going alone late at night).

How does the laundry room smell? Does it feel steamy?

REMARKS: Avoid rigid memorization. The student should understand the overall layout and the relationship of each location to others. Particularly, he should be able to go easily from *any* familiar location to *any* other familiar location. For example, if a problem occurs in the laundry room, he should be able to go directly to the superintendent's office *without* needing to go first to his own apartment. Practice this kind of thing, and build overall understanding of layout.

EXAMPLE 2: *OTHER AREAS AND FEATURES*

Some of the areas below are not present in all apartment houses. Also, a younger child might not go everywhere independently. Even a young child, however, should experience going there with someone else. As he grows older, he will naturally and easily learn to get there independently.

Elevator: See the Module, "Elevators."

Practice going to the same place by elevator and by stairway. Note that the elevator should not be used in case of fire.

Patio, playground, yard: Is the area common or divided?

See the Modules, "Back Yard Boundaries" and "Back Yard (Overall)."

Other hallways, stairwells, buildings, etc.: Depending on the student's age and the complexity of the development, the student should be at least somewhat familiar with the overall arrangement.

Go to a floor higher or lower than your own. Are the characteristics the same? (Number of stairwells, carpeting, etc.) Is there an apartment that is exactly above or below your own? What is the numbering pattern? If you came to this floor by mistake, how would you know it was wrong? (Notice any characteristics that are different. At the very least, your door key would not work.)

Visit various neighbors in their apartments.

Go on an errand to an apartment you have not visited before. Find it by understanding the numbering system or by asking directions. Do you need to count doorways, or are there other landmarks?

Walk all the way up and down a stairwell. How many floors are there? Are there apartments on all floors?

Walk all the way around outside the building.

Go in and out of every outside door.

If there is more than one building, go to each and enter at least briefly. Are the buildings all alike? Do they face the same compass direction? What is the address/numbering system? If someone came to your building by mistake, how could you help him find the right building?

Party Room: Even if the family does not ordinarily use the room, arrange to look at it. Someday there may be a function which the family does want to attend.

Walk around, with the cane, and look over the layout of the room. Find the coat closet, kitchenette, rest room, etc. Find a seat and sit down.

How is the room reserved? Is a special key needed?

Storage Locker: If a storage area is provided outside the apartment, the student should learn to go there. Lock and unlock it with the key. Alternatively, use a combination lock which has buttons or other features so that it can be worked by touch.

Roof: If there is a recreational area on the roof, the student should learn to go there. Discuss safety considerations (e.g., never climb on or over a railing.) Do the steps to the roof have unusual characteristics?

Balcony: Review safety, as for the roof. Feel the breeze. Can you hear sounds from down below? Discuss height in terms the student can understand. What is immediately above? Immediately below?

Consider allowing the student to reach the cane down through the railing and note that it does not touch the ground. (See also the Module, "Bridges and Overpasses.")

Security door with intercom and/or buzzer: Introduce a young child to the buzzer gently (from a distance the first time), to avoid possible fright.

The student learns how to open the door with his key, and what to do if the key is lost. He learns to use the intercom to let someone else in (following the policies of the manager and the family).

What is the policy about letting someone else in with you when you enter? (A blind person can be alert to whether others are present. He can open the door just enough so that others cannot slip in unnoticed. He can ask others where they are going.)

EXAMPLE 3: Visit another apartment house or condominium (not part of the same development). Note features which are different. A tour, as described below for someone who lives in a single-family home, is also valuable for the apartment dweller.

WHEN THE STUDENT DOES NOT LIVE IN AN APARTMENT OR CONDOMINIUM:

TEACHER PREPARATION:
Make arrangements with a resident or the manager before going. An apartment house is private property with security precautions.

EXAMPLE 4: Show the student around as much as practical, while he uses his cane and tours with little assistance. (See Examples above for possible areas to tour.)

Discuss how a person can quickly become independent around the building(s).

Go into an apartment and help the student understand that it is a complete home. Examine each room; compare with the student's own home.

Explain rent.

MODULE 17
UNFINISHED BASEMENT, "CRAWL SPACE," OR ATTIC

OBJECTIVE: The student will explore an "unfinished" attic or basement area. He/she will discuss its general characteristics and its relationship to the rest of the building.

AGE OF STUDENT: Preschool and up

PRIMARY SKILL EMPHASIS:
Structure of buildings
Floor plans
Varied terrain
Overhanging objects
Corners, turns, and angles
Detecting step-downs or drop-offs

ADDITIONAL SKILL EMPHASIS:
Sound direction and meaning
Air currents and echoes
Interpreting odors
Climbing, clambering, crawling, etc.
Flexibility and confidence
Weather and temperature

SEE ALSO (Other Modules):
   Bridges and Overpasses
   The Great Outdoors
   Rough Terrain
   Porch or Deck
   Utilities and Trash
   Poor Lighting Conditions
   What Is a "Room"?
   Outside and Inside the House

TEACHER PREPARATION: Arrange to visit an area where the student may safely go (at least part way) into an "unfinished" part of a building. If it is dirty, be sure that teacher and student wear suitable clothing. Consider bringing handwipes.

ACTIVITIES:

EXAMPLE 1: *CELLAR/BASEMENT*

Discuss basements with which the student is already familiar. Do they have regular, finished ceilings, walls, and floors? Explain that we will visit a basement area that is "unfinished"; the term does not necessarily mean that more work is really expected.

The student walks with his cane in the usual way to find the door to the basement. He walks down the stairs cautiously, using his cane extra-carefully. Stairs to such an area may have no railing on one side, no risers, etc. The student may examine some of the steps with his hands if they are a type he has not encountered.

Downstairs, note the sound of the cane when it taps the floor and then the wall: what are the floor and wall made of? Are there windows high in the wall? Why aren't they lower?

Walk around, noting various features. If the student is tall, could he hit his head on exposed pipes overhead? Discuss this possibility even with a small student. In an unfamiliar, unfinished cellar, a tall person may walk cautiously with one hand up to protect the head. But this posture should *not* be adopted in unfamiliar areas generally – only if the setting indicates the likelihood of overhangs or low ceilings.

Note odors, temperature, humidity, etc. Does the area ever have leaks or flooding?

What rooms are above you?

Do voices seem "hollow" or echoing? Note the sounds (or silence) when no one is talking.

Is the cellar used for storage or other purposes?

Discuss why some areas are left "unfinished."

EXAMPLE 2: *"CRAWL SPACE"*

If a "crawl space" (too low for an adult to stand up in) is available and safe, enter at least a short way. Have the student touch the ceiling (being careful of splinters), and note how low it is. If he can stand up straight but you cannot, have him touch you to observe your stooped posture. (Also, the sound of your voice will come from lower down than usual.) Note odors, temperature, humidity, etc.

CAUTION: Before entering such an area, be sure you know what is there. Such areas may have unexpected holes in the floor, sharp edges, nail points sticking through from above, and other dangers. Also, consider whether a young child might scoot away from you and then become frightened or confused; it could be hard to reach him and get him out. One solution is to hold the child's hand firmly and just barely enter for a brief moment. If behavior is very unpredictable, it is best not to approach such an area.

Under a porch or deck, there often is an area which is similar to a "crawl space" but is very safe and simple. See the Module, "Porch or Deck."

EXAMPLE 3: *ATTIC (WITH SOLID FLOOR)*

Explore an unfinished attic in a manner similar to exploring an unfinished basement.

An unfinished attic will probably have a very slanted ceiling. Hold the child up (or use a stool or ladder) so that he may touch as high as possible. Then help him follow the ceiling as it slopes lower. Can you follow it all the way to the floor, or is a partly-finished wall in the way?

Are there regular windows, or are there only air vents? Do pipes come up from below? Discuss their path and purpose. What rooms are below you?

EXAMPLE 4: *ATTIC WITH UNFINISHED FLOOR*

CAUTION: If the attic floor is unfinished (so that one must step only on certain boards and not on the floor at large), it is probably not safe for a younger student to walk there. Also, most teachers will not want to take a student into such an area (although a parent may).

In contrast, it is usually safe and easy for the student to go up and "take a peek," as described below. Note, however, that it is difficult for one person alone to assist an inexperienced student in climbing up a ladder and reaching through a trap door. Also, safety dictates that there should always be someone at the bottom of the ladder.

Poke your head in there: Even when it is unwise to actually enter an unfinished attic, it is usually safe and easy for a school-aged student to "take a peek." He can climb up the ladder and open the trap door. He can poke his head and upper body into the attic area and get the smell and "feel" of the attic. He can touch the flooring and understand why it is unsafe to walk on. All of this brings valuable experience and understanding. It can be a fascinating adventure which adds great interest to a lesson.

FOLLOW-UP: Compare the attics and basements of various homes, schools, and other buildings. (Discuss them if it is not practical to go there.) What is typical in your area? Note that in some locales, basements are difficult or impossible to build and maintain. In others, almost every building has a basement.

Exploring unfinished areas in regular buildings helps build flexibility for exploring caves, ancient ruins, etc., as in the Module, "The Great Outdoors."

MODULE 18
MORE IDEAS
For Lessons at Home
Indoors

AGE OF STUDENT: Preschool through primary grades

ABOUT THIS LIST:
Following is a list of objects, aspects, places, etc., around the home. Examining different things at various times helps assure variety and interest for the young child.

A given item may be incorporated into the actual lesson. (Example: The child is working on naming the various rooms. Whenever she names a room, she is also to find a piece of furniture and comment on its surface or texture.) Alternatively, a given item may serve as a "fun" end to a lesson. (Example: The child is asked to find and name each room in the house. When this task is accomplished, she is allowed to examine the top of the refrigerator.)

It is very interesting for a young child to examine and compare equivalent items in someone else's house – Grandma's windows, the neighbor's sink, etc.

REMARKS: Talk with the parent before opening closet doors or going anywhere not previously planned. There probably are many places which the parent does not wish children to get into at all. Also, the parent may be very uncomfortable about letting the teacher see areas that might seem "messy" or personal. Often it is better to suggest that the *parent* give the child a tour of certain areas. The teacher may wish to leave a "follow-up" suggestion after each lesson.

CAUTION: Always be alert for possible hazards. Examples include poisonous materials in the cleaning closet, hot pipes, sharp edges, etc. Also, be sure to use good safety practices when assisting a child to climb up and reach something.

IDEAS:
- Doorknobs, door handles (Are they all the same?)
- Exposed pipes (as, under the sink)
- Small access doors to plumbing, the attic, etc.
- Textures of various walls
- Textures of various upholstered furniture
- Different chairs and sofas (Sit on each one, and also examine each of its parts.)
- Steps
- Shutters, drapes, Venetian blinds, and other window treatments
- Fireplace
- Toys scattered around and/or stored
- The ceiling
- Brooms, vacuum cleaners, etc.
- Floor coverings – tile, rugs, carpet, etc.
- The top or upper part of something, such as the refrigerator, where the child ordinarily cannot reach
- Climbing under the table, behind the sofa, etc. (Discuss relationships such as *under* and *behind*.)
- Opening and closing various doors or windows
- Studying a picture on the wall (The child examines the frame tactually, and a verbal description of the picture is provided.)
- Air vents for heating and cooling

AT HOME
OUTDOORS

MODULE 19
BACK YARD BOUNDARIES

NOTE: This Module interacts closely with the following Module, "Back Yard (Overall)," which uses the same Figures and tends to have more complex examples.

OBJECTIVE: The student will recognize the boundaries of his/her back yard (or equivalent) at home. He/she will find each of three specific locations at or near a boundary, and return to the house.

AGE OF STUDENT:
Preschool and primary grades

PRIMARY SKILL EMPHASIS:
Boundaries
Landmarks
Orientation overall
Hills and inclines
Right and left
Varied terrain
Open space

ADDITIONAL SKILL EMPHASIS:
Corners, turns, and angles
Doors and doorways
Compass directions
Obstacles in path
Moving straight ahead
Correcting a path
Barefoot walking
Examining things tactually
Maps
Overhanging objects
Weather and temperature

FIGURE(S):
FIGURE 19-1: Yard #1
FIGURE 19-2: Yard #2

SEE ALSO (Other Modules):
Back Yard (Overall)
The Great Outdoors
From House to Curb
Obstacles: Noting Them and Proceeding
Walking Across Open Space
Outside and Inside the House
Utilities and Trash
Playground
Rough Terrain
What's Out There? (On the School Grounds)

TEACHER PREPARATION: Look around the home and yard with the student's family. Discuss boundaries, likely play patterns, and the child's present level of independence. Is it all right to walk into a neighbor's yard during instruction?

REMARKS: Most of these Examples assume a moderate-sized back yard which has a fence around most of the perimeter.

Also, this Module assumes the child is not yet independent in finding his way around the entire back yard, and that he will use the cane during this instruction. At another time, it may be decided that he will not use the cane in his own yard.

ACTIVITIES:
A. ALL BOUNDARIES CLEARLY MARKED

EXAMPLE 1: *BACK FENCE*
(*Preschool*)
Talk with the child about his back yard and what he enjoys doing there. Begin to elicit his understanding of the layout.

[This Example assumes that in Figure 19-1 the child is going between the house and the far back fence (west fence).]

"What is around the yard, and shows where your yard ends?... Yes, the *fence*.

"Today we're going to practice going to the fence and then going back to the house....

"Here we are at the back door. With your cane, walk straight ahead to the back fence. If there is something else in your way, just go around it."

Help the child, if necessary, so that he reaches the back fence (as distinguished from a side fence) fairly quickly. Be sure the cane taps the surface underfoot (with as good an arc as the child can now manage) and detects obstacles.

When the back fence is reached, note the sound when the cane strikes it. Help the child examine the fence with his hands. What is it made of?

Return to the house. Guide the child as much as necessary to see that he proceeds quickly and fairly directly. One good method is to place your hand on his shoulder and "steer" him gently, while he continues to tap the cane in front of him.

"Good! Here we are at the house. Notice how the cane taps the patio bricks. We'll find the back door.... I brought a stuffed bunny, and I put him here by the door. You may hold him for a minute.... Each time you come back to the house, we'll say hello to the bunny."

Help the child repeat the trip between the house and the back fence three times (or as judgment dictates). In this particular activity, see that he always reaches the far back fence (parallel to the back wall of the house). Emphasize walking fairly straight in spite of obstacles. Sometimes have the child point toward the house or toward the back fence. (Point with a finger in the conventional way, not with the cane.)

Observe what is at or near the back fence (if anything) – in this instance, rough ground, bushes, and the end of the vegetable garden.

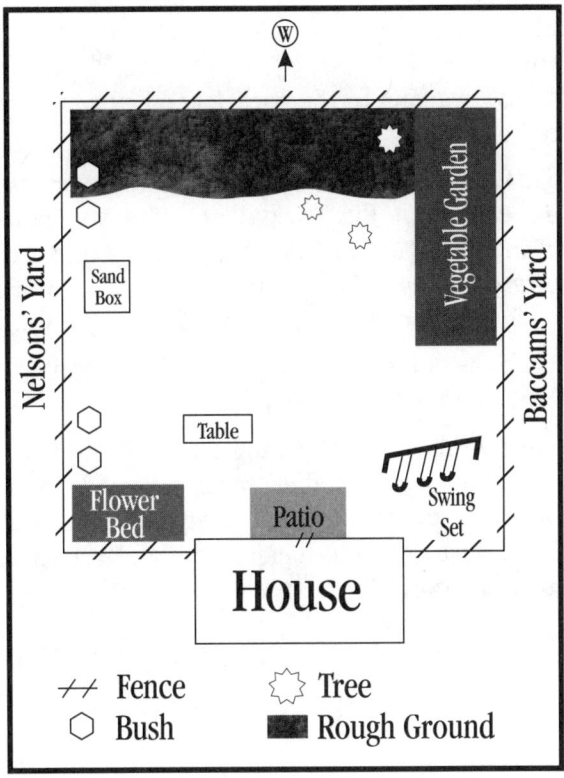

Figure 19-1
Yard #1

EXAMPLE 2: *PERIMETER*
(*Preschool*)
(Figure 19-1)

Walk around the entire perimeter of the yard, including the wall of the house. Note how the cane sounds in touching the fence, the side of the house, bushes along the fence, etc. Note other things encountered along the way, such as flower beds. Observe how the cane detects such things, and discuss whether the house or the fence is behind each.

Give a name to each side of the fence/yard (preferably names used in the household). For example, the four sides might be called:

"By the house"
"The Nelsons' side"
"The back fence"
"The Baccams' side"

Name each side as you pass it. Call attention to each corner.

EXAMPLE 3: SIDE FENCES
(*Preschool*)
(Figure 19-1)

Review walking to the back fence and returning to the house.

"Now, let's stand here a minute, pretending we just came out the back door. Can you point toward the Baccams' yard?.... Yes, it's that way, toward the *right*. Walk toward the right, and find the fence near the Baccams' yard...."

(Help the child find the right-hand fence quickly. Return to the back door.)

"Now we'll do the same thing with the Nelsons' fence. Point toward their yard.... Yes, it's to the *left*. Walk to the left and find their fence...." (Proceed to the left-hand fence, and return to the back door.)

EXAMPLE 4: TO AND FROM VARIOUS POINTS
(*Preschool*)
Figure 19-1)

Practice going to various parts of the fence and returning to the house. Frequently help the child point toward the house and then toward a particular area along the fence (e.g., petunias), to emphasize orientation.

[Note: This Module emphasizes locations around the perimeter. The "Back Yard (Overall)" Module emphasizes locations all over the yard, including "in the middle."]

End each session with enjoyable play in the yard.

EXAMPLE 5: WHICH WAY IS SHORTER?
(*Preschool and primary grades*)

Walk with the child to a specific location along the fence, less than halfway around. The sand box in Figure 19-1 is a good example.

"Now, suppose you are here and want to go in the house. Suppose you follow the fence—would you get to the house?... Let's try it. Which way should we go?"

In whichever direction the child chooses, assist him to follow the perimeter to the back door. Estimate the time taken, or use a stopwatch.

Return to the sand box. Point out that you could follow the fence in the other direction—would you reach the back door if you went around that way?

Discuss according to the child's maturity. Various levels of understanding include:

- Virtually no understanding of direction at all
- Rote memorizing (e.g., learning to follow the fence by the Nelsons' yard to return to the back door, but not grasping overall relationships)
- Understanding that following the Nelsons' fence is shorter, but not really grasping that a person *could* go around the other way to reach the door
- Beginning to realize that there are many possible paths of varying directness
- Mature understanding of the overall layout

Proceed around the perimeter in the other direction. Compare the time taken. Again, discuss at the level of the child's understanding. Try to help the child reach at least this level of understanding about the fence:

If you find the fence and follow it around, you will eventually reach the house no matter which way you are going. But you might go a long way roundabout. If you want to get to the house, it's best to think where you are and take the shortest way.

Depending on the child's understanding, include one more route between the house and sand box: walk directly between the two points, without following the fence. Include this whenever it fits best. If the child suggests it, do it immediately. If he does not suggest it, add it at the end.

ACTIVITIES:
B. BOUNDARIES NOT ALL MARKED

EXAMPLE 6: *VARIOUS CLUES POSSIBLE*
(*Preschool and up*)
(Figure 19-2)

Often a yard will have some tactual landmarks at or near the property lines, but substantial stretches without markers. In Figure 19-2, the house is on the east side of the yard; a hedge and garden extend part way along the north side; a shed is about halfway along the south fence; and there is nothing tactual to indicate the far back boundary (west). Several trees are scattered about the yard. A swing set is about 2/3 of the way back – closer to the north boundary than the south.

In a manner comparable to the lessons above, help the child practice walking to various places in the yard and back to the house. Help him form a mental map of the yard.

Walk with the student around the perimeter, guided by someone who knows where the boundaries are, to help him grasp the overall size.

Note that the yard extends beyond the hedge, beyond the shed, and beyond the swing set. From each of these three locations, walk to the west boundary and back.

The child needs to keep in mind where he is. He should pay attention to any sound or scent clues that may be present.

Walk to and from familiar landmarks in the neighbors' yards, so that if the child does leave his own yard unintentionally, he can figure out where he is.

The child may notice subtle differences which are missed by adults (especially sighted adults), such as a slight incline.

With experience, the student will learn to realize where he is and estimate distance.

See the Example below for additional help for a very young child.

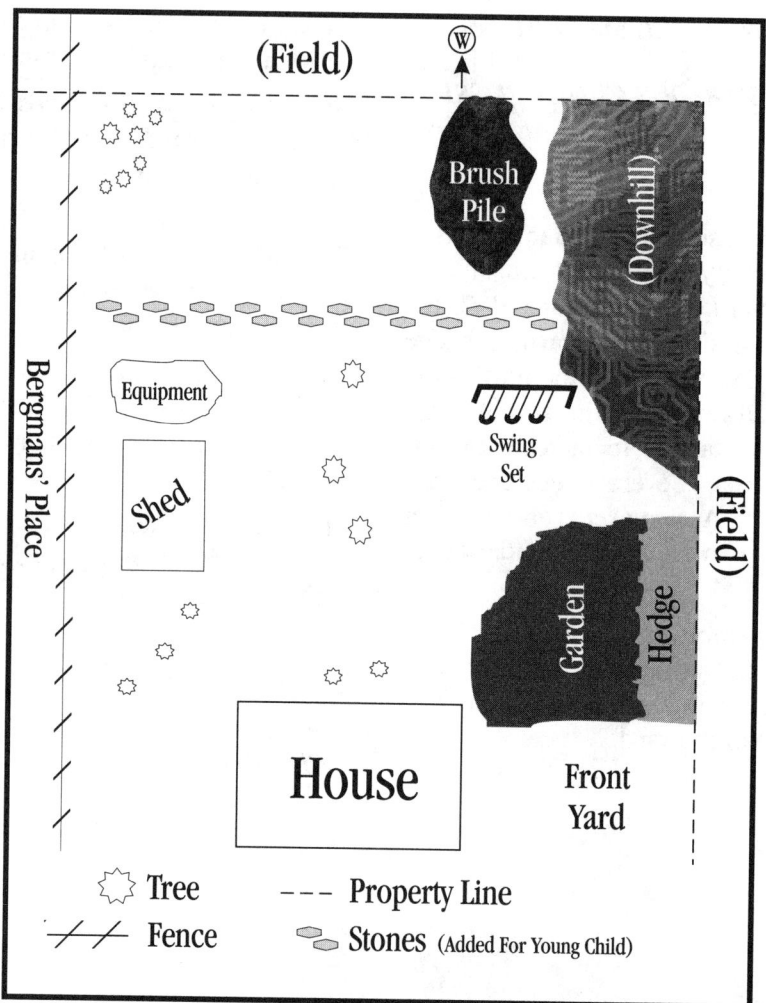

**Figure 19-2
Yard #2**

EXAMPLE 7: *HELP FOR A BEGINNER*
(*Preschool and primary grades*)

For a young beginner, learning to find his way around a yard without clearly-marked boundaries may take many months. Meanwhile, it is highly undesirable for someone to help him all the time. Even if supervision is required because of his age, he should be able to walk around without constant, direct help (physical or verbal).

Following are suggestions which can provide a degree of independence to an immature child.

If the yard has no fence, look for other boundaries (such as gardens, hedges, change of terrain, driveway, etc.) and work in a manner similar to the above Examples.

For a young child, if the edges of the yard are hard to detect, suggest the idea of placing some markers, temporarily or permanently. A good example is a row of decorative stones.

A similar idea can be used with a young child in a very large yard. Temporary markers could let him roam independently in a portion of the yard. The area can be expanded as he matures.

Encourage brothers and sisters, as well as other playmates, to show the blind child how to get around. Children sometimes seem to be "better teachers than the adults" – as long as they do not help too much in the wrong way.

VARIATION(S): In a yard with suitable terrain, see that the child walks barefoot at times.

RELATED PRACTICE:
Tactual maps: With a three-year-old, draw a raised square to represent the fence; place a large square of cardboard for the house, and a small one for the sand box. For a more mature child, provide more detail.

MODULE 20
BACK YARD (OVERALL)

NOTE: This Module interacts closely with the previous Module, "Back Yard Boundaries," which uses the same Figures but is in many respects more elementary.

OBJECTIVE: The student will discuss the overall layout of his/her back yard at home (or the equivalent). He/she will locate each major item in the yard, and will return to the house from any part of the yard.

AGE OF STUDENT: Preschool and up

PRIMARY SKILL EMPHASIS:
Boundaries
Open space
Landmarks
Obstacles in path
Correcting a path
Right and left
Corners, turns, and angles
Moving straight ahead
Varied terrain
Orientation overall

ADDITIONAL SKILL EMPHASIS:
Hills and inclines
Compass directions
Barefoot walking
Examining things tactually
Overhanging objects
Weather and temperature
Maps

SEE ALSO (Other Modules):
    Back Yard Boundaries
    Compass Directions
    Echoes and Air Currents
    The Great Outdoors
    Utilities and Trash
    Walking Across Open Space
    Playground
    What's Out There? (On the School Grounds)
    Rural Environment

FIGURE(S):
NOTE: The Figures for this Module are the same as those for "Back Yard Boundaries."

TEACHER PREPARATION: Look around the back yard, with a parent. Consider the most efficient ways for the student to learn to find each item, in view of his age and skill.

Talk with parents about (a) what the child is already familiar with in the yard; (b) what places, if any, he can already find independently; (c) what is most important for him to learn immediately.

ACTIVITIES:

EXAMPLE 1: *SEQUENCE OF SKILLS*
Often a child will already know how to find many or most individual items before the teacher comes to the home. In that case, much of this Module is unnecessary. However, the student may think of each item separately and fail to grasp the overall layout. Or, he may seem to understand the overall arrangement and yet have much difficulty finding particular places.

With a child of 8 or older, I usually follow the sequence listed below. As discussed in the Module, "Back Yard Boundaries," it is often best to name the directions in some way other than the points of the compass (e.g., "the Nelsons' side").

    – Walk around the perimeter while examining significant items (e.g, flower garden). At the same time, discuss things that are not at the perimeter (e.g., swing set).
    – Select a specific item and practice a logical path between it and the house. Then do the same for another item. In Yard #1, you might practice finding the sand box, flower bed, picnic table, and swing set – each individually in relation to the back door.
    – Practice going *between* any two of the

chosen items. The child may feel he must first go to the house before finding the other item. Help him get away from this pattern as soon as possible. As an easy example, in going from the picnic table to the swing in Yard #1, he can notice the edge of the patio instead of going all the way to the door.

– While continuing to practice as above for individual items, increasingly emphasize the overall layout. Consider making a tactual map.

– Promote overall flexibility. For example, in Yard #1, the child may be in the habit of always playing on the swing set first and then going to the sand box. Discourage rigid patterns.

With a younger child (approximately under 8 years), we may not examine the entire overall setting at first. We may not even go around the entire perimeter at first. Instead it may be best to start with finding particular items, and later help the child integrate the whole picture.

In Figure 19-2, a very young child might be eager to go to the swing set but tend to miss it and go too far west. A temporary guide (such as a row of stones) along the west boundary could be very helpful. Alternatively, such a marker line could be placed just beyond the swing set (as shown in Figure 19-2), not necessarily all the way to the west boundary.

Some families choose to place a guideline leading directly to the swing set. Railings or ropes are sometimes used; however, they have the strong disadvantage of encouraging dependence on something unusual and artificial. A better method would be a stone walkway to the swing.

EXAMPLE 2: *THE SAND BOX*
(*Preschool*)
(Figure 19-1)

A beginner may prefer to go along the perimeter to get to the sand box.

Turn left and follow along the house, then the edges of the flower bed, then the fence.

Soon, point out that a shorter route is possible. Come out the back door and proceed southwest at approximately the correct angle. Note the picnic table as you pass it. If you reach the Nelsons' fence and do not find the sand box, walk a bit in either direction. If you reach the rough ground, you are too far west. If you find the flower bed, you are too close to the house. With practice the youngster will easily go directly to the sand box, with very little correction needed.

When returning to the house, proceed in the equivalent manner. The patio makes it especially easy to know when you are near the door.

EXAMPLE 3: *THE SHED*
(*Preschool Through Primary Grades*)
(Figure 19-2)

Walk out the back door (facing west). Keep somewhat to the left, and look (with the cane) for the shed. The sound and feel will be distinctive when the cane tip finds the shed.

A beginner may choose to follow along the fence until the trees and shed are found; however, this should soon become unnecessary.

Examine the equipment west of the shed. If the student walks too far he will recognize the equipment and turn back.

Practice "making a mistake on purpose." Proceed west while keeping somewhat too far to the right, missing the shed and the equipment. The student learns to realize when he has walked so far that he must have missed the shed.

Carry out an actual errand. Get two large flower pots from the shed. Take them to the edge of the garden for the repotting job.

EXAMPLE 4: *THE SWING SET*
(*Preschool Through Primary Grades*)
(Figure 19-2)

Walk to the right, to the garden. Walk on west along the edge of the garden. Keep going essentially straight (not turning to follow the garden perimeter), and you will be headed for the swings. Arc the cane a little more widely than usual, looking for the support poles.

Listen attentively – a swing set usually jingles slightly in the breeze. Realize that if you go too far to the right you will go downhill. If you miss the swings and continue too far west, you should soon realize you have gone too far.

When a younger child is practicing this, allow him to swing awhile each time he makes a trip back and forth to the swings. If he has trouble but is making an effort, give help so that he succeeds at reasonable intervals and has a chance to play.

EXAMPLE 5: *BETWEEN THE SHED AND THE SWINGS*
(*Preschool Through Primary Grades*)
(Figure 19-2)

"Here we are at the shed...."

"Now, let's say that you want to play on the swings. You could, of course, go back to the house and then go to the swings. We practiced that. But there is a shorter and faster way...."

"Can you point toward the swing?.... I'll give you a hint. Right now we are facing toward the shed, and behind the shed is somebody else's yard. Whose yard?... Yes, it's the Bergmans'. So we know we don't want to go that way. And I gave you another hint a minute ago – we are not going to the house first. So, point toward the house and think, 'We are *not* going that way, either'...."

"Now, try again, please. Point toward the swings... Good!"

(Take hold of the child and help if necessary, so that he is facing and pointing toward the swing set.)

"I'll walk with you, and I'll help you the first time. Keep thinking about where we are. The shed and the Bergmans' yard are *in back* of us. We would find the hill going down if we went far enough, but we're not going quite that far...."

(As you talk, guide the child directly toward the swings. Gently tap the appropriate arm when you mention "left" or "right.")

"On our *left*, we are passing the field. If we went to the *right*, we would go back to the house...."

"Aha! Now what is your cane finding? Yes! This is a metal pole on the swing set. Now, we'll do that again – we'll go back to the shed and then find the swing again. When we find the swing next time, you may play on it."

Assist the child less and less as he practices going back and forth. At first help him go directly, to demonstrate the concept. Soon, however, it is important to let the child deviate from the "ideal" path, so that he learns to recognize where he is and correct his path.

REMARKS: These descriptions assume that the youngster will use the cane in the yard. We suggest that when a child is learning his way around the yard, the cane be used. Later it is an individual matter, depending on circumstances such as:

- How likely is it that the child will go into a neighbor's yard without wanting to return to the house for the cane?
- How large and complex is the yard, in relation to the youngster's age and experience?
- Are there many obstacles – especially, movable and unpredictable ones such as wheelbarrows?
- How well defined are the boundaries of the yard?

RELATED PRACTICE:

Tactual maps

MODULE 21
FROM HOUSE TO CURB

OBJECTIVE: The student will recognize the curb when it is found with the cane tip. The student will walk independently from his or her house to the curb and back.

AGE OF STUDENT: Preschool

PRIMARY SKILL EMPHASIS:
Street crossing
Open space
Varied terrain
Detecting step-downs or drop-offs
Sound direction and meaning
Boundaries
Landmarks
Sidewalk
Examining things tactually

ADDITIONAL SKILL EMPHASIS:
Structure of buildings
Right and left
Corners, turns, and angles
Open space
Orientation overall

SEE ALSO (Other Modules):
   Outside and Inside the House
   Street Crossing With Little Traffic
   Back Yard Boundaries
   Walking at Curbside
   Home Address

ACTIVITIES:

EXAMPLE 1: *TO THE CURB AND BACK*
(NOTE: This description assumes that the child is three or four years old, is just starting to use the cane, and previously had not moved confidently around her own yard. It also assumes that the distance to the street is quite short.)

Help the child to walk down the steps from her front door – the cane touching each step. Help her to recognize when the cane reaches the flat surface, and to understand that therefore she herself is almost down the steps.

"Now we're going to walk straight ahead to the end of your yard, all the way to the street. You know you don't go out in the street when you're playing, because a car might hit you. I'm going to help you know where to stop. Now, walk straight ahead – your cane will tell you if you're on grass or sidewalk."

Help the child recognize when the cane finds the step-down at the curb. Also note the change of sound in tapping the street surface. The child should also reach down and touch the curb with her hands. Listen for vehicles passing by.

"Can you point toward your house? Yes, it's back that way. Now, walk all the way to the house."

The student should find the front of the house with her cane (anywhere along the front). If she veers greatly, gently steer her (as, by putting a hand on her shoulder).

Repeat this (going back and forth between the house and the curb) as many times as appropriate for the child's attention span. Explain, for example: "We will do this three more times. Then we'll look at a very interesting pipe."

See that the child walks at least part of the time on the grass. Note that crossing the main sidewalk indicates that you are nearing the street.

When the child reaches the house the fourth time, ask her to walk to the corner of the house. (Direct her to a corner where there is a downspout from the eaves.) Examine that location and discuss the meaning of "corner."

Note the sound heard when the student strikes the downspout with the cane tip, and when she taps it with her hand; the downspout is made of metal. Talk about its purpose. The student examines it with her hands, up as far as she can reach, and down to the end at ground level. Where does the water go after it comes out?

CAUTION: Watch for possible sharp edges.

REMARKS: With appropriate practice, a child should be able to walk toward the street, stop at the curb, and return to the house, all independently.

Parents may choose to place a wind chime near the door for added orientation. (This is especially helpful in a relatively large yard, and therefore may be more appropriate in the back yard.)

An experienced blind person, in many instances, does not use her cane in her own yard. However, it depends on many factors – size and complexity of yard, likelihood of leaving the yard unexpectedly, personal preference, etc. As the child grows older, she may not ordinarily use the cane in her own yard. But at first it can be very valuable even in a small and simple yard.

FOLLOW-UP: Arrange for the child to examine the downspout again when water is running down.

EXAMPLE 2: *STRUCTURE OF CURB AND GUTTER*

STUDENT BACKGROUND: This Module assumes the student has had some introduction to finding curbs with her cane, and to walking on the sidewalk, but has not achieved independence and may not fully understand the concepts involved.

TEACHER PREPARATION: Look for a sidewalk with a curb close beside it. Note a location where it would be safe to sit down, and where it would not be especially dirty or wet. Look for a storm sewer grating which could be examined safely; consider the overall drainage patterns.

Possibly bring a moistened washcloth or paper towel for cleaning hands. Be sure the student will not be wearing her best clothes.

CAUTION: Young sighted children in good health commonly sit on the ground, and on the curb if safety permits. When watching a parade, adults sit on the curb also. A blind child should have the same opportunities.

However, individual circumstances should be carefully considered. If the child has special health problems, or constantly puts her hands in her mouth, touching the curb may be unwise. Also consider possible reactions from parents and preschool teachers; it may be prudent to talk with them beforehand.

****

Examine Curb and Gutter

"Today we're going to look for *curbs*. Every now and then we'll stop and find the nearest curb."

(Walk on the sidewalk for awhile and then stop.)

"Now point to the street beside us. Walk toward the street and find the *curb*. When your cane finds it, stop and tell me...."

"Yes, here we are at the curb. Now, today we are really going to look at it. We're going to do something we don't usually do. You shouldn't do this unless a grownup says it's OK, because you need to be sure that there aren't any cars too close."

Help the child to lay her cane down (not in the street) and examine the curb with her hands. See that it is possible to sit on the curb with one's feet in the street; compare to sitting on a bench. (Again emphasize that sitting here could be dangerous without adult guidance.)

Define and examine the *gutter* (with cane and/or hands). Is there a noticeable slope toward the curb? Discuss the drainage function; is any storm debris present now?

Various Locations

Wipe off dirty hands if necessary. Stand up, retrieve the cane, and walk back to the sidewalk. Note how the cane detects the grass "parking" strip, and then finds the sidewalk. Turn onto the sidewalk and proceed in the same direction in which you were originally walking.

Repeat all of this at least once at another point. Help the student understand that the street, with its curb, keeps going alongside as you proceed on the sidewalk.

Arrive at the corner. Find the curb at the crossing. While crossing the street [with assistance as necessary if the child has not yet learned independence]: name the *curb*, the *gutter*, the *middle of the street*, etc. Note the gutter and curb at the opposite side.

FOLLOW-UP: Examine a storm sewer grating, with further discussion of drainage. Explain that water goes through pipes underground and then into the river.

Examine various kinds of curbs and edges:
- Higher or lower curbs
- "Curb cuts" for wheelchairs
- A sidewalk immediately beside the street (with no grassy strip)
- Curbs made of various materials
- A grassy verge with no curb
- A ditch at the roadside

MODULE 22
HOME ADDRESS

OBJECTIVE: The student will state his or her house number and the name of the street. He/she will discuss the general concept of street addresses.

AGE OF STUDENT: Preschool

PRIMARY SKILL EMPHASIS:
Addresses
General travel (outdoors)
Street patterns
Understanding vision and partial vision
Traffic movement
Sidewalk
Maps

SEE ALSO (Other Modules):
Around the Block
Street Crossing With Little Traffic
From House to Curb
Driveways, Alleys, and Streets
Street Crossing With Little Traffic

ACTIVITIES:

While standing in front of the child's home, ask, "What is the name of this street? How do people know its name?"

After this is answered, continue: "Please go out to the big sidewalk and turn left. Walk all the way to the corner. I'll go ahead of you and call to you. I'll be standing by a pole when you get to the corner, and we'll talk about the pole."

Have the student approach the pole and touch it with her cane. "Is the pole made of metal? Notice how it sounds when your cane hits it."

Describe the sign. If possible, arrange for the child to reach up and touch it. Explain that it tells the street name in large letters, so that people can see it with their eyes. People can see it if they are walking, or if they are in a car and look out the window.

Locate the curb, and walk a short way along the curb (walking back toward the child's house). Repeat the name of this street.

Walk back to the corner; turn the corner and briefly walk along the curb beside the other street. What is the name of this other street? Explain (if it has not already been discussed) that actually the pole has *two* signs—one for each street. Do they face different directions?

Call attention to traffic, noting which street it is on.

Return to the child's home. What is the house number? Help the child touch the numerals if possible. Explain that they are large so that people on the sidewalk or in a car can see them with their eyes. Is the number lighted at night?

Recite the complete street address.

RELATED PRACTICE:

– Make a scale model of the street sign – i.e., a pole with a sign parallel to each street.
– Examine (or discuss) street signs at other corners.
– Walk to other homes in the same block and in another block. Examine house numbers when possible. Discuss the overall system of house numbers.
– Make a simple tactual map of the neighborhood.
– If the child is mature enough, discuss more advanced concepts, including:
 -Name of city and state
 -Complete address with zip code
 -Giving oral directions to the home (as when riding with someone unfamiliar with the area)

MODULE 23
PORCH OR DECK

OBJECTIVE: The student will name the outside features of typical houses, examine them where possible, and discuss how they relate to inside structure.

AGE OF STUDENT: Preschool through primary grades

PRIMARY SKILL EMPHASIS:
General travel
Stairs
Examining things tactually
Detecting step-downs or drop-offs

ADDITIONAL SKILL EMPHASIS:
Structure of buildings
Finding a seat
Doors and doorways
Sound direction and meaning
Air currents and echoes
Interpreting odors
Barefoot walking
Hills and inclines

SEE ALSO (Other Modules):
    Back Yard Boundaries
    Back Yard (Overall)
    Inside and Outside the House
    Home – Contents of Room
    What Is a "Room"?
    Unfinished Basement, "Crawl Space," or Attic
    Utilities and Trash

TEACHER PREPARATION: Look carefully at each porch or deck. What features are particularly interesting? Is there a place where the student could climb on and off without using the steps? Is it possible and safe to go underneath, at least for a short way?

ACTIVITIES:

EXAMPLE 1: *DETAILS OF ONE PORCH OR DECK*

"The Johnsons said we could go onto their deck today. Look with your cane for the second sidewalk to the left. Turn there and walk toward the house. When you find some steps, walk up onto the deck and look at it."

Note that the steps have no railings at the side; sweep the cane from side to side enough to avoid stepping off sideways.

Note the sound of the cane tapping the wooden floor. It sounds different than on an indoor wooden floor.

Find the door leading inside. If possible, walk in briefly and note what room opens onto the deck.

Walk around the perimeter of the deck, noting its size. Is there a railing?

Examine planters or other features. Sit on each chair or bench. A triangular corner seat may be a new experience.

Look for places where it is easy to get off and on without using the steps. (Reach over the edge with the cane to verify height.) Practice getting off and on at various places – climb, jump, or simply step. (Some blind children believe this is never possible.)

Go underneath to experience how it feels. Is it cool? Does it smell musty? Tap the underside of the wooden floor (probably with the hand, not with the cane). Are things stored underneath?

EXAMPLE 2: *COMPARE OTHERS*

In a similar manner, examine and compare various kinds of porches and decks.

Explore a deck that is high above ground level, with many steps leading up. Note the guard rail. Understand that stepping off would cause injury. Stand upright underneath.

Walk around on a large porch that has a roof over it. Can you easily step on and off at many different places?

Explore an enclosed porch which has screening or windows. Why is it called a porch, even though it has walls and a roof?

Examine an entrance which has no porch or deck. Are there steps, a welcome mat, or other typical features?

MODULE 24
OUTSIDE AND INSIDE THE HOUSE

OBJECTIVE: The student will walk around the perimeter of the house, both inside and outside, while discussing relative positions and spatial relationships.

AGE OF STUDENT: Preschool through the primary grades

PRIMARY SKILL EMPHASIS:
Floor plans
Structure of buildings
Orientation overall

ADDITIONAL SKILL EMPHASIS:
Corners, turns, and angles
Doors and doorways
Sound direction and meaning
Varied terrain
Landmarks
Right and left
Compass directions

SEE ALSO (Other Modules):
   Outside and Inside the School
   What Is a "Room"?
   Porch or Deck
   Back Yard Boundaries
   Around the Block

TEACHER PREPARATION: If possible, have someone assist by staying inside when the student is outside, and vice versa. This person could be another child.

REMARKS: Even though the child may not normally use his cane in his own home and yard, it is helpful to use it in this lesson. He may be moving in areas where he ordinarily does not go (e.g., a garden). Also, he will be working with important concepts (e.g., corners) and integrating them with cane usage.

ACTIVITIES:

Student inside
Emphasize, "We are *inside* the house now."
Walk around inside at ground level, name each room, and open at least one window in each room.

Student outside
"Now your brother, Jason, will stay inside and go to each window like we just did. We will go to the front door and go *outside*. We will walk along outside the house, touching the house. Each time we come to an open window, we'll talk to Jason about what is inside."

Have the student walk along the outside of the house, with the cane touching the wall with each arc. Locate each window by any of several methods: (1) You announce it yourself. (2) The person inside calls out. (3) The student finds it by using clues already learned (e.g., the dining room window is behind the apple tree). (4) The student continually slides his hand along the wall, looking for windows. (This alternative, often called "trailing," is sometimes used excessively or inappropriately. However, this is one situation where there is a clear reason for it.)

At each window, talk to the person inside and name the room.

Continue all around the house. Note additional landmarks, such as gardens, as the cane finds them.

When the back door is found, open it and step in momentarily. Name the room. Continue all the way around the house. Then go back in the front door and confirm that you are back where you started.

Were there any interior rooms that had no windows?

VARIATION(S): Repeat with reversed roles. The other person goes around outside, while the student and teacher talk to him from inside.

Repeat at another familiar house.

For a multi-story house, repeat for each floor. When outside, bend down to talk through basement windows; shout upward to talk through upstairs windows.

REMARKS: With a preschool-aged child, it may be best to work with only part of the house during a given session.

MODULE 25
UTILITIES AND TRASH

OBJECTIVE: The student will examine and discuss features of utility systems (e.g., water pipes and meters) and trash collection. He/she will carry a bundle to where the family's trash is placed out.

AGE OF STUDENT: Preschool through primary grades

PRIMARY SKILL EMPHASIS:
Structure of buildings
General travel
Daily living skills
Interpreting odors
Examining things tactually

ADDITIONAL SKILL EMPHASIS:
Carrying things
Floor plans
Maps
Responsibility and citizenship
Weather and temperature
Traffic movement

SEE ALSO (Other Modules):
  Outside and Inside the House
  Back Yard Boundaries
  Back Yard (Overall)
  Carrying Things
  Unfinished Basement, "Crawl Space," or Attic

TEACHER PREPARATION:

See Cautions.

If you are a teacher working with a child in his home, ask the parents' approval beforehand. They may not want a very young child to know where certain things are, lest he be tempted to tamper with them.

At a school or in an apartment house, check with the custodian before going into an area ordinarily restricted; do not work with valves or circuit breakers unless the custodian is present. In a private home, it is best for the parent to turn valves, turn circuit breakers on and off, change fuses, etc.

CAUTION: Examining water arrangements is usually safe even for a young child, if care is taken to avoid hot pipes. Examining electrical or gas arrangements, however, involves danger. With a very young child it may be best to examine only the water system.

Look beforehand at each item, and consider whether it would be safe and appropriate for the student to examine it.

ACTIVITIES:

EXAMPLE 1: *WATER*

Turn the water on and off at two or more faucets, and discuss the importance of water. Take a drink.

Discuss where the water comes from. "Big pumps get it out of the river. It comes here in a big pipe under the ground. Little pipes bring it into the house.

"We have to pay money for water. How does the water company know what your family should pay? There is a *meter* that shows how much water you used. Let's go look at it.

"Go out the back door and turn right. Go around the corner to the pansy bed. I'll help you look behind the pansy bed today." When the child arrives at the location, help him find the meter with its pipes. Discuss the path of the water. Describe the numbers on the meter.

"Suppose we needed to fix a pipe. We'd need to turn off the water at an extra place, or else it would keep coming out while we were fixing the pipe. Go to the laundry room, and I'll show you something interesting....Here is a place where we could turn off all the water for the whole house." (Help the student examine the valve and its connections.)

Direct the child to a fixture which has an individual extra shutoff (e.g., a sink with a valve on each incoming pipe underneath).

When the child arrives, show him a valve. Help him close it and demonstrate that no water will come out when the faucet is "turned on" at the usual place. Help him turn the valve back on and see that the faucet works as usual.

EXAMPLE 2: *ELECTRICITY*

Proceed in a manner similar to the above, doing as much as is appropriate for the child's age. Explain the meter. Examine circuit breakers or fuses, and also the master switch. Actually turn off a circuit breaker or remove a fuse (See Caution, above), and observe that certain lights and appliances will not work. Restore circuit breaker or fuse. Is there a diagram of each circuit?

EXAMPLE 3: *GAS*

Proceed in a manner similar to studying the water system. It may not be practical to turn any gas off; however, discuss how a pilot light can be re-lighted.

Explain that this is "natural gas"—not a liquid, but rather "a special kind of air." It is not the same as gasoline, which is also called "gas." Obtain a scented card from the gas company, to demonstrate the odor of natural gas. Discuss safety and emergency procedures in case gas is smelled.

EXAMPLE 4: *TRASH COLLECTION*

CAUTION: Young children may be fearful of loud, sudden, unfamiliar noises. Also, a strong and unpleasant smell may be upsetting. If the arrival of the trash truck is to be observed, stand well back from the curb at first. Walk closer only if it seems appropriate.

Observe safety precautions around moving trucks and machinery.

If a young child does not keep his hands out of his mouth, avoid allowing him to touch dirty surfaces. Consider carrying a hand-wipe packet.

At Home

Empty the wastebaskets and carry trash to the outdoor trash can. If carrying a sack, use the cane normally. If using two hands on the container, the cane can be brought along and perhaps used partially. (See the Module, "Carrying Things.")

Examine the trash can as much as appropriate. Walk around it and tap it with the cane. What is it made of?

Place trash can(s) at the curb for pickup. (If the container is too large for the child to carry, he can observe others moving it, and he can examine the container again when it is at the curb.) Is trash sorted for recycling?

If possible, approach the curb when the trash-collection truck is arriving. (See Caution, above.) Greet workers and observe the collection. Note sounds, including the backing-up signal. Note odors.

Other People's Trash

Arrange to walk to a neighbor's home. Go to where their trash containers are kept. What are these containers made of? Is an odor noticeable? Where are they placed at the curb? If you were visiting here and helping with the trash, how would you find the cans and take them to the curb?

Examine trash containers and procedures at school.

Locate a large dumpster outside a business. Touch it with the cane. What is it made of? Discuss commercial collection.

EXAMPLE 5: *ADDITIONAL OPPORTUNITIES*

Many other features around the home and nearby lend themselves to lessons in a similar vein. Below are a few examples:

- Telephone system
- Utility poles
- Drain spouts on the house
- Storm drains, gutters, etc.
- Street signs of various kinds
- Mail and package delivery
- Delivery of large purchases (e.g., furniture)
- Fire hydrants

RELATED PRACTICE: Make a tactual picture of each meter, with a movable pointer.

On a simple tactual map of the house and/or yard, indicate pipes or meters.

Examine systems and meters in other homes and other buildings.

Visit the water works, the gas company, the electric company.

MODULE 26
MORE IDEAS
For Lessons at Home
Outdoors

AGE OF STUDENT: Preschool through primary grades

ABOUT THIS LIST:

Following is a list of objects, aspects, places, etc., which are typically found outside around the home. Examining different things at various times helps assure variety and interest for the young child.

A given item may be incorporated into the actual lesson. (Example: The child is practicing finding key locations in the back yard. Each time she finds an item as directed, she and the teacher pause to examine textures found there.) Alternatively, a given item may serve as a "fun" end to a lesson. (Example: The child is asked to find and name five key locations in the back yard. When this task is accomplished, she is allowed to climb on the old tree stump.)

It is very interesting for a young child to examine and compare equivalent items in someone else's yard – Aunt Lou's rock garden, the neighbor's shed, etc.

Cane usage is appropriately practiced even when the child frequently stops to examine things by touch.

REMARKS: Talk with the parent before opening doors or going anywhere not previously planned. There probably are many places which the parent does not wish children to get into at all. Also, the parent may be very uncomfortable about letting the teacher see areas that might seem "messy" or personal. (A good example of both problems might be the inside of a shed.) Often it is better to suggest that the *parent* give the child a tour of certain areas. The teacher may wish to leave a "follow-up" suggestion after each lesson.

CAUTION: Always be alert for possible hazards. Examples include poisonous materials in a storage area, gas or electric motors, sharp edges, etc. Also, be sure to use good safety practices when assisting a child to climb up and reach something.

IDEAS:

- Vine, trellis, summer house
- Hedge (How do you get around or through it?)
- Vegetable garden
- Flower garden
- Rock garden
- Shed or other outbuilding
- Swings and other play equipment
- Tricycles, bicycles, riding toys
- Pipes and eave spouts
- Yard ornaments
- Textures of various walls
- Trees and bushes (fruit-bearing and otherwise)
- Examining various *parts* of plants – roots, stems, leaves, flowers, seed pods
- Noting textures of various plants, or plant parts – rough, prickly, soft, velvety, etc.
- Moss, lichens
- Patio chairs, lawn chairs, etc. (Sit on each one, and also examine each of its parts.)
- Picnic table or patio tables
- Steps
- Shutters and other window treatments
- Fireplace chimney
- Fences
- Surface of patio, driveway, etc.
- Hills and inclines
- Barbecue facilities
- Opening and closing various doors
- Tree stump
- Utility meters
- Varied terrain – grass, sand, gravel, mulch, wood chips, bare dirt, cement, etc.

- Short, mowed grass
- High, unmowed grass or weeds
- Shovels, rakes, hoes, etc.
- Lawn mowers, leaf blowers, etc. (See Caution, above. Guide child's hand to examine safe portions of machine.)
- Old-fashioned cellar door
- Root cellar or other underground storage
- Seasonal or weather-related items, such as dry leaves or ice

AT SCHOOL
INDOORS

MODULE 27
ORIENTATION INSIDE NEW CLASSROOM

OBJECTIVE: The student will examine the general layout of [the classroom.] He/she will independently find each of four specific locations.

AGE OF STUDENT:
Preschool through elementary school (See Examples)

PRIMARY SKILL EMPHASIS:
Orientation within a room
Obstacles in path
Finding a seat
Floor plans
Landmarks

ADDITIONAL SKILL EMPHASIS:
Doors and doorways
Right and left
Corners, turns, and angles
Communication and instructions
Stowing cane

SEE ALSO (Other Modules):
Home – Contents of Room
What Is a "Room"?
Routes for New Buildings and New Classrooms (Early Elementary Grades)
Routes for New Buildings and New Classrooms (Upper Grades Through High School)

TEACHER PREPARATION: It is important for both the student and the itinerant teacher to get acquainted with the classroom teacher as soon as possible. This is reassuring for everyone, and heads off many potential problems and worries.

This matter is discussed in detail in the *Handbook for Itinerant and Resource Teachers of Blind and Visually Impaired Students*, by Willoughby and Duffy – particularly in the chapters "Starting Anew Each Time" and "Your Professional Role." It is vital that the classroom teacher(s) and the specialized teacher(s), as well as the student and parents, discuss arrangements well in advance of the new term. If you teach only travel, ask the teacher who handles general arrangements to join you.

REMARKS: Arrange to enter the classroom for actual practice when the class is not present. Ask permission to look inside a desk or two.

Inquire what rest rooms the class uses, what exit doors are used to go to buses, the playground, etc. Ask about customary names or descriptions for parts of the room – for example, "front wall" and "back wall," "reading corner," etc.

CAUTION: If there is any doubt about the grade/class placement for the following year, avoid saying, "This will be your room next year." Instead, describe the room with an objective label (e.g., "Mrs. Norton's room"), and imply that the lesson is routine practice. Alternatively, wait until placement is decided.

ACTIVITIES:

EXAMPLE 1: *KINDERGARTEN STUDENT PREPARING FOR FIRST GRADE*
For a young child, try to arrange several visits before class is begun in the new room. Give the child a general overview, and start to teach him independence in the most important places. At least one visit in the fall, shortly before classes start, is highly desirable even if intensive work was done in the spring. After class starts, work with the classroom teacher to be sure the child achieves and maintains independence.

Introduction: "There are a lot of desks in here. In kindergarten you sit at tables; but first graders have desks. Just one person sits at each desk.... Walk on in, to the middle of the room." (Guide the child in the right direction if necessary.) "Find a desk and sit down."

Help the child lay his cane under the desk, and examine the desk to note such features as a rigidly attached chair. Allow him to open the desk and lightly examine the other student's possessions without disturbing them. Ask the child to move to at least one other desk, and repeat.

Describe the general arrangement of desks—straight rows, groups of four, etc. The child examines at least one grouping or row.

The doorway: "Now, we have moved around a lot. Let's think where the door is." Help the child as necessary, and go to the door. Walk back and forth between the doorway and a nearby desk.

Four walls: Starting from the door, walk around all four sides of the room. Describe or examine, at least briefly, each feature that is notable. Call attention to turning each corner, and name the new wall in some way: for example, "This is the *front* of the room. Most of the desks face toward this wall. Mrs. Norton usually stands here when she talks to the whole class."

Walk around again, more quickly, analyzing the overall layout.

Other features: If there are other important features not yet examined, go to each of them and discuss their location. Example: "We are at the *back* of the room right now. Find the wall....Go to the *front* of the room and I'll show you another interesting thing." (Have the child use his cane to go around desks and other obstacles. Help if necessary so that he reaches the front of the room fairly directly.)

"When Mrs. Norton is at the front, sometimes she sits down. She has a high stool so that she can easily see the class, and so they can hear her well. Walk toward me and you'll find it." (Allow the child to examine the stool and sit on it briefly.)

Find the teacher's desk. Where is it in relation to the door, the students' desks, etc.? Does the teacher often sit there during class?

Permanent vs. changeable features: Note things that will surely be the same next year, such as the walls themselves and the door. Call attention to other things that will probably not change—e.g., large bookshelves and heavy cupboards.

Explain that some things may be different next year. Examples include the desk arrangement, animal cages, and movable easels.

(Note: in talking with the teacher, assure her that you do *not* expect that the room arrangement will remain precisely the same.)

EXAMPLE 2: *OLDER STUDENTS*

When an elementary-school student will have one main classroom, orientation should be carried out in a manner similar to the above, but in an age-appropriate manner.

It should not be necessary to explain basic concepts. Instead, briskly help the student examine the overall layout, especially any differences from previous familiar arrangements. Examples include desks in groups rather than in rows; the door at the back instead of the front; a fire exit leading directly outside.

In middle school and high school, it becomes less helpful to examine specific rooms beforehand. Usually, the main work is in learning to find the room itself. The student will easily learn where his desk is, and any other major points, when the class actually meets.

For a specialized room such as a science laboratory or industrial arts, detailed examination beforehand continues to be important for independence.

FOLLOW-UP: As noted at the beginning of this Module, the student should meet each new teacher in person. This may occur in the course of the travel lesson, but other meetings may need to be planned.

With a young student, probably the itinerant teacher will meet at a separate time to discuss details of arrangements such as transcribing. At higher levels, however, arrangements may be discussed with the student present. This prepares the student for making his own contacts in college and on the job.

REFERENCE(S):
Willoughby and Duffy. *Handbook for Itinerant and Resource Teachers of Blind and Visually Impaired Students,* pp. 363-376, 401-410.

MODULE 28
ROUTES FOR NEW CLASSROOM
Early Elementary Grades

OBJECTIVE: The student will walk independently between his/her own classroom and all areas of the school building where students of this age ordinarily go.

AGE OF STUDENT: Kindergarten and early elementary grades. (This Module is written in a style suitable for a six-year-old.)

FIGURE(S):

FIGURE 28-1: New Classroom and Rest Rooms

PRIMARY SKILL EMPHASIS:
General travel (indoors)
Orientation overall
Floor plans
Corners, turns, and angles
Landmarks
Right and left
Doors and doorways

ADDITIONAL SKILL EMPHASIS:
Sound direction and meaning
Structure of buildings
Compass directions

Correcting a path
Stairs

SEE ALSO (Other Modules):
Playground
Rest Rooms at School
Orientation Inside New Classroom
Lunchroom and Kitchen
Routes for New Buildings and New Classrooms
Alternate Routes Within a Building
Errands
Fire drills
Doors and doorways
Description of Basic Techniques

ACTIVITIES:

REMARKS: These Examples assume that the student has attended (or is now attending) kindergarten in this building, and is now preparing for first grade. (See Figure 28-1) It assumes that he has learned his way to and from the following locations in relation to the kindergarten room: front door (to buses); office; lunchroom/gym.

ROUTES FOR NEW CLASSROOM (Early Elementary Grades)

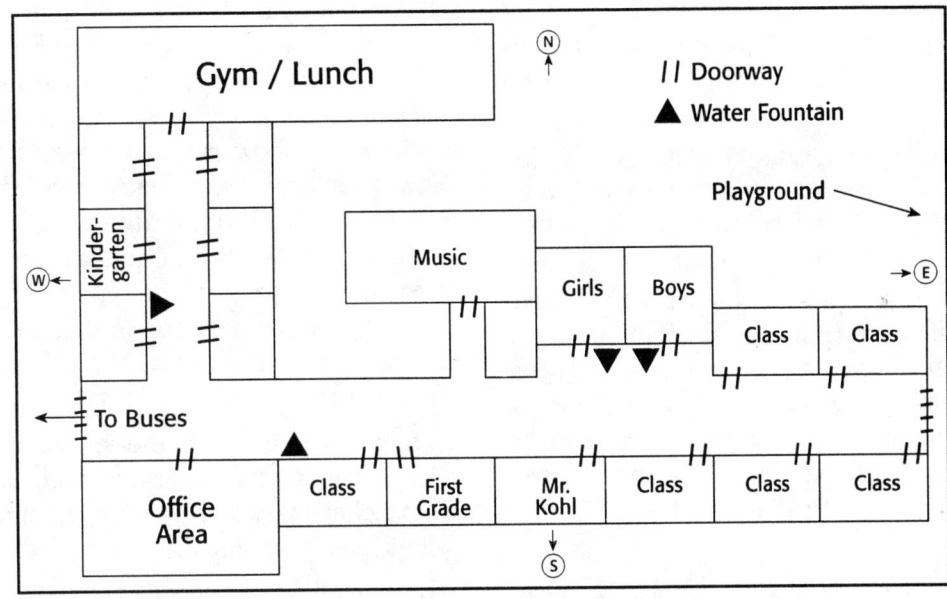

Figure 28-1
New Classroom and Rest Rooms

EXAMPLE 1: INTRODUCTION

Ask the student to go to the front door of the school (near the bus loading area) independently. Then ask him to follow you (listening to your voice and footsteps) as you go to the first grade room. Note the following points:

- We walk straight ahead, rather than turning left toward the kindergarten.
- We pass the familiar office on our right.
- We pass a drinking fountain.
- On the right, we pass one classroom door which is not first grade.
- The second door (on the right, after the office) is the first grade.

"Think about how we got here. Can you point back toward the front door, where you go to the bus? ... Let's go there again, and we will think about how you can find the first grade yourself, from the front door...."

"Go out the front door and come in again. Stand with your back to the front door. Point to the hall that goes to your kindergarten room. You could also go that way to the gym."

"Now point straight ahead. That's the way to the first grade. Remember, we will pass the office, a drinking fountain, and one extra door."

"You already know how to find the office. Go past the office, and tell me you're passing it. Then find that fountain, and get a drink if you like...."

"Good! Here's that fountain. Now keep going and count two doors to find the first grade room."

The child continues to practice this route as needed. An independent student, even at this age, may need very little practice.

EXAMPLE 2: TWO HALLWAYS

Return to the front door of the school. Discuss the route to the gym: Turn left, proceed past the kindergarten, and go all the way to the end of the hall. Practice this and return to the front door.

"Now we're going to the first grade room again. When we get there we will think about how to turn around and go to the gym from there."

At the first grade room, elicit as much understanding of the return route as possible. If necessary, explain it all yourself, and then explain it again as you walk to the gym with him. "Yes, you need to go back toward the office and the front door. Then what?...You'll need to turn toward the kindergarten and go on to the gym.

When we go there from here, it will be a *right* turn. Let's practice. You go toward the front door by yourself, and I'll help you know where to turn."

Help the student understand that (as he goes west toward the front door) he will need to turn right, into the hall that leads north. The first time (and several times if needed), you may choose to tell him where to turn, and then have him walk independently to the familiar gym (noting when you pass the kindergarten). Later, show him how to keep to the right in the first-grade hallway and watch for the place to turn. Sounds, air currents, and/or caning the wall will indicate when he has reached the turn.

Explain, if necessary, that the "gym" is also called the "lunchroom" and is converted by placing or removing tables. (See also the Modules, "Lunchroom and Kitchen" and "Lunchtime.")

Discuss compass directions at some point, though not necessarily at first. In this example, the child can learn that the first-grade hall goes east and west; the front door is at the west end and the playground door is east. The kindergarten hall goes north and south; the office is at the south end, and the lunchroom is north.

Also practice walking between the kindergarten room and the first grade room.

EXAMPLE 3: *INSIDE THE NEW CLASSROOM*

Actually entering the new classroom is exciting, and may be used as an incentive for learning the hallway routes. The Module, "Orientation Inside New Classroom," offers detailed suggestions.

EXAMPLE 4: *MUSIC ROOM*

(See Figure 28-1) This example assumes that kindergartners have music in their own classroom, and the student is not familiar with the music room.

"In kindergarten, Mrs. Sails [kindergarten teacher] teaches music. But in first grade, you'll have a different teacher for music, and a special room. Today we'll practice finding that room.

"Show me again where the first grade room is....Good.... Now cross to the *other* side of this hall—we can call it the north side of the hall. We're going to go east toward the playground...Show me which way that is....Yes. Now, your cane has already found that there is just a little bit of wall in this direction, and then a big space. We have found the little hall that goes to the music room. Turn left...Here we need to look for the door straight ahead.... This is a short hall, and the music room is the only room here."

If there is a class in the music room, listen awhile to enjoy the music and begin to recognize the teacher's voice. Note that the music was an added clue in finding the room.

Arrange a time to enter the room and explore it as described in the Module, "Orientation Inside New Classroom." Let the child briefly play an instrument that is not easily damaged—e.g., maraca or triangle.

Practice going back and forth to the first grade playground. (See the Module, "Playground.")

EXAMPLE 5: *INTEGRATION OF SKILLS*

Consider all of the locations where first graders are likely to go. Probably this will include: front door to buses; main office; rest rooms; water fountain; gym; library; lunchroom; music room; playground. If the child has already gone to these same places previously, examine how the route differs in relation to the new room. Practice random routes from any of these locations to any other.

Help the student think of the whole picture, rather than rigidly memorizing. For example: "Let's stand by the first-grade door, here, and pretend we're just coming out. Point to your right....is that the way to the gym?...No! It isn't. We went that way when we were looking at the first-grade playground. We will need to go to the *left* to get to the gym... Go there now, please. When you get there we will play 'catch' for five minutes."

MODULE 29
REST ROOMS
AT SCHOOL

OBJECTIVE: The student will locate an appropriate rest room. He/she will enter, take care of personal needs, and return to the classroom independently.

(Objectives for daily living skills may also apply.)

FIGURE(S): NOTE: Refer to the Figure in the immediately previous Module, "Routes for New Classroom: Early Elementary Grades."

AGE OF STUDENT: Kindergarten and up (See Examples)

PRIMARY SKILL EMPHASIS:
General travel (indoors)
Right and left
Compass directions
Doors and doorways
Orientation within a room
Corners, turns, and angles

ADDITIONAL SKILL EMPHASIS:
Daily living skills
Correcting a path
Floor plans
In a crowd or a line
Stowing cane

SEE ALSO (Other Modules):
  Routes for New Classroom (Early
      Elementary Grades)
  Routes for New Buildings and New
      Classrooms (Upper Grades Through
      High School)
  Orientation Inside New Classroom
  Alternate Routes Within a Building
  In a Crowd
  Doors and Doorways

CAUTION: It is a very personal matter to enter a rest room, discuss what is inside, and use the facilities. If you and the student are of opposite sex, your lesson should go only as far as the door. If orientation inside the rest room is needed, someone of the same sex should assist. (A possible exception would be for preschool children or a medical setting.) The counselor, nurse, classroom teacher, or any congenial staff member of the same sex might help.

REMARKS: The need for a rest room is one of the most important and basic needs for any child at school. Yet discomfort and suffering are all too common, as shown in "Blindness-What it Means in the Mind of a Blind Child," by Ramona Walhof (See *References*). That article includes a poignant example of needless suffering due to no one's realizing that the child could not find the rest room independently.

Consider what kinds of rest rooms the student has already experienced. The Examples for first grade assume that the kindergarten had small one-person rest rooms, and that first graders will use a much larger one.

If the student is a boy, be sure he has learned how to use a urinal, and how to unzip his fly instead of lowering his pants.

If at all possible, practice for the new school year during the spring, or before school opens. Independence on the first day of school means a great deal.

Consider whether mature vocabulary needs to be taught. A young child may need to learn to substitute "bathroom" or "rest room" for "potty."

These descriptions assume that the teacher is a woman and the student is a girl. (See CAUTION note above.)

ACTIVITIES: Refer to the Figure in the immediately previous Module, "Routes for New Classroom: Early Elementary Grades." A hallway runs east and west, with a playground exit at the east end. On the north side of the hall, one passes the following as one proceeds from west to east: the large north-south hallway leading to the gym; a small hallway going north to the music room; a large alcove with water fountains and rest room entrances; and two classrooms. When a person enters the alcove with the fountains, he or she finds the rest room doors facing south, with the girls' on the left (west) and the boys' on the right (east).

On the south side of the hall, the student's own classroom is opposite the music hallway (although the first-grade *door* is a bit west of the music hallway); Mr. Kohl's door is opposite the girls' rest room; and other classrooms are east of Mr. Kohl's.

EXAMPLE 1: CLASSROOM TO REST ROOM
(*First grade*)

The student turns right from her classroom door, and walks east to find Mr. Kohl's door with her cane. She crosses the hall and finds herself in the entryway to the rest rooms. (The two doorways are set back from the hallway, in a kind of an alcove. Also in this alcove, between the two individual doors, are water fountains.)

The student keeps to the left far enough to be sure she is not entering the boys' room. Especially at first, finding the extreme lefthand end of the entryway may be necessary in being certain to avoid the boys' door.

During the first lesson or two, help the child to examine the boys' doorway, so that she understands where it is. Do this when other students are not present, in order to prevent giggling and misunderstanding. With practice, the child learns to note the beginning of the entry area, and then keep left toward the girls' doorway.

Go on into the girls' room. Encourage the student to look around and identify sinks, stall doors, etc. She can find each with her cane and then verify by touching with her hand. Open at least one stall and touch the bottom of the stool with the cane, to verify that it is there.

Mention where to place the cane while sitting on the toilet. It could be laid on the floor; however, sometimes a rest room floor is wet or dirty. The cane can usually stand in the corner of the stall.

Help the student verbalize the layout of the room—e.g., stalls on the left, sinks on the right, as you enter.

Explain that, in contrast to the one-person rest rooms in kindergarten, several people may be in this rest room at one time. Young children usually are not particularly self-conscious about this, but be sensitive to the possibility. The student should practice closing and opening the door to a stall from the inside, and understand that it is customary to close the door. Help her learn to walk along and examine each door to see if it is locked.

Wash hands. Note where the soap, towels, and wastebaskets are. (Are the wastebaskets movable or in fixed locations? They can be found with the cane, or perhaps casually with the foot if very close by.)

Practice going back and forth to the classroom.

Some young children may continue to need assistance for awhile in a large rest room. Practice may also be needed in walking back and forth under crowded conditions. Suggest to the classroom teacher that another girl might act as a "buddy" for awhile if necessary. This help should be phased out soon.

EXAMPLE 2: VARIOUS WAYS TO THE REST ROOM
(*First grade*)

Practice another approach. Starting from the first-grade door, the child crosses the hall immediately, then turns east, and notes the side hall going north toward the music room. She proceeds past that branch hallway, using her cane to find where the wall resumes. Soon she finds the wide opening which leads to both rest rooms. The girls' entrance is reached first.

Sighted students in this setting may very naturally proceed in a diagonal from the classroom to the rest room. The blind student may proceed this way, too, in time. (It may be well to mention, as the student gains experience, that this is all right.) To begin, however, it is best to cross straight over at a selected point.

Consider the possible confusion of mistaking the music hallway for the rest room entrance. How do these locations compare? How do they smell and sound different? If you did actually start down the music hallway by mistake, how would you soon know where you were? How would you correct your path and proceed to the rest room?

EXAMPLE 3: *BETWEEN REST ROOM AND PLAYGROUND*
(*First grade*)

Practice going between the rest room and the playground. Children will probably be encouraged to use the rest room while going to or from recess.

When coming in the east door, you pass two classrooms (on the north side) and then find the bathroom area. Emphasize that the rest rooms will be on your *right* as you go west, and that you will come to the boys' room *first*.

Where are the drinking fountains?

EXAMPLE 4: *OTHER REST ROOMS*
(*First grade*)

Are there other rest rooms that might be used by first graders—near the gym or lunchroom, for example? If so, practice there in a similar manner.

EXAMPLE 5: *FOURTH GRADE*

Show the student the location of the rest room and its surroundings, in the same general way as for a younger student, but using mature terminology. Brief practice should be sufficient if the student is experienced in general travel skills. A short discussion may be enough if none of the areas are new to the student.

(*NOTE: Help of a personal nature should be from someone of the same sex. See Caution note near the beginning of this Module.*)

If the rest room has a sanitary napkin/tampon dispenser, examine it and discuss how it works. (If there is no dispenser, take the opportunity to mention where sanitary supplies could be found if needed. If there are no dispensers, the nurse or secretary almost certainly has supplies.) Consider whether the student is getting adequate guidance about menstruation; help to arrange for more information if needed.

EXAMPLE 6: *OLDER STUDENTS*

A student should learn immediately where *all* the convenient rest rooms are, for maximum flexibility and convenience. Don't let your student restrict herself to one "favorite" rest room.

A girl should find out where the napkin/tampon dispensers are; they may be only in certain rooms. Many girls are very self-conscious about managing and disposing of tampons or napkins; be sure your student knows how and where to do this. See that she is acquainted with the small disposal baskets which sometimes are in toilet stalls, in addition to regular wastebaskets.

(*NOTE: Help of a personal nature should be from someone of the same sex. See Caution note near the beginning of this Module.*)

It is helpful to understand where the rest rooms for the opposite sex are located. If this is not known, the student may approach one in such a way as to appear to be entering.

REFERENCE(S):

Walhof, Ramona. "Blindness—What it Means in the Mind of a Blind Child."

MODULE 30
FIRE DRILLS

OBJECTIVE: During a fire alarm, the student will use his/her cane and exit from any area of the school with no more help than is commonly given to other students of the same age.

AGE OF STUDENT: Preschool and up (See individual examples)

PRIMARY SKILL EMPHASIS:
Emergency procedures
Orientation overall
Doors and doorways
Floor plans
Communication and instructions
Stairs
Flexibility and confidence
Responsibility and citizenship
In a crowd or a line

ADDITIONAL SKILL EMPHASIS:
Attitudes toward blindness
Structure of buildings

SEE ALSO (Other Modules):
>Emergency Exits (In Various Buildings)
>Exterior Fire Escape
>In a Crowd
>Walking in a Line of People
>Alternate Routes Within a Building
>Description of Basic Techniques (Including Stairway Technique)

TEACHER PREPARATION: Learn the policies and routes for fire drills at the particular school. Explain to teachers that a blind student should need no more help than other students in an emergency. Emphasize that the cane is important and useful in this situation as in other situations; arrange to provide practice as needed.

Be sure no one assumes that the blind student should use another route "for the handicapped." She should walk out in the same way and at the same place as others.

ACTIVITIES:

EXAMPLE 1: *FIRE DRILL WITH CLASS*
(*Kindergarten and up*)

Talk with classroom teachers about fire drills. They may assume that the student would be assisted by others and would not use the cane. Explain that the student should indeed use the cane, with other assistance being phased out as quickly as possible.

Teachers may fear that the cane would trip others during the crowded, tense drill. Show the student and the teacher how the cane should be pulled up closer in a crowd.

A beginner in fourth grade or above should use the cane in fire drills immediately. If necessary, she might be given extra help on a temporary basis, but the cane should be carried and used as much as possible even at first. The same is true of a youngster in the lower grades who has used a cane for some time.

When a primary-grade youngster is just starting to use a cane, the discussions under the Example, "Class of Very Young Children," below, may apply.

Sometimes it is said, "She can't find the cane quickly enough, so she needs to go on without it." On a given occasion, any person may need to leave something in the interests of time and safety. A good comparison is shoes. If a student is playing a game and her shoes are far across the room, she may need to go without them on this occasion. But ordinarily the shoes will be worn. A blind student's cane is even more vital than shoes; it should ordinarily be within arm's reach and be kept as a matter of course. It is *not* comparable to the matter of leaving books, purses, and other personal items which do not relate to mobility. The cane enables the blind person to exit safely on her own. If the cane continually "cannot be found quickly" or "is out of reach," it is improperly placed.

Be sure the student has the skill and understanding to go out independently even if not with a class. (See Example 2, below.)

EXAMPLE 2: *DRILLS ANYWHERE IN THE BUILDING*
(*First grade and up*)

This instruction is important when the student has gained some independence in walking around the school.

By this time, she has experienced fire drills with her own class. She has learned to keep her cane within reach, ready for use at any time, and to use it appropriately as she walks out with the class.

Discuss how fire drills are carried out from the student's classroom(s). Then ask, "Suppose you were on an errand to the office, and the fire alarm went off. Would you go back to your room, to go out with your own class?"

Discuss the concept of "going out the nearest door." Explain that you will have some "practice fire drills." You will announce "Fire alarm!" and the student will hurry outside in a simulated drill.

Go to the office area. Note the nearest door. Announce "Fire alarm!"

When the student has proceeded outside to a reasonable distance from the building, stop for discussion. Explain that in a real drill, another teacher would have greeted and assisted the child soon. Probably that teacher would have helped her rejoin her own class for roll call.

Walk around the school and find the main exits. Discuss which rooms are near each exit. Practice going out various doors and walking to a safe distance from the school.

Walk around inside the school. At unpredictable intervals, announce "Fire alarm."

Explain that from now on during *any* lesson inside the school, you may give the imitation alarm and the student must go out. This might even occur during a Braille lesson. One never knows when an emergency will occur; this is one reason why the cane should always be kept handy.

The student should understand these principles:
- Do NOT spend time in going back to your own room or looking for your own class. Get out of the building as fast as possible.
- Often another class will immediately appear, walking out in a line. It is appropriate for you to join that line. You can follow them to the nearest exit efficiently.
- Regardless of whether another class appears, proceed immediately to the nearest exit you can find, and go out. Keep going until you are quite some distance from the building.
- If a staff member (not just your own teacher, but any staff member) tells you what to do during a drill, do what is asked.

EXAMPLE 3: *CLASS OF VERY YOUNG CHILDREN*
(*Preschool and kindergarten*)

Talk with teachers about fire drills. Discuss the child's current abilities in relation to the general principle that the cane should be used in fire drills.

The overriding consideration is safety in an emergency. Therefore, the ideal procedure may not always be possible at first. A young beginner may be so inexperienced that the cane really is more of a problem than a help in a fire drill. Also, if the cane is being used only part of the time, it may not be immediately available. Thus sometimes at this age it is best to wait awhile.

Help others *avoid* saying, "The cane would be in the way," "You don't need it for a fire drill," "The cane won't help," etc. Instead the message should be, "We will do things this way now, and later you'll learn to use the cane."

As the travel teacher, talk with the child about her understanding of drills. (Note: Be careful not to frighten a very young child who may think a real fire is expected for sure. Say, "We are very careful not to have any real fires. But we are going to *pretend* there is a fire, so we know what to do about it. This is *not* a real fire, just pretend.")

Even if the child will not yet use her cane in an actual drill, carry out a simulated drill (individually) with the cane. Explain that later it will be used independently in drills with the class.

As the child gains in skill, see that the cane is phased in for fire drills – certainly by first grade.

REMARKS: Routine fire drills are often announced ahead of time to the staff, though not to the students. You may decide to be present just before a drill. (Confer with the classroom teacher beforehand if you plan to do anything more than observe and go out with the group. Also, be prepared with a plausible explanation to students for being there, in order to avoid revealing the planned drill.) Then observe carefully (assisting, if appropriate, with a very young student.)

RELATED PRACTICE: Prepare in a comparable way for any other drills applicable to your region – tornado, earthquake, etc.

MODULE 31
DOORS AND DOORWAYS

OBJECTIVE: The student will use appropriate cane techniques to find a door or doorway and proceed through it.

AGE OF STUDENT: Preschool and up (see Examples)

PRIMARY SKILL EMPHASIS:
Doors and doorways
Posture, grip, gait, and arc
Floor plans

ADDITIONAL SKILL EMPHASIS:
General travel (indoors)
Carrying things
Air currents and echoes
In a crowd or a line
Landmarks
Structure of buildings
Right and left
Orientation overall
Corners, turns, and angles
Correcting a path

SEE ALSO (Other Modules):
Doors Closed or Open
What Is a "Room"?
Rest Rooms at School
Posture, Gait, and Arc
Description of Basic Techniques
Right and Left
Obstacles (Noting Them and Proceeding)
Carrying Things
General Overview – Buildings

FIGURE(S):
FIGURE 31-1: Using Cane to Find Door(way)
FIGURE 31-2: Vertical Cane Finds Knob

CAUTION: When standing close to a door to discuss or examine it, take care that someone on the other side does not open it quickly and hit you.

ACTIVITIES:

REMARKS: Locating doorways (as well as perpendicular sidewalks and other things to one's side) can be done by arcing the cane as usual but extending the arc a little farther to one side to contact the side of the hallway or building. The touch on the opposite side should be in the usual place. It will be necessary for the traveler to walk close to the wall and touch it with the cane tip on that side of each arc. (See Figure 31-1.) Note that when one is *not* looking for a doorway, one should *not* hug the wall.

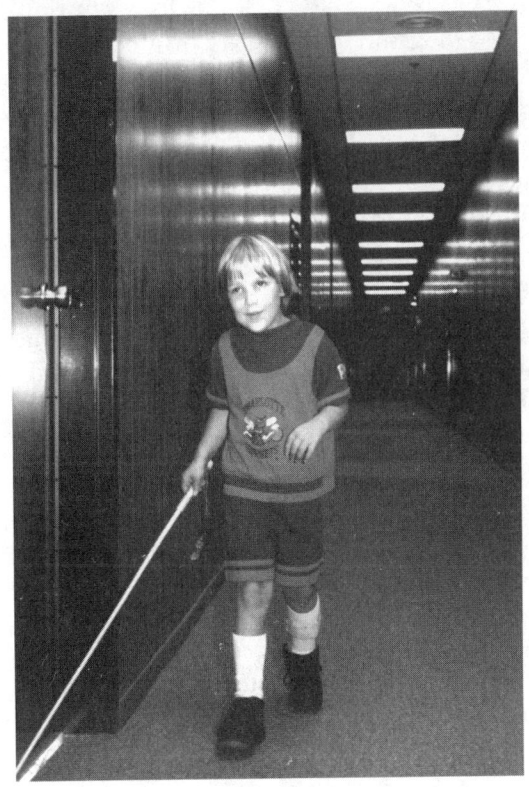

Figure 31-1
Using Cane to Find Door(way)

EXAMPLE 1: *A KINDERGARTNER WHO IS JUST BEGINNING*
"Walk straight ahead here – there's plenty of room. Show me how your cane moves.....Good! You're sweeping it from side to side, in front of one foot and then the other foot.

"We're just walking down the hall, not looking for anything at the side, and most of the time your cane won't touch the wall. We're just walking along. Go to the end of the hall, turn around, and stop...."

"Now I'd like you to practice looking at the wall with your cane. Sometimes there's a reason to do that. This time, keep close to the wall on your right. Each time your cane goes to the right, tap the bottom of the wall." [Physically assist the child as necessary, and proceed for a short way along a straight wall without any doors.]

"What is this wall made of?... How does it sound when your cane taps it?...

"Now, pretty soon your cane will find something different in the wall. Tell me when you find it." [Assist the child, if necessary, to find and recognize the door.] "This is the door to a classroom. Your cane made a different sound in tapping it, because the door is *wood*. Also, the door is set back a little ways into the wall. That's easy to find, isn't it? Now, keep going—and each time you find a door, tell me it is a door....

"Now you've found three doors by yourself—great! Turn around and look for doors on the other side of the hall. We'll count three of them. When we find the third one, we'll go in. It's the fourth grade, and they're at recess. We'll go in and look at their shell collection."

REMARKS: A very young beginner may need several sessions before she can use the cane independently to find doorways. At first you may need to move the cane for her. Soon she should be able at least to announce when the door is found, and in time she will control the cane independently.

EXAMPLE 2: *BEGINNER–UPPER ELEMENTARY SCHOOL*

Proceed essentially as for the kindergartner, but use more mature wording. The amount of practice described above is probably enough for one session for a young child, and it ends with a "fun" activity. With an older beginner, a longer practice session is appropriate. Any relaxation at the end should be age-appropriate.

An older beginner should learn to find doorways during the very first lesson(s).

EXAMPLE 3: *CONTINUED PRACTICE*

Review general principles in walking past doorways.

If one is not imminently looking for a doorway, it is usually not desirable to cane the wall with every step.

When caning the wall to look for a doorway, the cane should touch the wall (or door) each time it is tapped to that side. However, it is important to keep arcing to *both* sides because obstacles may be present.

Finding the door with the cane is better than feeling with one's hand; it gives a better appearance, and leaves one hand free to carry things.

The student should be able to follow directions to various rooms (in a familiar area or not) in terms of doorways. For example:

- "Go to Miss Johnson's room. Then go on toward the cafeteria and find the second door on your left. Tell me what room that is."
- "Walk south in the main hall. Find the second classroom past the front entrance." [The student notes that a storage-closet door "doesn't count." It is not set back into the wall as classroom doors are. Also, it is not spaced the normal distance from the next classroom.]
- "Mr. Nathan's room is the eighth door on the right after the main front entrance. Go there and find it by counting eight doors. Give Mr. Nathan this box." [Note: Frequently have the student carry a sizeable object while looking for doorways, to discourage groping with the free hand.] "Then come back and tell me what you noticed that would let you find it an easier way next time, instead of counting so many doors."

Look for ways to find a given doorway without counting a large number of doors. For Mr.

Nathan's room, above, suppose that a hallway branches off to the left, across from the fifth door; it is easily noticeable in regard to echoes and air currents. Therefore, the student needs only to count three doors after that. A comparable clue almost always can be found to prevent the necessity of counting a great many doors. Examples include changes in floor surface; bends or irregularities in the hallway; a water fountain; the odor of the physics lab; etc. Also, if the room is at the far end of the hall, it might be faster to go to the end and turn around.)

EXAMPLE 4: *MULTIPLE DOORS SIDE BY SIDE*
(*Preschool and primary grades*)

Select a location where at least two doors are side-by-side, leading to essentially the same place. The main front entrance to the school is probably an example. The cafeteria or gym may be another. Note any rules about which door to use (e.g., keep to the right).

The example below assumes that the front entry has four doors side-by-side.

"I'm going to show you something about the main front door. First I'd like you just to practice going out. Go out the main front door, go to the flagpole, and come back in."

Does the student realize that actually there are several doors side-by-side? Discuss this, along with the fact that people often say "the front door" (singular) when they actually mean the set of four doors together.

Note which door(s) the student has most often used.

Help the student start at one side and count the doors. One way to do this is to hold the cane vertically against the first door and then slide it along (still holding it vertically). It will encounter each door handle. Note that this is also one way to find the handle or knob on a single door. (See Figure 31-2.)

Prop all four doors open. The student walks past them and counts the open doors; this makes it particularly clear that there are indeed four. Examine the pillars or posts between doors.

The student starts at one side and walks in one doorway, out the next, in the next – slalom fashion. Close the doors and repeat.

Discuss why there are so many doors. (Large numbers of people go through at the same time. There may also be an element of decoration and symmetry.)

"Our school does not have a rule about which of these doors you use. But you need to know that there are more than one. If one door sticks, you can use another. Also, when you go through different doors you'll be a little bit more to the left or right when you get through. For instance, if you go in through this right-hand door, you'll be very close to the office, which is on the right as you go in. Each of the others is a little more to the left, and a little farther from the office. Now, please practice going into the office through two different doors. Start with the right-hand door. Go to the office and come back out here. Then do it again with another door. Mrs. Kohler knows you'll be doing this. She'll be happy to see you come in."

Review the concept of right and left in relation to turning around. The "far right-hand door" when you go in becomes the "far left-hand door" when you come out.

Emphasize that usually a person should *not* take time to count doors or otherwise be concerned about which of the four doors is used. But it *is* important to understand that there are (or might be) several doors side-by-side.

Note: An older student should not need detailed practice in relation to multiple doors. But she needs to understand the concept, and it is well to verify understanding occasionally. An experienced student might benefit from deliberately going through the leftmost door and walking some distance, then doing the same with the rightmost door, to examine the range of space included.

Note any special features, such as a railing between the two middle doors.

Call attention to multiple side-by-side doors in businesses, theaters, etc.

REMARKS: Consider mentioning to teachers that your student may practice finding doors without actually entering. Also, she may cane the door while going by.

If someone in a room does invite the student to enter, you or the student would shake your head or say "Thanks, we're just practicing."

FOLLOW-UP: Practice in places other than the student's own school, so that she becomes accustomed to various kinds of doors and doorways.

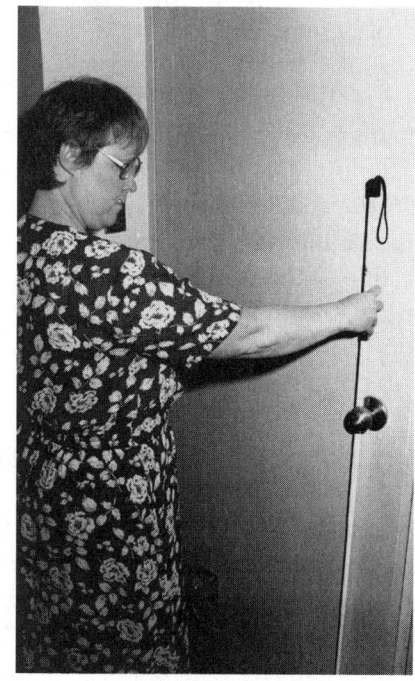

**Figure 31-2
Vertical Cane Finds Knob**

MODULE 32
DOORS CLOSED OR OPEN

OBJECTIVE: The student will use appropriate cane techniques to find a door or doorway and proceed through it.

AGE OF STUDENT: Preschool through primary grades, with review and expansion of experience thereafter

PRIMARY SKILL EMPHASIS:
Doors and doorways
Orientation overall
Obstacles in path
Posture, grip, gait, and arc

ADDITIONAL SKILL EMPHASIS:
Carrying things
Corners, turns, and angles
Emergency procedures
Floor plans
Flexibility and confidence
Landmarks
Right and left
Structure of buildings

SEE ALSO (Other Modules):
   Doors and Doorways
   What Is a "Room"?
   Carrying Things
   Rest Rooms at School
   Elevators
   Unexpected Drop-off or Step-Down
   Obstacles (Noting Them and Proceeding)
   Posture, Gait, and Arc

TEACHER PREPARATION: Carefully consider the student's level of understanding. Beyond kindergarten, a student usually will need only an admonition not to assume that a given door will always be open (or closed), and plenty of experience in various situations. On the other hand, a preschool child may need very basic practice, as described in the Example, "Basic Concept Development."

CAUTION: When standing close to a door to discuss or examine it, take care that someone on the other side does not open it quickly and hit you.

Think about where you (the teacher) will be while the student goes through a door. With a young child or in a public place, be careful that the student is not on the other side of the door when she needs help from you.

REMARKS: Avoid confusion or distraction due to two people going through at once. You might say, "Often it is polite to hold the door open for someone else. But during lessons I would like you to pretend I'm not here, so that you can practice going through doors alone. I will go through ahead, or I'll come along behind, but I'll open the door for myself."

ACTIVITIES:

EXAMPLE 1: *FIRE DOORS*
(*Primary grades and up*)

Most modern buildings (other than one-family homes) have "fire doors" in the hallways. They are normally open. With a fire alarm, however, the magnetic device holding fire doors open will release, and the doors swing shut. This blocks off a portion of the hallway to retard the spread of a possible fire.

An inexperienced blind student may not realize the doors are there, or may assume that they never close. If they do close, she may be confused.

Show the student the fire doors and discuss their function. Are there two or four doors across the width of the hallway? Are there narrow pillars between them? (Such pillars demonstrate the importance of arcing the cane correctly when walking in the hall.) Explain the magnetic device.

If possible, give the student experience with finding the fire doors closed. Go through them and be certain that the student is not disoriented. Re-emphasize that one should not assume that things will always stay in the same position.

EXAMPLE 2: *A LOCKED DOOR*
(*Elementary grades*)
(NOTE: Arrange beforehand with the principal or custodian before opening a door that is normally locked, even if you know where the key is kept. Be careful about security precautions: e.g., do not tell the student where the key is kept.)

"We say that Miss Ann's room is the second door on the right. To get there we go past Mrs. Brown's room first. But there really is another door along the way here, and we hardly ever talk about it. It's never open. Let's go look at it."

The student locates the door with her cane. She tries the knob and verifies that the door is locked.

Explain that this is the custodian's closet, and you have borrowed his key with permission to look inside. The student takes the key and unlocks the door. Examine the shelves, the cleaning supplies, and the large sink. Why is the door kept locked?

The student closes the door, locks it, and tries the knob to be sure it is locked.

Find the custodian. Return the key with thanks.

EXAMPLE 3: *DOOR WITH HAZARD*
(*Intermediate Grades and above*)
(NOTE: Some persons have advocated special doorknobs and/or special floor surfaces to indicate "danger" to blind persons. This is unnecessary and misleading. If there is true danger to everyone except trained workers (such as high voltage), the door should be locked. If the "danger" is something which a mature person can handle, such as a fire escape, the blind traveler should be assumed to be responsible for herself, just as the sighted person is. A person using a cane skillfully is in no more danger than others are. A young child – blind or sighted – should be accompanied.)

Discuss the fact that some doors have, or might have, a potentially dangerous situation behind them. Often such doors are locked, but an error could occur.

Elevator doors are a good example. Practice approaching an elevator door, entering, and going to the desired destination. A malfunction, though very unlikely, could conceivably cause a door to open when the car is slightly too high or low, or even absent. The cane should always touch the floor of the car before the person steps inside.

Go to a loading dock and walk outside. Good cane usage will find the drop-off easily. (See also the Module, "Unexpected Drop-off or Step-Down.")

Sometimes a door will have a sign, "Danger – Employees only." If there is really a severe danger (e.g., high voltage), the door should be locked. But a blind person (who would not see a sign) should always be alert to surroundings, and use the cane well.

Discuss possible situations such as:

- At the telephone company, you go through a door that you believe leads into the business office. Inside, however, there is a loud buzz of machinery and a peculiar odor. You are apprehensive that you might have entered an equipment room by mistake. You return to the hall, go to the next room, and ask directions again.
- In a hotel, you open a door which you thought would lead into a branch hallway. You feel a blast of outside air. You realize that this is the fire escape, and do not go out.
- A more complicated variation of the situation above: You start to step through the door and realize it is the outdoor fire escape. But the door suddenly blows shut and locks behind you. You knock loudly on the door, but no one rescues you. You walk gingerly down the fire escape, muttering unprintable remarks under your breath. You finally reach the sidewalk, walk around to the front door, and re-enter – thankful that the temperature is

not below freezing and you did not drop your cane. You resolve to prevent being locked out in the future.

EXAMPLE 4: *FINDING DOORWAYS*
(*Kindergarten and primary grades*)

Discuss the idea that we should not assume a given door will always be closed or always be open, despite what may be customary. Give examples.

Walk in and out of two or more classrooms. At each doorway, note whether the door was closed or open. Briefly examine the structure of the door, the threshold, the doorstop, etc.

Walk down the hallway. Stay at the side, using the cane to check for doorways. (Note: it is advisable to carry a book, briefcase, etc., in the free hand, to ensure that the cane will be relied upon. Note the importance of being able to carry something comfortably in the free hand.) At each doorway, determine with the cane whether the door is open or closed. Go into the fifth room, noting whether the door was open or closed.

EXAMPLE 5: *OUTSIDE DOORS*
(*Kindergarten and primary grades*)

Are the outside doors to the school usually closed or open? Examine an outside door – its overall structure, and how it could be propped open.

Walk in and out while the door is held open. Repeat with the door closed so the student must open it. If there are multiple doors side-by-side, note that one may be open while another is closed. The student should realize this possibility. However, it is *not* worthwhile to attempt always to find an open door if there is one. This is true even though other students may say, "Hey! This door is open!" It is usually more efficient simply to find a door, and then open it if necessary.

EXAMPLE 6: *BASIC CONCEPT DEVELOPMENT*
(*Preschool*)

A very immature child may have only a partial understanding of the concept of open vs. closed. For kindergarten age or below, it is well to emphasize the general concept with activities such as these, at least briefly. A particularly immature child may need more than one session of concept development, along with other types of practice.

Give the student a closed box. Discuss the fact that it is *closed;* then *open* it. Pass the box back and forth, taking turns opening and closing it. Provide a small toy and demonstrate: Can we place the toy inside while the box is closed? While the box is open?

Take the toy along, and in a similar manner demonstrate the open and closed states of a drawer, a cupboard, the refrigerator, etc. Notice what moves when the item is opened or closed. Especially examine the door on the cupboard, refrigerator, etc. Examine the handle, the catch, and the hinges. Discuss the similarity to a door leading into a room.

Door is closed: Go to the classroom door, which is closed. Note the sound of the cane finding the (wooden) door. Examine the door and compare it to the doors on the cupboard and the refrigerator. Note the handle or knob, the catch, and the hinges. Touch the bottom, the left side, the right side. Reach as high as possible and talk about the top.

"Can we walk through now? No, we have to *open* the door."

Open the door, walk through, and close the door again. Proceed some distance away and come back to the door. Find the door with the cane; open it; walk through to a given spot. Repeat this as many times as appropriate for the child's ability. Keep discussing whether you are in the hallway or in the classroom.

Door is open: Open the door and discuss ways to keep it standing open if desired. Is there an automatic closer which will hold the door open if we adjust it? Do we need to get a doorstop? Shall we have a classmate hold it open? With the door staying open, practice going in and out as above. The cane finds the doorway, the door standing open beside us, and other clues which tell us we are going through the doorway.

How to tell which: "Now, suppose you come to the door and you aren't sure whether it is going to be closed or open. How can you tell? Let's try it. Miss Ann will stay here, and she will open or close the door for a little game. It won't be the same every time. Now you will walk back and forth between your desk and the hallway, just as you have been doing. But this time when you get to the door, you will say whether it is closed or open. If it's open, you say 'open,' and just go on through. If it's closed, you say 'closed,' and then you open it and go through. When you have done that six times we will be finished and you may pick out a scented sticker for your chart."

(Note: If Miss Ann is silent whenever she does not change the position of the door, the child can easily hear whether the position is being changed. Miss Ann should–in the tradition of other games–ostentatiously make sounds with the door *every* time, to camouflage what is actually being done.)

Note: Ordinarily, a student beyond the preschool level should not need help with the actual concept of open vs. closed. However, the activities in this Example can make practice enjoyable for students in the early grades.

MODULE 33
LUNCHTIME

Note: This Module emphasizes obtaining a lunch, eating, and clearing up. The Module, "Lunchroom and Kitchen," discusses touring the lunchroom and kitchen, and learning to find one's way around.

OBJECTIVE: The student will bring or select his/her lunch, eat, and clear up, with only minimal (if any) assistance.

AGE OF STUDENT: First grade and up (Also preschool/kindergarten, where applicable, with more assistance as appropriate for age)

PRIMARY SKILL EMPHASIS:
Orientation within a room
Carrying things
Obstacles in path
Finding a seat
Stowing cane
Correcting a path
Floor plans
In a crowd or a line
Purchase or transaction

ADDITIONAL SKILL EMPHASIS:
Finding a person
Corners, turns, and angles
Flexibility and confidence
Interpreting odors
Sound direction and meaning
Human guide
Daily living skills
Responsibility and citizenship
Etiquette

SEE ALSO (Other Modules):
    Lunchroom and Kitchen (Overall Layout
       and Procedures)
    Errands
    Restaurant
    Walking in a Line of People
    Human Guide
    Carrying Things
    In a Crowd
    Obstacles: Noting Them and Proceeding
    What Is a "Room"?
    Walking Across Open Space

TEACHER PREPARATION: If possible, observe an actual lunchtime before instructing your student. Seemingly minor details become important when large numbers of people are hurrying to eat in a short time. Also, the words or signals which determine food choices, and which control seating and behavior, may seem obscure. Ask an experienced staff member to walk through with you and explain. When a student will be eating in a different lunchroom the next term, practice beforehand if at all possible. For example, practice with a kindergartner in the spring before first grade. If a class of young children goes in a group to eat a sample meal during the previous term, the blind student should have individual practice in addition.

ACTIVITIES:

EXAMPLE 1: *GENERAL TOUR*
If possible, examine the lunchroom before the school term begins. The kindergartner who will eat hot lunch in first grade, and the fifth grader who will be at the Middle School next year, should tour the new lunchroom in the spring. For a new student who moves in, include the lunchroom in the overall tour of the school.

EXAMPLE 2: *TICKETS AND LUNCH COUNT*
The Module, "Errands," provides detailed suggestions about errands around the building, such as buying a lunch ticket.

In many schools, students wishing to eat hot lunch must buy tickets ahead of time. Also, a "lunch count" is typically taken early each morning—perhaps with choices among "hot lunch," "salad bar," "milk only" (with one's own sack lunch), etc.

Taking the count to the office from each classroom may constitute another errand.

A menu is available—usually posted on the wall and also read over the public address system.

EXAMPLE 3: *GETTING UTENSILS AND FOOD*

Your student should learn exactly where to find items he should pick up by himself—typically napkin, straw, and silverware. (Note that for economic and/or behavior control reasons, many school lunchrooms serve the most minimal of utensils. For example, there may be only spoons or only forks. There may be no straws.) Teach the student to get his utensils with the least possible fingering of other utensils.

With a conventional cafeteria line, the staff behind the counter can easily describe the food, and explain the choices (if any). A blind student (presumably knowing the menu ahead of time anyway) normally will not need an extra person to help him through a familiar line. If others gain information visually (e.g., reaching for peaches vs. pineapple), he can simply ask someone behind the counter, or another student in the line.

More and more schools offer a self-service salad buffet with many ingredients and many choices. More assistance may be needed here. However, familiarity with a particular setup often enables the student to help himself while asking only a few questions.

Carrying a tray requires practice and planning. Practice carrying the particular trays used—perhaps at first empty, then variously loaded. Experiment with different positions, including bracing the tray against the body. Often the cane can be used fairly normally, either in a completely free hand or using a few fingers.

A "full load" varies according to circumstances. Some schools use flimsy paper plates and no actual tray; others use solid plastic tray/plates that hold everything firmly. Some often have soup, others never. Distance and route from serving window varies.

Help your student plan independence without unreasonable balancing acts. A tray without soup, carried for a moderate distance by an experienced student, usually does not require help. If a flimsy tray with a bowl of soup must be carried across a large and crowded room, it is probably reasonable to ask for help. But neither of these situations require help during the entire lunch period. Occasional minimal assistance is reasonable as needed; constant help is not.

EXAMPLE 4: *FINDING A SEAT*

Younger students often enter in a line by classes, accompanied by a teacher. Often they proceed together all the way to a table, sitting in a prearranged pattern. The blind student can follow the group. Teachers and other students should give verbal direction as needed.

Older students typically go as individuals and select their own seats. Often a blind student will go with a friend (as do many sighted students), and assistance is readily available if needed. But an individual blind student, in a complex and busy lunchroom, may find it hard to find a desirable seat. It will not be the same from day to day, because students sit in varying places.

Ask advice from the counselor when your student is starting out in a new, large lunchroom. Probably at first it will be best to go to lunch with a classmate—a friendly student recruited by the counselor if the blind student is not well acquainted. Help your student work out his own arrangements as time goes on. Avoid the extremes of (1) constant attention by people who assume that no independence is possible, and (2) a lonely, nervous student who dreads lunch hour.

Justin, in seventh grade, continually sat with a clique of girls who ignored him. He always went to the nearest table, and he had no idea where to find anyone more friendly—not even a group of boys among whom he would be inconspicuous. Don't let this happen to your student.

EXAMPLE 5: *WHERE TO PUT THE CANE*

Two principles will settle most questions about where to put the cane while eating lunch: "Use it as much as possible, even if in a non-standard way"; and "Keep it with you at all times."

As described above, often a person carrying a loaded tray can use his cane, at least partially. Even if he cannot actually use it, he can carry the cane prominently along with the tray. This accomplishes three important things: (a) the cane is in his hand and ready whenever it can be actually used; (b) the cane lets others know that the student is blind, so that they are less likely to zip across his path and expect him to see them; (c) the cane comes along to be placed under the seat and remain with the student.

When the student is seated, usually the best place for the cane is under the table. It is, however, necessary to keep it out of busy aisles. This is very easy with long benches at picnic-style tables. With smaller tables, it may require more thought, but is not difficult. Help your student analyze the traffic patterns and the shape of the tables, and to ask other students whether the cane is sticking out.

If the student happens to sit next to a wall, there is no innate harm in standing the cane against the wall. I discourage this, however, because people will tend to assume it is the *only* good arrangement. (They erroneously conclude that the student *must* sit by a wall or corner, or that the cane must be placed some distance from him.) The floor, on the other hand, is always available.

Other Modules have further suggestions about stowing the cane—notably "School Bus" and "Orientation Inside New Classroom." This is a very simple matter which, unfortunately, can cause quite a fuss if not anticipated.

EXAMPLE 6: *EATING SKILLS*
Methods for eating, along with other skills of daily living, are beyond the scope of this book. Orientation and mobility in the lunchroom, however, naturally brings up the subject.

Use this opportunity to note whether skills are age-appropriate. Work on any weaknesses (preferably in private) if it is within the scope of your job. Otherwise, discreetly pass on information to parents and other teachers who can work on it.

EXAMPLE 7: *AFTER LUNCH*
Typically, students deposit trash in containers; scrape garbage from hot-lunch trays or plates; deposit trays or plates to be washed; and exit the lunchroom—all according to a specific, ordered path and sequence.

Head off the incorrect assumption that the blind student will need constant help, and/or will not accomplish everything (cannot scrape garbage off his plate, for example). Again, if there are weaknesses in daily living skills, see that instruction is provided.

Go to the lunchroom when a crowd is not present, for practice without embarrassment or pressure. But it is also important to assist or watch during an actual busy, crowded lunchtime. Look for hints to give your student—e.g., there are extra trash barrels by the vending machines.

Carrying a tray after lunch is usually much easier than beforehand, but may still require planning. Any remaining food or drink may spill easily. A formerly closed container may now be open and messy (e.g., half-eaten applesauce from a sack lunch). A small plastic bag in the lunchbox, pocket, or purse can prevent a messy balancing act.

REFERENCE(S):
Willoughby and Duffy. *Handbook for Itinerant and Resource Teachers of Blind and Visually Impaired Students*, pp. 285-296.

RELATED PRACTICE:
Daily living skills

MODULE 34
LUNCHROOM AND KITCHEN
Overall Layout and Procedures

Note: This Module discusses touring the lunchroom and kitchen, and learning to find one's way around. The Module, "Lunchtime," discusses actually obtaining and eating a lunch.

OBJECTIVE: The student will bring or select his/her lunch, eat, and clear up, with only minimal (if any) assistance.

AGE OF STUDENT: Preschool through primary grades

PRIMARY SKILL EMPHASIS:
General travel (indoors)
Stowing cane
Finding a seat
Carrying things
Examining things tactually
Orientation within a room
In a crowd or a line
Landmarks
Obstacles in path
Purchase or transaction

ADDITIONAL SKILL EMPHASIS:
Doors and doorways
Daily living skills
Etiquette
Sound direction and meaning
Finding a person
Interpreting odors
Open space

SEE ALSO (Other Modules):
>Lunchtime
>Fire Drills
>Errands
>In a Crowd
>Restaurant
>Routes for New Classroom
>What Is a "Room"?
>Obstacles: Noting Them and Proceeding
>Walking Across Open Space

TEACHER PREPARATION: Look around the kitchen and lunchroom to note points of interest and possible hazards. Arrange for a kitchen tour at a time convenient for the staff.

REMARKS: Classes of young children often tour the kitchen, but usually only once. During the rushed lunch hour, there is little chance for exploration.

Sighted students of all ages see beyond the counter into the work area. But if appropriate opportunities are not arranged, the blind student may have little understanding of kitchen procedures and layout. This Module promotes understanding of the environment, with varied practice in use of the cane.

STUDENT BACKGROUND: Discuss what has already been learned about food preparation and school lunches.

ACTIVITIES:

EXAMPLE 1: *LUNCHROOM TOUR*
The student learns (or reviews) walking independently to the lunchroom. Example: Turn right when going out the classroom door. Walk briskly, not caning the wall, until sound and air currents tell you that you have entered the large open lobby. Turn right and proceed down that hallway. Cane the right-hand wall as necessary to find the lunchroom doors.

Smell the food cooking (or note lingering scents after lunch).

Enter the lunchroom when other students are not eating. Independently find a table and take a seat. (If the class always sits at the same table, practice going and coming from that one. But also practice going and coming from at least one other table.) Practice leaving the lunchroom from at least two different tables. Practice going directly to the door, and also via the dirty-plate discard area.

Go to the kitchen door or window and greet the cooks. Anticipate (or recall) the kitchen tour.

Walk independently around the perimeter of the lunchroom. Name each door or other feature, with help as necessary. Examples: kitchen doors; window for serving; window for dirty trays; storage closet; hallway doors; stage; fire exit; cooks' office; teachers' lunchroom.

If tables fold up when not in use, ask the custodian to demonstrate, with the student touching the tables enough to understand the procedure.

CAUTION: Do not attempt to fold or unfold large tables without the custodian's help. Large, folding tables may move or pinch in unexpected ways. This is especially true with tables which fold up into the wall or closet.

EXAMPLE 2: *KITCHEN TOUR*

The student walks to the lunchroom independently with her cane. She goes to the kitchen door, introduces herself and the teacher, and asks for a tour.

Smell the food cooking, or note lingering odors after lunch.

Use the cane as much as practical when walking around in the kitchen; however, it may be laid on the floor or placed against the wall when the hands are continually examining various items.

Help the child examine meaningfully such things as those listed below. Discuss size in comparison with home equipment. If certain things are unsafe to touch, explain why.

- Oven: How many shelves? Reach in to feel depth and width. Feel the shelves. How many ovens are there?
- Stove top: How many burners? Gas or electricity?
- Sinks: Note the size. Examine the garbage disposal, sprays, etc.
- Storage cabinets
- Refrigerators and coolers
- Electric mixers, blenders
- Large mixing bowls, measuring cups, and other containers
- Look at some containers of packaged or canned food.
- Large spoons and other utensils
- Examine the serving line from behind the counter. Are there steam tables?
- How are lunch tickets processed?
- Examine the trash can while it is clean.
- Trace the path that dirty trays or plates follow for washing.
- Dishwasher

FOLLOW-UP: Send a thank-you note to the lunchroom staff. A young child may dictate for the teacher to write in Braille; a somewhat older student writes her own letter in Braille. (The teacher provides a version in inkprint for the reader.) An older student may type the note.

At home, the student examines equivalent utensils and equipment and thinks about size comparison.

MODULE 35
WALKING IN A LINE OF PEOPLE

OBJECTIVE: In a waiting line (such as for buying tickets), the student will move along appropriately from the end of the line until reaching the front, without touching people with his/her hands.

OBJECTIVE: When his/her class is walking single file, the student will walk along without assistance, at any given point in the line.

AGE OF STUDENT: Preschool and up
(Note supplementary suggestions for youngest students)

PRIMARY SKILL EMPHASIS:
In a crowd or a line
Sound direction and meaning
Finding a person
Etiquette
Meeting the public
Purchase or transaction

ADDITIONAL SKILL EMPHASIS:
Communication and instructions
Attitudes toward blindness
Carrying things
Daily living skills
Flexibility and confidence
Responsibility and citizenship
Human guide
Stowing cane

SEE ALSO (Other Modules):
  In a Crowd
  Lunchtime
  Fire Drills
  Errands
  Walking Independently While Following Someone
  The Airport

FIGURE(S):
FIGURE 35-1: Pencil Grip

FIGURE 35-2: Slow-Moving Line

ACTIVITIES: *SLOW-MOVING LINES*

EXAMPLE 1: *MOVING ALONG WITH THE LINE*
Introduce or review the shortened-up ("pencil grip") position for use in crowds. (See also the Module, "In a Crowd.")

The tip of the cane should be only about one step in front (or even less, in a very slow-moving line). The grip is modified (see Figure 35-1), and may be below the handle. The arc is not generous.

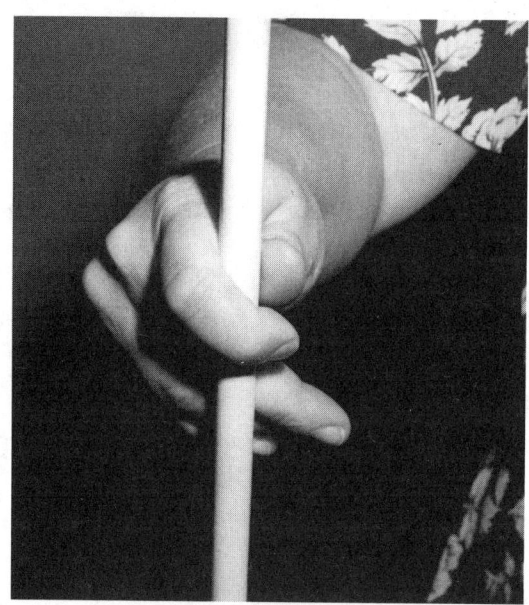

**Figure 35-1
Pencil Grip**

Discuss examples of slow-moving lines. Most typical in the school setting are lines for drinking fountains, lunch tickets, and lunch service. Such a line ordinarily moves so slowly that regular rhythmic arcing is not appropriate. Instead, the student should hold her cane nearly vertical, with the tip gently touching the heels of the person ahead from time to time.

Seek out such lines and ask the student to join them. (If the currently available line is not for something actually desired, the student may complete an errand for someone else, take a nominal drink, etc.)

EMPHASIZE THAT THE HANDS ARE NOT TO BE USED FOR POSITIONING ONESELF IN LINE. Position and motion can be judged by use of the cane (as above), by listening, and by conversation.

With a beginner, sometimes the teacher should proceed alongside her as she moves up the line. The teacher may physically help the student move the cane appropriately and stay behind the same person. The teacher may also call attention to sound clues.

Most commonly, a line proceeds on a level surface. Sometimes, however, it snakes up or down a stairway, over a curb, etc. Although regular, rhythmic arcing is not normally used in a slow-moving line, judicious continual use of the cane prevents unfortunate stumbles.

See Figure 35-2.

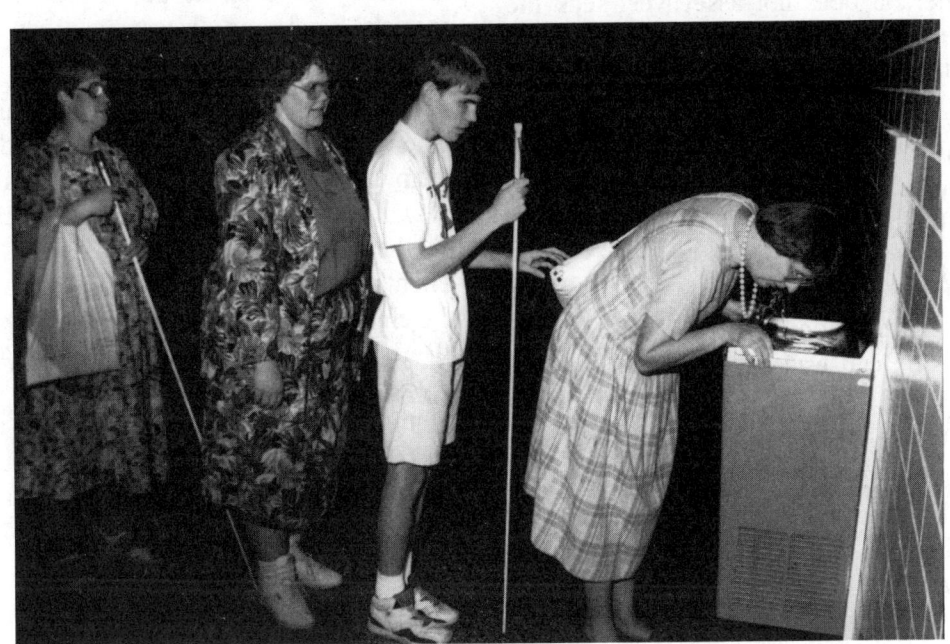

**Figure 35-2
Slow-Moving Line**

EXAMPLE 2: *REACHING THE FRONT*
Help your student be alert to approaching the front of the line.

With a drinking fountain, the water may be heard (though not always, in a noisy environment); the front person will stop talking and bend over to drink. In a ticket line, the clerk's voice becomes closer and closer.

When the front of the line is actually reached, use of the hands often is appropriate. The student will reach for the fountain, touch the ticket counter, pick up a lunch tray, etc. Again, however, the cane should help determine that the front actually has been reached. The cane tip should touch the wall or counter ahead. The handle may touch the fountain or the counter.

Especially with younger students, it may be wise to remind staff to speak to the blind student by name. Beyond the earliest grades, however, the student herself should assertively determine when she is being spoken to. If a clerk says, "OK, next," or "What can I do for you?" the student can ask "Am I next?" or "Did you mean me?"

Demonstrate options for using or stowing the cane at the front of the line. For example:

- Place it on the floor. This could be crossways in front (along the wall or counter), or parallel to the line.
- Hold it loosely in the crook of one arm
- Simply pause while holding the cane normally (if both hands are not needed for the task in question)
- Change to a different position or procedure with the cane. For example, "Lunchtime" gives suggestions for carrying a tray and a cane together.

EXAMPLE 3: *WHERE IS THE END OF THE LINE?*

If a blind person does not assertively seek the end when entering a line, misguided "courtesy" often will place her near the front.

When a high school student approaches a familiar lunch line, she knows how it is structured (e.g., the end is somewhere in front of the north lockers, with students proceeding past the ticket window and through the double doors). The voices of students in line can be heard. The student can go to the appropriate area and listen attentively. She can walk along beside the line toward the rear, with the cane tip sometimes gently touching other students' feet.

However, especially in an unfamiliar or irregular line, it can be hard to discern where the end is. Simply asking, "Is the end that way?" (while pointing) and/or "Is this the end here?" may suffice. However, misplaced courtesy still may cause someone (especially an adult) to say "right here" and usher the blind person into the middle of the line. Especially in public, some creativity is advisable.

My husband (who is blind) says, "I want to get them to give me the information I need, instead of their telling me just what they want to tell me. If I can get the information I want, then *I* can make the decision as to where I should be; otherwise, I am compelled to accept the decision they make *for* me.

"I try to get them to focus on giving me information, rather than on trying to get me to do what they have decided I should do. I may accomplish this by asking, 'Are you the last person in line?' I then make sure I get *behind* the person I am talking with; and if he is not the last one, I proceed toward the end of the line."

EXAMPLE 4: *SUPPLEMENTARY SUGGESTIONS FOR YOUNG BEGINNERS (Age 8 and under)*

A student over 8 – even a beginner in terms of techniques – understands the concept of a single-file line. A very young child, however (or an older student with special problems), may need instruction in the concept itself.

Place several stuffed animals, dolls, etc., in a line on the floor. Help the student position herself at the end, and then at the front. Examine the animals' heads and discuss how they all face the front.

When a very young child is first learning, tell the other children that the student needs to touch them today. Walk with the student along a line of waiting children, and help her touch each one on the arm (with her hand) as she passes by. Then position her in the line. Help her touch the child ahead (with her hands) as you explain, "Beth has her back to you. She's *in front* of you in the line." (NOTE: This activity should *not* include feeling faces or examining the other child's whole body.) Help the student turn around and touch the child behind her, with similar explanation.

After organized practice with the concept of a single-file line, the child should learn to use the cane for positioning.

A child's age should not become an excuse for continual touching of others' bodies. Even three-year-olds are ordinarily admonished, "Keep your hands to yourself!" It should be the same for a blind child. At age 3 or 4 we *tolerate* more touching of other people (along with more noise, silly behavior, whining, etc.) than we would with an older child. But we continue to shape behavior toward greater maturity.

ACTIVITIES: *FAST-MOVING LINES*

EXAMPLE 5: *GENERAL TECHNIQUES*

Many aspects of walking in a brisk line are similar to waiting in a slow-moving one. However, additional techniques and understanding are needed.

A "pencil grip" for the cane is called for, as above. (See also "In a Crowd.") The cane should be near-vertical or somewhat extended, depending on circumstances. If it were extended far out, in normal position for fast walking, it would tend to trip others and require too much space.

The student must listen in an alert manner to recognize how fast the line is moving. Speed may increase or decrease, or the line may stop suddenly.

Remind your student that gentle, controlled arcing of the cane is important for the comfort of the person ahead. "He doesn't want you *whacking* his heels," you might say with some humor. Occasionally ask other students for feedback on appropriateness and comfort. Gentle tapping is a necessary accommodation and should be accepted by classmates; but hard "whacks" are an uncomfortable imposition. Continually remind students that touching others with the hands is neither appropriate nor necessary.

EXAMPLE 6: *SUPPLEMENTARY SUGGESTIONS*
(Age 8 and under)

A child under 8 may take quite awhile to master the skill of walking in a line. For awhile, at least, it may be necessary for her to take another child's arm and walk beside him even though the rest of the line is single file.

Keep working toward the point where the child can walk alone in line, however. If she cannot yet do so all the time, probably she can sometimes. Seek out opportunities such as:

- Proceeding single file in a waiting line which is moving very slowly.
- Walking single file when the class is moving rather slowly, but taking someone's arm when they move briskly.
- Walking first in line, receiving extra help from the classroom teacher
- Receiving some guidance from the child behind
- Walking single file for short, familiar distances, but taking someone's arm for longer distances
- Walking at the end, where the student can continually correct possible wavering without needing to consider students behind

EXAMPLE 7: *ANY POSITION IN THE LINE*

As mentioned in suggestions for younger children, a beginner may find the front of the line an easy position to manage. The others are following behind *her*, and she can easily receive help from the adult leader.

The very end of the line has advantages also. There is no one behind to be bothered if the blind child wavers or lags. Following others is especially easy when the whole group is ahead.

Such simplifications should be for beginners only, however – and even then not all the time. Being first in line may be a privilege coveted by others. Remaining always in any particular position implies lack of competence and is very restrictive. Ordinarily, an experienced blind student should be able to go along in any position in line. Also, she should not depend on a particular friend walking behind or in front of her.

An exception does occur if the area is particularly confusing or noisy. (Example: The sixth-graders are touring a place of business. There are many people around, and it is hard to sort out voices.) When appropriate, the blind student should take someone's arm or otherwise receive extra guidance for a limited time. (See also "Human Guide.")

EXAMPLE 8: *STOP-AND-GO*

A moving line may suddenly stop, or slow down greatly. Careful use of the cane and alert listening allow the student to manage this.

Sometimes a class lines up, waits, and then proceeds on a signal. This is especially common in elementary school. For example, after recess the class might line up at the door, then proceed inside when the playground aide waves them on.

This is a very simple situation which even a young child can quickly learn to handle. But it is necessary to practice the skill of using the cane to notice movement of the feet of the child ahead, and to practice listening to voices and footsteps.

Often the signal is an audible whistle, bell, or spoken command. If the customary signal is visual, the specialized teacher may want to ask that sound be included. For example, the playground aide might say, "Go ahead, First Grade," as she waves them on in.

EXAMPLE 9: *NOT ALWAYS SINGLE FILE*

Sometimes a line reaches a certain point and then dissolves, rather than proceeding farther as a controlled line. On the way out to recess, for example, students typically go wherever they please after their class leaves the building.

Another variation is a "line" which is imprecise and not single file. A group waiting for a public bus is a good example.

FOLLOW-UP: As your student progresses, seek out additional opportunities and variations. Examples typically found at school include:

- Entering or leaving the school building
- Water fountains
- Proceeding together as a class to a different room (e.g., the second grade going to gym)
- Lunch tickets
- Lunch service
- Tickets or sign-up for school play, ball games, special activities, etc.
- Waiting by the teacher's desk (students wishing to ask a question during a study period)
- Library checkout
- Proceeding to or from recess
- Waiting for the school bus

Following are typical examples away from school:

- Tickets
- Waiting for a public bus or other transit
- Rest rooms (a line outside or inside the rest room)
- Vending machines
- Checkout/service counter in a place of business
- Waiting for a door to open (e.g., at a popular business just before it opens)
- Entering a theater

MODULE 36
ERRANDS

OBJECTIVE: The student will independently complete age-appropriate errands to the office and other locations where classmates routinely go – at least one errand per week, with the destination not always the same.

AGE OF STUDENT:
Independent errands: Kindergarten and up.
Readiness activities: Preschool.

PRIMARY SKILL EMPHASIS:
Carrying things
Communication and instructions
Finding a person
General travel (indoors)
In a crowd or a line
Landmarks
Purchase or transaction
Orientation overall

ADDITIONAL SKILL EMPHASIS:
Doors and doorways
Daily living skills
Etiquette
Examining things tactually
Orientation within a room
Responsibility and citizenship

SEE ALSO (Other Modules):
> Alternate Routes Within a Building
> Asking Directions And Figuring It Out
> PUBLIC BUILDINGS (SPECIFIC EXAMPLES) Modules
> Carrying Things
> Doors and Doorways
> Fire Drills
> Walking in a Line of People
> Routes for New Classroom
> In a Crowd

TEACHER PREPARATION: Explain to school staff members, as necessary, that the student will be learning to run errands. Check on staff responsibilities and schedules, and avoid "practice" errands at inconvenient times. Ask classroom teachers to tell you about errands students routinely do, and others that might occur occasionally.

Find out where the pickup/delivery points are for the U.S. mail, interschool mail, teachers' mailboxes, and any other relevant services such as films. Consider placing tactual labels in selected places. With a young or immature child, see that there is something in his teacher's box, so that he may deliver it. ("Plant" something yourself if necessary.)

If mailboxes are in a restricted area where students do not ordinarily go, be careful. If students commonly knock on the door and hand something in, teach your student to do this. If students never go there, take a student in only to teach an important concept, and only with the agreement of persons inside. (Staff do not like to be observed by students when they take off their shoes, tell adult jokes, or otherwise "let down their hair" in the lounge.)

See the "Caution," below, about the controls of the public address system.

ACTIVITIES:

EXAMPLE 1: *GENERAL ERRANDS AT SCHOOL*

Typical examples of errands include:
- Buy lunch ticket (for self or a teacher)
- Take lunch-count list to office or lunchroom.
- Get mail from teacher's mailbox.
- Pick up or return a film.
- Deliver object or message to office.
- Deliver object or message to lunchroom, custodian, etc.
- Deliver object or message to another classroom.
- Go to playground or rest room and look for classmate who may be dawdling.
- Return books to Media Center

Help the student practice each type of errand, beginning with those most commonly done and/or the easiest. Try to have the student actually deliver an object or message while practicing. A very young child might enjoy simply *showing* a favorite toy to the secretary when he has learned to find the office.

Buying a lunch ticket is especially valuable practice. If the student brings his lunch or eats at home, he might get the teacher's ticket.

Your student should know what to do if no one seems to be present at the destination.

- Listen to determine whether someone is there but busy. In that case, wait silently for your turn.
- If no one responds after a reasonable time, say the person's name aloud in a questioning tone – e.g., "Mr. Smith?" or "Is anyone here?"
- If there still is no response, leave the item in a conspicuous place or take it back to the sender, as directed.

EXAMPLE 2: *MAIL AND MESSAGES AT SCHOOL*

REMARKS: The number of lessons and amount of time spent is extremely variable according to circumstances.

If the child is young and/or the route is particularly valuable practice, many lessons and much time might be devoted. Delivery errands are enjoyable, with high prestige, and thus provide excellent motivation and variety.

For an older student, one quick lesson may suffice. Also, different levels of knowledge are appropriate for different ages.

Concept development: Discuss the general concept of delivery of packages and written messages. Discuss the U.S. mail, the interschool mail, and any other relevant services.

Teachers' mailboxes: Accompany the student to the teachers' mailboxes. Note the location of the student's own classroom teacher's box. Is there anything in it? Can we deliver it?

Note how this particular mailbox can be distinguished from the others. (Count over from the end, find the Braille label, etc.)

Deliver the mail to the classroom teacher.

Films, etc.: Go to the pickup point for each of the other services (e.g., films). Discuss what kinds of deliveries are made. How is the pickup point identified? (Tub, table, sign, etc.)

Integration: Practice going to and from each delivery point. As appropriate, count doorways, note landmarks, ask permission from the librarian, etc. Complete an errand with guidance.

Regular, independent errands: When the student is able to complete errands independently, provide practice and inform the classroom teacher. See that the student takes a turn at typical errands.

RELATED PRACTICE: Correspond with a "pen pal" in another school. Send letters through the school mail or U.S. mail. A very young child might dictate a letter to be Brailled and sent with tactual art work.

EXAMPLE 3: *PUBLIC ADDRESS SYSTEM*

REMARKS: This activity is exciting and motivating for younger children. Also, it helps the child to understand the environment in general and hence to improve overall travel skills.

Always arrange this activity by talking with the appropriate staff member(s) *before* telling the student about it. See also Caution, below.

CAUTION: The controls for the public address system are delicate and ordinarily off-limits to students. With an immature child, it may be unwise to allow him to touch the controls at all, or even to get near them. He might merely speak into the microphone, or even just stand by while someone else talks.

In the classroom: Listen to announcements in the classroom. Learn where the classroom loudspeaker is; examine it if possible.

Where does it come from? At a time which the teacher has arranged, walk independently to the office. Find the doorway with the cane and walk in. Ask the secretary if we may use the P.A. system.

Follow the secretary to the P.A. control area. Set the cane down and examine the switches and microphone. Are there separate switches for each room and for All Call?

Hold the microphone and speak to the classroom. A very young child might simply say, "Hello, this is Marc." An older student might give an actual announcement.

If reverse communication is possible, listen to the classroom for a reply.

Thank the secretary. Walk back to the classroom independently.

FOLLOW-UP: Keep teachers informed as the student learns skills. Ask them to make a point of sending the blind child on his share of errands. With proper training, the blind student should have the same duties as others.

Over time, be sure that errand-running is maintained. Each year, check that the student continues to run errands as others do (not accompanied by another student).

MODULE 37
ALTERNATE ROUTES
WITHIN A BUILDING

OBJECTIVE: The student will walk between two given points by two different routes (which are not necessarily equivalent in length). He/she will discuss the overall layout and the concept of alternate routes.

AGE OF STUDENT: See Examples

PRIMARY SKILL EMPHASIS:
Orientation overall
Compass directions
Right and left
Floor plans
Flexibility and confidence
General travel (indoors)

ADDITIONAL SKILL EMPHASIS:
Doors and doorways
Corners, turns, and angles
Emergency procedures
Orientation within a room
Parallel and perpendicular
Correcting a path
Structure of buildings

SEE ALSO (Other Modules):
Routes for New Classroom (Early Elementary Grades)
Routes for New Buildings and New Classrooms (Upper Grades Through High School)
Fire Drills
Outside and Inside the School
General Overview – Buildings

FIGURE(S):
FIGURE 37-1: School Office Complex
FIGURE 37-2: An Unusual Connection
FIGURE 37-3: Parallel Hallways

TEACHER PREPARATION: Look around the school for places where alternate routes to a given destination are possible. (One route will usually be longer, but the concept is important.) If nothing else, note where a person could go outdoors and then come back in another door to reach the destination.

Look for connections directly between rooms, as well as connecting hallways. Note paths that are not ordinarily used by children, or may not be within the experience of the blind student. (Ask permission if you consider opening something which is normally closed, or taking a student into an ordinarily forbidden area.)

STUDENT BACKGROUND: Most of these examples assume that the student is already familiar with the usual routes.

However, when an experienced student is becoming acquainted with a new building, he should analyze patterns immediately (numbering systems, stairwells, hallway connections, etc.)

ACTIVITIES:

EXAMPLE 1: *INTRODUCTION AND DISCUSSION*
Walk to a chosen destination and back, by the usual route.

In a manner appropriate for the student's age, discuss why a person might want to use a different route – obstructions, crowding, repair work, desire for variety, a complex errand, etc.

Can the student think of an alternate route in this instance? If so, proceed with it even if it is not very efficient. Compliment the student for thinking of it. Then, if there is a more efficient alternative, practice it also.

Discuss whether the alternative routes are ordinarily permitted for students. (It can be helpful for the student to go with the teacher into an area usually "off-limits" for students, as an aid in understanding the layout.)

Include practice with landmarks, counting doorways, noting terrain, etc. How are you certain that you really did arrive at the chosen location?

This work is especially important in a large school where, for example, two long parallel halls are connected at intervals by short connecting halls. The student needs to grasp the overall picture.

Analyze the pattern of room numbers. In a multi-story school, the first digit usually reflects the floor number. In a one-story school, often various wings or areas will have distinctive first digits. At the very least, the numbers increase in a certain direction.

EXAMPLE 2: *OFFICE COMPLEX*
(*Preschool and primary grades*)
(Figure 37-1)

This Figure shows a typical administrative office complex. Students ordinarily enter the main office through either of two doors from Hallway A, which runs north and south along the west side. They buy lunch tickets and conduct other business at a long counter, rather than walking through this large open area among the staff members' desks. Certain other rooms open off this area; however, students are expected to enter those rooms from another hallway.

South of the open area is the principal's inner office. It also has a door to Hallway C, which runs east and west along the south side of the complex.

On the east side of the complex are four small rooms. From north to south they are: nurse's room, counselor's office, teachers' workroom, conference room. The first three are accessible both from the open area and from Hallway B, which runs north and south along the east side of the complex.

The conference room, in the southeast corner, is accessible only through the principal's office, the workroom, and Hallway C.

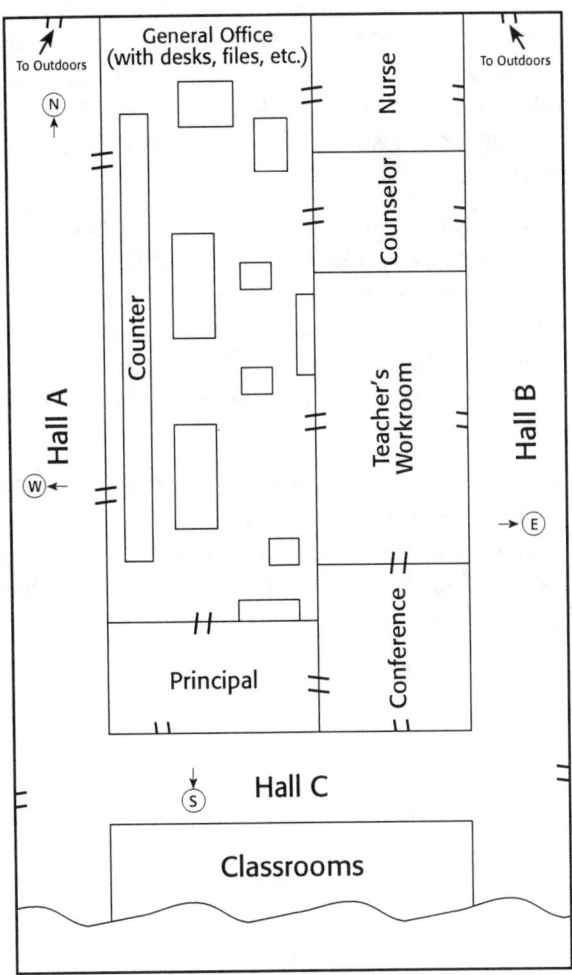

Figure 37-1
School Office Complex

Exploring

Consider the nurse's room. It is accessible from the large open area of the office complex, and also from Hallway B. Children ordinarily enter only from Hallway B. But sighted children, when at the counter in the general office, see through and know about the inner connection.

Have the student go to the nurse's room in the usual manner (via Hallway B). Greet the health aide. Then (without explaining the inner connection) ask the student to go to the office and greet the secretary.

When the student is at the counter in the office, confirm that he arrived correctly by the conventional route (out the east door of the nurse's room, south in Hallway B, West in Hall C, north in Hall A, and through the west doors of the open area). Then announce, "There is a shorter way between here and the nurse's room. You didn't use it because students don't go that way without permission. Do you know what the short way is?"

If the child cannot explain, ask, "Forget about walls for a minute. Imagine you could go through walls magically. Point toward the nurse's room." Orient the student if necessary. When the direction is understood, explain that there is a connecting door and it will be explored today.

Explain that today there is permission to go through the open area and explore. Help the student go in the correct direction, looking for a door. When he arrives, he verifies that he has indeed found the nurse's office.

Discuss how a blind person can learn of such connections:

> When you are in the nurse's room, often you can hear the secretary talking or hear office machines running.
> Understand the overall floor plan and realize what rooms are back-to-back. Recognize that rooms sometimes have connecting doors.
> If a blind person is a staff member, he would walk around in the office area without special permission, and use such connections routinely.

In a similar manner, examine the alternative entrances to the counselor's office, workroom, conference room, and principal's inner office.

Study a simple tactual map of the entire complex.

Note another alternative route between the nurse's room and the general office. A person could go outdoors at the north end of Hallway B, and then come back in at the north end of Hall A.

EXAMPLE 3: *AN UNUSUAL CONNECTION*
(*Preschool and up*)
(Figure 37-2)

At the north end of the main hallway are a few steps leading down to the gym entrance. Just before the gym entrance, a small hallway branches off to the east; on its north side are doors to the Instrumental Music room. This room, however, is actually part of the stage for the gym (which doubles as an auditorium).

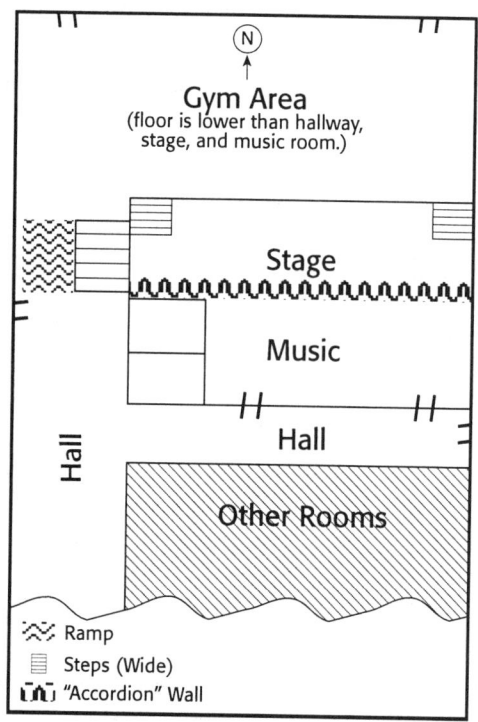

**Figure 37-2
An Unusual Connection**

How Does This Connect?
The instrumental music class meets in a room that is actually part of the stage for the gym. However, a sturdy movable "accordion" wall is nearly always in place, forming the north side of the room. Students enter from the hallway on the south side of the room.

On the other side of the movable wall is another part of the stage, often used in connection with the gym. The gym floor is down a few steps, at a slightly lower level.

If your student is not in instrumental music, first have him explore the music room (when the class is not present). He enters and takes a seat. Then he walks around the perimeter noting the hall door, the window, and the accordion wall. If rhythm instruments are available, let the student play some of them briefly.

Next, go to the gym in the usual manner – through the hall and down the steps. Examine the outer stage area.

Go back to the music room (via the hallway). Examine the movable wall. How can we tell it is movable? If possible, open the wall slightly and walk through: good cane usage will find the edge of the stage easily. Walk down from the stage to verify that you are indeed in the gym. Walk back up onto the stage and into the music room.

Depending on the child's maturity, repeat and continue to explore the area.

REMARKS: In the above example, if opening the wall is not advisable, someone might talk to the student through it. ("I am on the stage in the gym.")

A student who is in the instrumental music class should already understand the movable wall to a degree. Gym activities would often be heard through it. The teacher would sometimes comment. Nevertheless, the student would benefit from actually opening the wall and walking through.

EXAMPLE 4: *ALTERNATE ROUTES BETWEEN ROOMS*
(*Preschool and primary grades*)
(Figure 37-3)

This Figure shows parallel hallways and a typical system of room numbers. Hall N (at the north) and Hall S run east and west, with classrooms opening onto them. Hallway W is at the west end, running north and south; it opens onto the west playground and onto halls N and S. Hall E, at the east end, is similar. The administrative office is at the north end of Hallway E; the main front entrance to the building opens onto Hallway E from the east.

Room numbers increase from east to west. On the north side of Hallway N are Rooms 101-105; 102 is Mrs. Arnes' room. On the south side of Hall N are 106-110. Along Hall S, Rooms 111-115 are on the north side; the Music room is 112. Rooms 116-120 are on the south side.

All classrooms are of equal size. Thus, 101 is across from 106; 102 is across from 107; etc. Also, 107 (on the south side of Hall N) is back-to-back with 112 (north side of Hall S).

A real building is unlikely to be quite this precisely regular, but comparable characteristics are typically found.

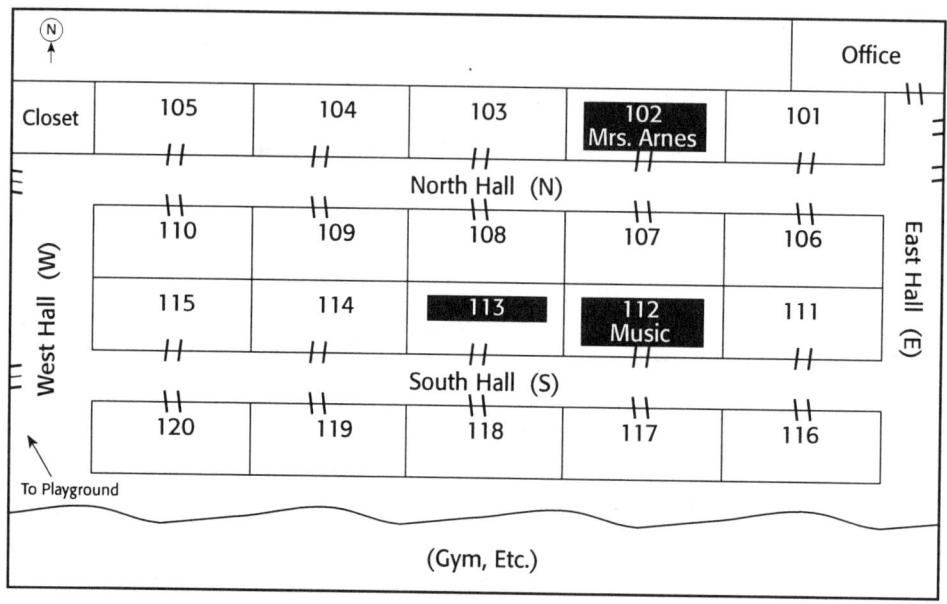

**Figure 37-3
Parallel Hallways**

Where Are We Now?

Assume that the student's own classroom is 102, Mrs. Arnes' room. The class goes to music in 112. Ordinarily they go in a group via Hall E; the student can also go alone.

Starting at Mrs. Arnes' room, ask the student to walk to the music room and back. [Assume that he goes via Hallway E.]

Standing in front of Mrs. Arnes' room again, comment, "Good—that is how we usually go, and it's the shortest way. Now let's suppose that the hallway between us and the music room—near the office—is being fixed. It's all torn up and we can't go that way. Can you tell me another way to get to the music room?"

Proceed to Music via the west hallway (supply the idea if the student cannot). Note that the distance is somewhat farther, though not greatly so. Talk about other possible reasons why a person might choose to go that way.

To emphasize the overall layout, walk all the way around in a rectangle, noting when you pass the music room. Do this again in the reverse direction.

EXAMPLE 5: *WITHIN A ROOM*
(*Preschool and kindergarten*)

A young and inexperienced child may need similar practice within one room. For example, at preschool he may have learned to walk from the door to the toy shelves along one particular path, and he may fail to realize there are other possible approaches.

EXAMPLE 6: *OVERALL LAYOUT*
(*First grade and up*)

Refer again to Figure 37-3. Again assume that the student's own classroom is 102.

Walk around and discuss the arrangement of the rooms. (The amount and kind of analysis should be tailored to the student's maturity.)

Main hallways run east and west. In each set of numbers, the smallest number is farthest east.

Rooms 101-105 are on the north side of the first hall (the hall farthest north), and 106-110 are on the south side of the first hall. Rooms 106-110 are back-to-back with 111-115. (There are no direct connections between the rooms that are back-to-back.) Rooms 111-115 face a second hallway (farther south).

Walk back and forth in the north hallway. Note that in each of rooms 101-105, there are windows on the north side, and the south side of each room has a door facing the hall. Rooms 106-110 have doors facing north toward the same hallway; there are no windows.

Go to the south hallway. Consider rooms 111-115. They have doors facing south onto the south hallway; there are no windows.

Recall or introduce the "Rooms back-to-back" Exercise, below.

A tactual map is especially helpful when a student first starts analyzing the arrangement of several rooms. However, the experienced student should also be able to grasp a complex layout mentally, rather than always requiring a diagram. Someone may ask how a blind person can do this when he cannot "visualize." Avoid pointless discussion, and simply assure everyone that it can easily be done. ("Each person has his own way of arranging things mentally" is a good statement.)

EXAMPLE 7: ROOMS BACK-TO-BACK
(*Kindergarten and up*)

Again refer to Figure 37-3 and assume that the student's classroom is 102.

When no class is present, enter Room 112 (Music). Go to the north wall and ask, "If we could go through this wall, where would we be?"

Emphasize that rooms 111-115 are back-to-back with rooms 106-110. If you could "go through the wall," you could walk through one of those rooms, then through another room, and be in the north hallway.

You are in 112, and would (in imagination) be going through 107. Upon walking on out of there, you would be across the hall from 102. (A short route, indeed, between the Music room and Mrs. Arnes' room!)

Go back to the north hallway and stand in front of 102. Enter 107, go to the south wall, and establish that the music room is beyond it.

With a young child, try to arrange to hear sounds from the music room as a confirmation. If a class is in there, perhaps music can be heard. Alternatively, arrange for someone to knock on the wall in response to your knock.

Depending on the student's maturity, consider analyzing the numbering relationship for the entire two rows (Room 111 is behind 106, and so on).

Also, consider where you would be if you could "go through" the *side* wall of a room. For example, if you are in 112, what is on the other side of the west wall? To many young learners, this is not at all obvious – even when they know how to go from 112 to 113 via the doors.

REMARKS: Even though "going through the wall," as above, cannot provide an actual alternative route, it provides important insight and understanding.

Continually watch for other examples where you might discuss what is on the other side of a wall. This includes a discussion of what is outdoors. Sighted students see through the window, but an inexperienced blind student may have no idea what is out there.

Real-life numbering systems and layouts are rarely as well-ordered as in this sample. It is important, however, to point out patterns even when they are imperfect.

EXAMPLE 8: ALTERNATIVE FIRE EXITS
(*First grade and up*)

Review the standard fire exit from a given location. Find an alternative exit in case the usual one is blocked. (There may be an official designation.)

RELATED PRACTICE: Study a tactual floor plan of the school.

REFERENCE(S):
Richard Mettler. *Cognitive Learning Theory and Cane Travel Instruction: A New Paradigm*, pp. 121-144.

MODULE 38
ROUTES FOR NEW BUILDINGS AND NEW CLASSROOMS
Upper Grades Through High School

OBJECTIVE: The student will walk independently to find his/her current classrooms and all common locations where students usually go, in any sequence. He/she will follow directions to an unfamiliar location with minimal help.

AGE OF STUDENT: Fourth grade and up

PRIMARY SKILL EMPHASIS:
General travel (indoors)
Orientation overall
In a crowd or a line
Compass directions
Floor plans

ADDITIONAL SKILL EMPHASIS:
Stairs
Communication and instructions
Structure of buildings

SEE ALSO (Other Modules):
> General Overview – Buildings
> Alternate Routes Within a Building
> Fire Drills
> In a Crowd
> Auditorium or Theater
> Routes for New Classroom – Early Elementary Grades

FIGURE(S):

FIGURE 38-1: Floor Plan, Central Junior High School

TEACHER PREPARATION: Walk around in all major areas of the building beforehand if at all possible. Examine a map. Ask about locations where students commonly go, and about any conventions or rules about traffic patterns (e.g., an up-only staircase). Form a good mental image of the building as a whole, and plan how to explain it.

Consider the building's complexity in relation to level of skill. How much can realistically be learned in each practice session? How many sessions can be held before classes begin?

REMARKS: This Module assumes that the student is experienced in general travel skills. It assumes the student has classes in several different rooms, and the rooms may be different each term.

If at all possible, begin practice during the previous spring or summer.

When a blind student practices routes in a building which she may attend soon, questions are likely to surface. Contact at least one staff member (probably the principal or counselor) before starting. It is very important that this be handled well, to encourage smooth planning and prevent awkward misunderstandings. If you teach only travel, ask the itinerant teacher to join you in making contact and discussing general arrangements.

As you begin the first lesson, introduce the student to the principal and other key personnel. Consider meeting with all the staff, well before the end of the year. Discuss general arrangements, and explain that the student will be practicing travel.

At the very least, contact the principal or counselor and be sure that he/she understands general arrangements and plans. Ask this contact person to explain to others. Suggest how a written or verbal memo might be worded. For example:

> To All Staff
> For Your Information:
>
> The itinerant teacher from Student Services
> will come occasionally this spring with a
> blind student who is practicing travel with a
> cane. The student is Terri Carlson, who
> will be in seventh grade next year. Terri is

in regular classes at Central Elementary, with support services; she uses Braille and tape recordings.

Many students already know Terri from elementary school. If students ask, please explain that Terri is blind and will be attending here next year; she is learning her way around the building. If they ask why her eyes are covered, explain that this helps her rely on the cane rather than on inadequate vision. (She only wears these "sleep shades" during actual lessons, and not at other times.) Please explain as needed, with a matter-of-fact tone which conveys information rather than pity or concern.

The itinerant teacher (Doris Willoughby) and Terri will be pleased to get acquainted as time allows. However, students and staff should avoid interrupting during a practice session.

If you have questions about arrangements for next year, please contact Mr. White or Ms. Garner (or Mrs. Willoughby at Student Services). An IEP meeting in late April will fine-tune arrangements for seventh grade.

ACTIVITIES:

EXAMPLE 1: *NEW BUILDING*
NOTE: The amount of practice needed by individuals varies greatly. For many older students, the detailed practice described below (spread over several sessions) would be unnecessary; one or two sessions with overall orientation would be sufficient.

Regardless of the amount of practice needed, it is vital that the student learn "mental mapping" skills. This is aided by use of an actual map, however simple – a large piece of paper the appropriate shape, with tactual marks or pieces of cardboard on it, can be sufficient.

Overall verbal description is also important. For Figure 38-1, one might say:

> This building faces east. The longest hallway runs north and south; it is often thought of as being in two parts, the north hallway and the south hallway. There is also a hall running east and west.
>
> Classrooms are located along all the hallways. The gym and the auditorium are at the far south end.
>
> The main entrance is in the middle of the east face. As you come in the main entrance, the principal's office is on your left. On the right is a lobby area with informal seating.
>
> When you come in the front door, there is a stairway almost straight ahead (to the right of the hall which goes west). Downstairs, the lunchroom is under the office complex. Upstairs, the library is above the office complex.
>
> The second floor and the basement have very few regular classrooms, and they are all in the east-west hallway.
>
> Room numbers start with 1, 2, or 3, according to floor level. (The main floor has the 200's.) Then, the *second* digit in the room number will be 1 or 2 for the north hallway, 3 or 4 for the south hall, and 5 or 6 for the east-west hall. So, room 255 would be on the main floor, in the east-west hall. Odd numbers are usually – though not always – on the west or north side of a hallway.

A mature student may find that such a description, with a brief practice session, is sufficient orientation. With a less mature student, it is important to build such a description during several sessions, as she gains in understanding.

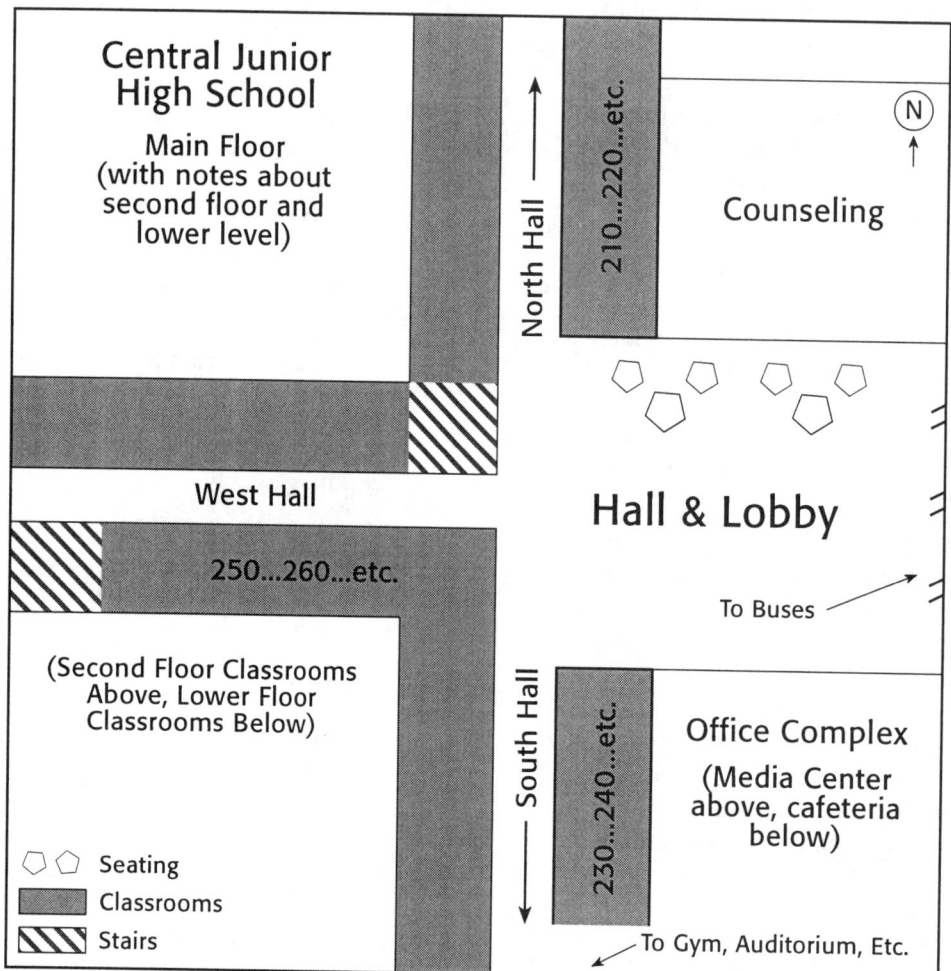

**Figure 38-1
Floor Plan
Central Junior High School**

Lesson 1: Introductory Tour
Go in main entrance, and proceed to office. Greet secretary and counselor. Leave message of greeting for principal. Tour building overall, with counselor as tour guide. Discuss overall pattern of hallways and room numbers. Greet a few people and briefly converse.

Before leaving, practice route between bus loading area and office.

Lesson 2: Upstairs (300's)
Student walks independently from bus loading zone through main front door to office. Each time, the student will tell the secretary when she and the instructor are entering or leaving the building.

Practice the following routes:

a. Go up the east stairs, walk all the way west on the upper floor, then come down the west stairs and return to the office. Note that stairs continue down to the ground floor (below first floor); use cane carefully.

b. Go up east stairs again. Go straight ahead into media center. Locate large counter, where library assistants can be found. Introduce yourself to a library assistant. Go back out into hallway, and return to office via the east stairs.

c. Repeat *b.*, except return to office by west stairs. While passing through hallway, discuss what rooms are there.

Lesson 3: Three Levels
a. Walk from the office, up the east stairs, to the door of the media center. Return to the office. Note that the stairs continue down below first floor.

b. Go to the east stairway again, and proceed down to the lowest floor (100's). At the bottom of the stairs, the lunchroom is ahead and slightly to the left. Tour the lunchroom area, with the teacher or counselor explaining traffic patterns. Greet the head cook.

c. Go back up the stairs to the main floor (200's). Turn west and walk through the hallway; discuss what rooms are there. How does the numbering compare to the rooms upstairs?

d. Go up the west stairs. Proceed east to the media center and to the counter inside. Ask whether Phil, a friend who helps in the library, is present; if so, take a few minutes to converse.

Lesson 4: North-South Hallway, with Gym
a. Walk north from the office area, past the stairway, and proceed to the outside door at the far north end. Discuss what kinds of classes are here; analyze the numbering system. Return to the office area.

b. Proceed south from the office area, to the gym. Are there any classrooms nearby? Note outside doors nearby.

c. The student independently follows directions to certain locations in relation to north-south hallway. For example: "Mr. Hancher's resource room is at the far north end – the last door on the right as you approach the outside door. He is expecting you to stop in and say hello. Go there and visit briefly. Then meet me back at the counselor's office."

Lesson 5: All Current Classrooms
Use an actual (or sample) complete schedule of classes. Walk through the schedule in the given sequence, including lunch. Note any handy clues that can save time (e.g., the entrance to room 213 is more recessed than most, and often a loud air blower can be heard nearby).

Go to the same rooms in a different order.

Note convenient rest rooms.

Lesson 6: Busy Hallways
By this point, some practice probably will already have occurred while halls and stairways are crowded. But if timing has not allowed this, it is important to arrange it.

Review the technique for pulling the cane up to a more vertical position when walking in a crowd.

Are some clues less usable when halls are crowded and noisy? (For example, perhaps the air blower cannot be heard.) Is there a need to modify one's path, to avoid missing clues or being swept past one's destination?

If the student is already used to crowded halls in her present school, relatively little work may be needed. But for her first experience with large numbers of students moving individually (as opposed to each class walking together in a line), practice is very important. Otherwise, the student may become fearful and overwhelmed.

Even if it requires special arrangements, find a way to accustom the student to crowds. If you really cannot ever work when classes are changing, perhaps you could work at the end of the day when everyone is hurrying out. Perhaps you can visit a different school or a busy mall.

Lesson 7: Office Area and Review
Analyze the relationship among various places in and near the administrative office: general office area with secretaries; principal and assistant principal; nurse's room; counseling area. Note that the counseling area is on the other side of the main front entrance, and that the lobby area (with seating) is an informal gathering place for students.

Practice going between a given classroom and a specific destination in the office area.

Lesson 8: Continued Practice and Discussion
Continue practicing as needed. Emphasize integrated understanding of the overall layout rather than memorizing routes.

Work as much as practical during the term which precedes a change, and/or during the summer. Review intensively just before the end of vacation. As school begins, watch for areas needing practice or troubleshooting

Provide at least minimal familiarity with each major areas of the building, even if the student will probably not go there regularly this particular year.

Discuss likely problems or misunderstandings. Probably someone along the way will suggest (or even direct) that the student should take extra time, be accompanied, rely on the elevator, etc. Discuss how to deal with such comments, both from students and from staff.

Examine additional locations and features such as:

- Other outside doors, including emergency exits
- Other rest rooms
- Complete tour of the gym, including dressing rooms (with tour guide of same sex)
- Detailed examination of traffic patterns and seating in lunchroom
- Ramps: Especially note if there is a "parallel path" situation where the hallway goes up or down slightly (e.g., one side of the hallway consists of a few steps, and the other side of the hall consists of a ramp going to the same place).
- Telephones
- Places where students gather informally
- Vending machines
- Study halls
- Elevators (it is desirable to know where they are, even when one will not be using them)
- Teachers' lounge (May students knock and ask to talk with a staff member?)
- Detailed tour of media center, with its conference or study rooms
- Tornado shelter areas
- Auditorium (See also "Auditorium or Theater" Module.)

REMARKS: If it should prove impossible for the student to become comfortably independent before school starts, it may be necessary to provide a guide and/or allow extra time at first. However, there should be a clear plan for phasing this out. It is important to talk with staff about methods for walking independently in busy hallways; otherwise it may be thought impossible.

EXAMPLE 2: *NEW SCHEDULE WITH LITTLE CHANGE*

A new class schedule in the same building may involve very little change. Perhaps new classrooms are close to the previous ones and are already familiar to the student.

An experienced student may need no help from the cane travel teacher. She will simply get her schedule, consider the sequence, and practice once or twice on her own. Any confusion is easily handled by inquiry and practice.

A less experienced student will benefit from guided practice with the travel teacher. Help her blend the new situation with the knowledge and skill she already has. Practice the new schedule in normal sequence; but emphasize overall understanding, and practice other sequences also. Look for helpful clues and aids to efficiency. Practice with halls busy and with halls empty.

If at the beginning of the previous term the student needed help or extra time, work to see that such accommodations are now needed less or not at all.

EXAMPLE 3: *NEW SCHEDULE WITH MAJOR NEW ROUTES*

Sometimes a new schedule includes a major area where the student has had little or no experience. Perhaps some classes are on the third floor; in the fine arts wing; in the outside annex; etc.

Treat this as though it were a "new building," and use some of the suggestions given in Example 1. If possible, begin well before the previous term ends.

This points up the desirability of gaining at least slight familiarity with *all* areas of the building as soon as possible. This includes areas where the student does not expect to have classes until later, or even where she never expects to go. One can never tell when a sudden need to go there may arise; and the more background the student has, the less adjustment and new learning would be required.

EXAMPLE 4: *REMODELING OF FAMILIAR BUILDING*

When a student goes to a new building or a different area, everyone usually recognizes the need for orientation. But when remodeling or other major changes are made in a familiar building, re-orientation is often neglected or incomplete.

An Embarrassing Omission

Melanie quickly learned her way around the high school, walking to ninth grade classes independently. Her tenth grade schedule was similar, and she needed little help from me. Her parents and teachers easily showed her what she needed to know.

The following summer, a new wing was built at the west end. The first and second floors were extended, adding several new classrooms on each floor, as well as a new media center. When Melanie began eleventh grade, she assured me she had no problem with her new schedule. Her cousin had shown her the new rooms; she had been in the media center; the new addition was very nice.

In December, I happened to go upstairs with Melanie. Afterward I asked, "Shall we go back down the west stairs or the east stairs?" After a stunned silence she asked hesitantly, "What do you mean ... the west stairs?"

Despite three months in the new wing, Melanie had no idea it included a new stairway and two exits.

This gap in knowledge was embarrassing to Melanie and to me—and also to the interested and caring counselor when she noticed our extra practice.

Nowadays I not only *ask* whether the student is familiar with a new area; I do some direct checking.

MODULE 39
MORE IDEAS
For Lessons at School
Indoors

AGE OF STUDENT: Preschool through elementary school

ABOUT THIS LIST:

Following is a list of objects, aspects, places, etc., found in a typical school. Examining different things at various times helps assure variety and interest for the young child. Many other suggestions appear in the Modules in this section (AT SCHOOL, INDOORS), and are not necessarily duplicated on this list.

A given item may be incorporated into the actual lesson. (Example: The child is working on walking between her classroom and the office. Each time he arrives and names the room, he is to go in, locate a piece of furniture, and comment on its surface or texture.) Alternatively, a given item may serve as a "fun" end to a lesson. (Example: The child is asked to find and name certain rooms. When this task is accomplished, he is allowed to play with stuffed animals in the library.)

Be alert to interesting things that are seasonal or temporary. If something would be especially valuable for your particular student (e.g., observing a piano tuner), inquire ahead and make an appointment.

Cane usage can be practiced even when the child frequently stops to examine things by touch.

REMARKS: Check with the principal and/or custodian before going where children do not ordinarily go, or allowing the student to touch something which is ordinarily forbidden. This is especially true when there are safety hazards. Also, avoid bringing a child into the teacher's lounge without advance planning; the staff expects privacy in the lounge. Ask permission before bringing a child into another teacher's classroom, even when it is vacant, and be scrupulous about not disturbing anything.

CAUTION: Always be alert for possible hazards. Examples include poisonous materials in the cleaning closet, hot pipes, motors, sharp edges, etc. Use good safety practices when assisting a child to climb up and reach something. Seek assistance if needed. (Example: Ask the custodian to accompany you and the student in touring an unused basement area which might contain hazards.)

IDEAS:

- Puppets and toys in the counselor's office
- Live animals in the science room or other classrooms
- Live plants, especially if blooming
- Storage rooms (Old chairs and desks may seem mundane, but can be quite fascinating to a child.)
- Vending machines
- Ramps
- Benches
- The teachers' lounge (See Remarks, above)
- A long, straight, easy walk in a hallway (confidence-building for a beginner)
- Stuffed animals or puppets in the media center
- Toys in the kindergarten or preschool room
- Interesting objects on the desk of the principal or another staff member (See Remarks, above)
- Tornado shelter (Possibly the student has been there for drills but never has had the chance to examine the entire room.)
- Crawl space or unused area
- Construction or repair (See Caution)
- Band or orchestra practice (Stand near the door and listen)
- A piano tuner (Go toward the sound. Ask the tuner if he/she has time to show and explain the procedure.)

MORE IDEAS (At School, Indoors)

- Portion of the building used by a different age group (If the child will soon move up into the age group in question, this is important preparation.)
- Doorknobs, door handles (Are they all the same?)
- Exposed pipes (as, under a sink)
- Textures of various walls
- Texture of various furnishings
- Different chairs and desks (Sit on each one, and also examine each of its parts.)
- Steps
- Shutters, drapes, Venetian blinds, and other window treatments
- The ceiling
- Brooms, vacuum cleaners, etc.
- Floor coverings—tile, rugs, carpet, etc. (How is the gym floor different?)
- Gym equipment
- Opening and closing various doors or windows
- Studying a picture on the wall, especially one with historic or symbolic importance (The child examines the frame tactually, and a verbal description of the picture is provided.)
- Air vents for heating and cooling
- People to meet
- Crawling under or through something
- Floor or baseboard which gives an unusual sound when tapped with the cane
- Onstage or backstage

AT SCHOOL
OUTDOORS

MODULE 40
SCHOOL BUS

OBJECTIVE: [For a student who regularly rides a bus] The student will walk to and from the correct bus independently. He/she will board, select a seat, and leave the bus with no more assistance than is customary for other students. (He/she may ask directions as needed.)

[For a student who does not usually ride a bus] The student will examine the general structure and arrangement of a school bus. He/she will board a bus, take a seat, and leave the bus with minimal assistance.

AGE OF STUDENT: All ages

PRIMARY SKILL EMPHASIS:
Doors and doorways
Finding a seat
Stairs
In a crowd or a line
Stowing cane

ADDITIONAL SKILL EMPHASIS:
Street crossing
Daily living skills
Detecting step-downs or drop-offs
Sound direction and meaning

SEE ALSO (Other Modules):
Public Buses
In a Crowd
Doors and Doorways
Walking In a Line of People
Meeting a Car
Urban Rapid Transit

TEACHER PREPARATION: It may or may not be possible for you, the teacher, to assist the student on her very first trip. Talk with parents and bus personnel. (Note: Consult the school principal before giving directions to bus drivers. The principal may wish to participate in the discussion.) Discuss cane usage and placement. Mention that blindness should not affect where a child should sit on the bus.

As soon as possible, conduct lessons as below, as needed. Review each year or whenever changes occur. Arrange to spend extra time practicing as needed—probably by having the student leave class a few minutes early for a lesson while the buses are waiting.

STUDENT BACKGROUND: A young or immature child who has not previously ridden a bus needs explanation and reassurance. Be sure she understands:

- Where the bus will load/unload near her home, and how she will get to and from her home.
- Where she will sit (Will she have an assigned seat, or may she choose?)
- The bus driver will help any student who has a problem or is lost.
- Where the bus will unload/load near the school, and how she will get to and from the building.

An experienced student preparing for a new route will need to know:

- The name or number of the bus or route.
- Her own address, with directions if it is hard to find.
- How to go to and from the bus at each end of the route.
- What to do if she waits a long time and the bus does not arrive.

ACTIVITIES:

EXAMPLE 1: *PREPARING TO RIDE*
Practice getting onto the bus. Walk alongside, with the arc of the cane extended enough to look for the bus doorway. Also listen for the driver's voice, and hear the motor idling, to aid in orientation.

Greet the driver and verify that this is the correct bus.

Walk up the steps with the cane, noting that the first step is high.

Using the cane, walk down the aisle and take a suitable seat.

Place the cane appropriately. It may be laid on the floor (pointing toward the front and back of the bus, and not extending into the aisle). It may be placed between the seat and the wall. Or, the student may hold the cane semi-vertically against the body with the tip on the floor.

Walk to the back of the bus and sit in the extreme rear seat. Examine the emergency door. Walk through the bus and practice sitting in various seats – on each side of the aisle, in window seats vs. aisle seats, etc. Examine the windows; are students permitted to open and close them? Are there emergency exits in the side of the bus?

Review rules for bus behavior.

(Optional): Sit in the driver's seat and examine some of his/her controls.

Get off the bus. The cane finds the steps, noting the long step to reach the ground. Good cane usage prevents tripping over the curb or unexpected obstacles.

EXAMPLE 2: *TO AND FROM THE BUS, AT SCHOOL*

Practice the route to and from the schoolhouse door. If there is a choice of doors, practice with each one.

When leaving the school, consider how to find the right bus. Does it always stop in the same place? Or is it in a lineup, and do sighted students look for the bus number?

Suppose that the blind student rides on Bus #8, which will be in a line of several buses near the gym. When she finds the doorway of a bus that may be the right one, she should ask whether it is #8. If it is not, she might seek directions as to where #8 is, or simply keep going and ask at each bus. In time she will probably learn various helpful facts about the lineup – e.g., if she finds #15, then #8 is probably the next one forward.

It is often helpful to ask directions from other passengers who are waiting. They may easily spot a given bus in a lineup. However, assistance can easily be overdone; other students should give information as needed, *without* undue physical assistance.

Especially with a younger student, the driver may call her name as she approaches. However, even a young child should start to learn a more mature approach which does not depend on any one person.

Sometimes the student might arrive at the lineup area before her bus arrives. Alert your student to this possibility. If other people are there, they will explain. If no one is there at all, she should simply wait.

EXAMPLE 3: *TO AND FROM THE BUS, AT HOME*

In a similar manner (if needed), practice the route to and from the bus at the home end. A very young child may need instruction even if the bus is right outside the door.

If an older student has always had the school bus come right to her home, consider changing to a stop on the regular route. This provides valuable independence and experience.

EXAMPLE 4: *IF THE STUDENT DOES NOT USUALLY RIDE THE BUS*

A student who comes to school by other means should, nevertheless, become familiar with buses. Arrange for her to practice boarding a bus and sitting in various seats.

This is excellent readiness for learning to use public transportation. Also, review techniques before the class goes on a field trip in a school bus.

RELATED PRACTICE: Ride a public bus (even if the student is at the "readiness" level on this task).

MODULE 41
MEETING A CAR

OBJECTIVE: The student will go to a location where he/she is to meet a vehicle, verify that the driver is the person expected, and enter.

AGE OF STUDENT: Preschool and up

PRIMARY SKILL EMPHASIS:
General travel (outdoors)
Communication and instructions
Sound direction and meaning
Finding a person
Traffic movement

ADDITIONAL SKILL EMPHASIS:
Attitudes toward blindness
Flexibility and confidence
Understanding vision and partial vision
Sidewalk
In a crowd or a line
Parallel and perpendicular
Street crossing

SEE ALSO (Other Modules):
School Bus
Asking Directions And Figuring It Out
In a Crowd
Distinctive Sounds
Walking Toward a Sound
Visually Confusing Appearance
Errands
Street Crossing With Little Traffic
Street Crossing With Lights (Basic Skills)

REMARKS: Even if a student is not regularly picked up at school by someone in a car, it is important to discuss these methods during the elementary years. All students will meet cars from time to time, particularly as they get older.

STUDENT BACKGROUND: Before accomplishing this task independently, the student needs a degree of travel skill and a degree of mature judgment. Nevertheless, a very inexperienced young child can be guided through the task and gradually accomplish more and more of it alone.

CAUTION: Discuss the points listed below under "Teacher Preparation" in detail with parents and classroom teachers.

Emphasize that although partial vision may be helpful, it is *not* safe for the child to rely solely upon vision.

Also note techniques for avoiding confused identity or deliberate impersonation.

TEACHER PREPARATION:
Inquire whether the child is regularly picked up by someone in a car (at school or elsewhere). If so, help them make arrangements conducive to the blind child's independence. Mention these points:

– A fully sighted child may stand still, survey a line of cars, note a particular car, and then run over to it. This is not appropriate for a blind child.

– A fully sighted child may "walk around and look for Grandma's car." A blind child may do this, but needs a specific plan. Ideally, he would go to a particular location (e.g., the southwest corner of the block). However, there may be many parents waiting in cars, so that a person cannot be sure of having the same spot each time. One solution is to go slightly farther from the school, so that the area is not crowded. Another idea is for the child to walk back and forth periodically in a particular area, waiting for the driver to greet him.

– The driver may honk lightly in a particular pattern (e.g., twice). However, the student should also verify identity in an unambiguous way. He should realize that someone else may honk in the same pattern. Also, in some situations honking may be inappropriate.

– A child with considerable useful vision, in

a non-complicated situation, may find vision helpful. For a child with very little vision, trying to identify cars visually is more confusing than helpful. In any case, positive identification by voice is vital. Parents may not understand at first that a partially-sighted student does not see detail of vehicles or faces as others do, and should not rely on vision alone.

- It is best for the driver to speak to the child first. But the child should be alert for the possibility of someone else's calling him, and be coached about ways to verify identity.
- As a child gains maturity, he should realize that disguised voices and attempted deception are possible. Many families have codes for checking identity; these are more commonly used on the telephone or in third-party messages, but can also be used by a blind child in person.
- If the child is the first to speak, he should *not* say, "Is that you, Grandma?" (That makes it too easy for a stranger to attempt impersonation.) Instead he might say "Hello, there!" and wait for a response.

ACTIVITIES:

EXAMPLE 1: *A BEGINNER WITH HELP*
(*Kindergarten*)

Perry is a kindergartner with little vision. He will be picked up by his grandmother at 11:30 each school day. The cane travel teacher has discussed details with Perry's parents, the grandmother, and the classroom teacher.

It is agreed that Perry will walk to the south end of the block and wait for Grandma at the corner. The area is not crowded at this time, and there is very little traffic.

At first, an adult goes with Perry each time. (The travel teacher can do this on Tuesdays, and on other days another staff member will go.) The adult reminds Perry about cane usage as he walks down the front steps of the school, and about general posture and arcing as he proceeds down the block. She helps him remember to turn left at the bottom of the steps, to stay on the sidewalk, and to recognize if he reaches the curb at the south corner. Usually Grandma has already arrived and calls out to Perry as he approaches. The staff member says, "That's Grandma's voice, isn't it? Go ahead." Perry then gets into the car independently.

After three weeks, Perry is doing well with little assistance. It is decided that no extra adult is required: the teacher who watches all the kindergartners as they leave will watch Perry as well. (The south corner can easily be seen from the front of the school.) On Tuesdays the cane travel teacher will also watch and will give suggestions and reminders.

EXAMPLE 2: *INDEPENDENCE*
(*First grade and up*)

The next year, Perry is in first grade. He is dismissed at 3:00 along with most of the other students in five grades. Many parents and relatives wait in their cars along the block and in the adjoining parking lot.

It is decided that Perry will walk to the south corner as before. However, now Grandma may be anywhere along the block. (An arriving car tends to get at the end of the line and move up as others meet their children and depart.) Perry walks along rather slowly, listening for his grandmother's voice and/or a particular honk. If he reaches the south corner, he turns around and walks back to the school entrance, then repeats if he still has not found her. (Other children are doing essentially the same thing, although their way of looking is different.)

Occasionally Grandma has difficulty parking in the usual area. She may park somewhere else and walk over to get Perry. Or, she may wait until there is less traffic.

All the children, including Perry, have been instructed to return inside the school if they wait a long time and their ride does not arrive.

For the first few days, an adult watches Perry carefully to be sure he makes connections. Thereafter he needs no extra help.

RELATED PRACTICE: Review procedures for stowing a cane quickly and efficiently when entering a vehicle.

Also emphasize that, when leaving a car, it is important to check the ground with the cane before actually stepping out.

FOLLOW-UP: When riding in a car or bus, even a young student should begin to understand the route taken. This matter is discussed in detail in the Module, "Public Buses." Don't let your student view such trips as nebulous passages comparable to the Star Trek™ Transporter!

REFERENCE(S): Castellano, Carol. "Serena Can Wait at the Bottom of the Hill."

MODULE 42
PLAYGROUND

NOTE: This Module deals specifically with play areas. The Module, "What's Out There?" deals with the school grounds overall.

OBJECTIVE: The student will go to any of [5] chosen locations on the playground, play independently, and return to the building.

AGE OF STUDENT: Kindergarten and elementary grades

PRIMARY SKILL EMPHASIS:
Orientation overall
Varied terrain
Open space
Stowing cane
Climbing, clambering, crawling, etc.
Boundaries
Examining things tactually
Obstacles in path
Landmarks

ADDITIONAL SKILL EMPHASIS:
Doors and doorways
Hills and inclines
Maps
Air currents and echoes
Weather and temperature
Sound direction and meaning
In a crowd or a line
Etiquette

SEE ALSO (Other Modules):
Routes for New Classroom (Early Elementary Grades)
Outside and Inside the School
What's Out There? (On the School Grounds)
Walking Across Open Space
Rough Terrain
Back Yard Boundaries
Back Yard (Overall)
The Great Outdoors
Walking In a Line of People

FIGURE(S):
FIGURE 42-1: First Grade Playground

TEACHER PREPARATION: Look over the playground. Note popular play areas and equipment, as well as other landmarks. Inquire what door(s) the class will use, and where (or whether) they will assemble before coming back in.

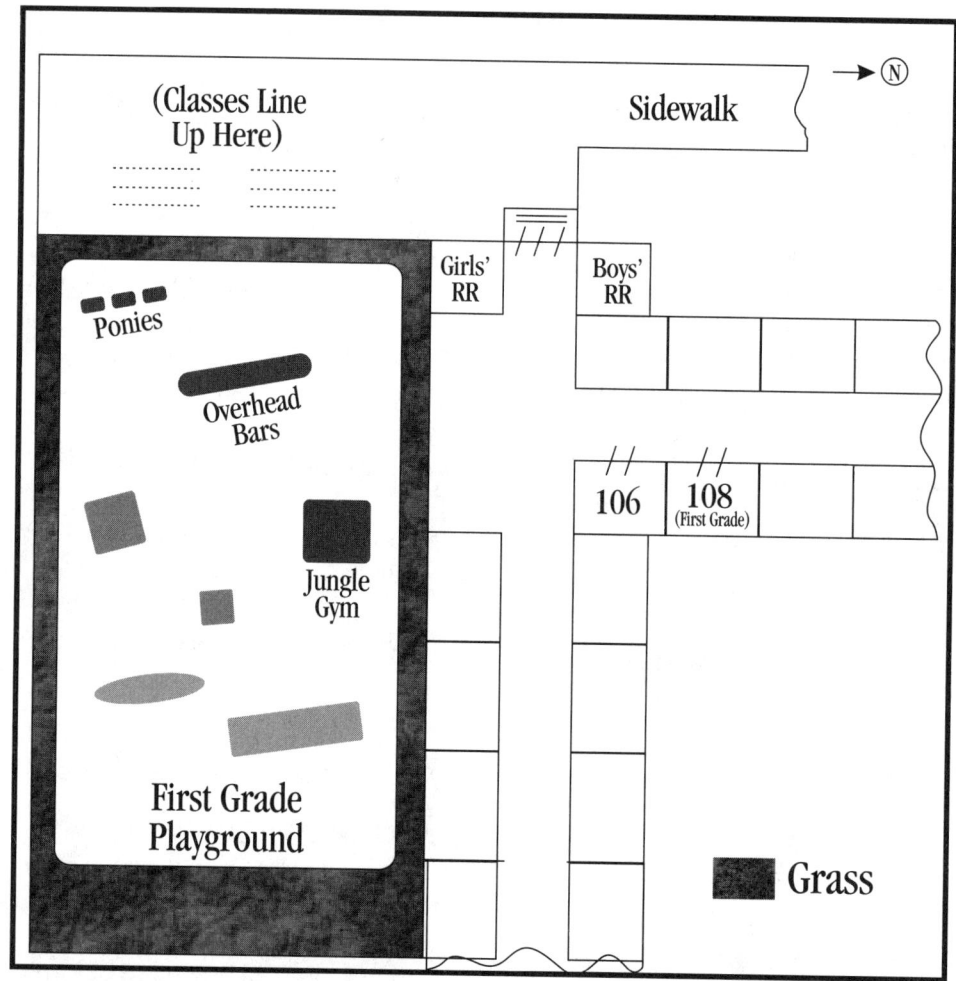

Figure 42-1
First Grade Playground

ACTIVITIES: See Figure 42-1.

EXAMPLE 1: *GETTING ACQUAINTED*
If possible, introduce the child to the playground before he begins to play there with a group. This example describes a kindergartner who will play in a new area in first grade.

"We're going to look at the playground you'll use in first grade. This is very exciting!"

Start at the first-grade room (the room itself having been explored during a different session).

"Stand with your back to the first-grade door and pretend we're just coming out of there. Now, we turn left to go to the outside door. The outside door will be on our right....Keep to the right and use your cane to look for the way out."

The child finds the area leading to the rest rooms, noting that the boys' room is on the right and the girls' on the left. He finds the exit door and goes outside. (Actually, there are multiple doors side by side.)

Emphasize the skills of knowing left and right, and of using the cane to arc correctly while touching the wall with each arc to search for the door.

Outside, the child goes down a few steps. Note good cane usage in detecting and going down the steps.

"Turn left on the sidewalk. Now, as we walk along we will soon notice a lot more wind blowing....Feel that?...That means we are past the end of the building, and we are at the playground. The first-grade playground is on your left.

"Today I will go to some things to play on, and you can follow my voice. Let's start with the jungle gym. Follow me...."

Keep talking as the child follows you to the jungle gym and finds it with his cane. He sets his cane down and plays on the equipment for a short while.

Repeat with two or three other pieces of equipment, as the child follows you to each and then plays there.

"In first grade, each time recess is over, the teacher will stand on the sidewalk and blow her whistle. I'll do that for practice today, and you come over to me...."

Go to the sidewalk. Imitate the sound of a playground whistle or blow a real one. Keep talking as the child comes to you and "gets in line."

"Today I kept talking to you after the whistle so you would know where I was. Next year you will hear the children all running, and can follow them. Also, you will know the way after you practice."

Practice re-entering the building. Note that directions are the reverse of what they were when you went out.

Find the correct rest room. Probably students will go there after recess.

Return to the first grade door and notice that it is the second door on its side of the hall.

Practice in a manner similar to the above on several occasions. Each time, show the student another part of the playground. Build familiarity, but do not expect understanding of the entire layout at this time. If time permits, do teach the child to walk independently between the first grade and one particular location on the playground. For example: Turn left as you leave the door, then turn left again at the corner of the building. Walk at the edge of the grass. You will soon reach the jungle gym.

EXAMPLE 2: *SPECIAL CONSIDERATIONS*

Some playgrounds have areas requiring special attention, often involving safety. Examples include a street without a fence; a deep window well; a swing set.

Quickly acquaint the blind child with any such things. He should learn where each item is and how to recognize it, and he should receive the same strong cautions that others get. (Examples: always stop at the grass which adjoins the curb; never climb onto or over the railing around the window well.)

Some equipment, such as a swing set, is safe when approached carefully and used right, but can be dangerous otherwise. Problems may include approaching busy swings from the front or the back, or swinging wildly sideways.

Teach the student how to approach a swing set from the side, using general orientation and listening. Be sure he knows how to swing (and pump) normally. Provide a way for him to get his turn when others are present. For example, other children might tell him when it is his turn, and show him which swing is free. Or, perhaps everyone could wait in line at one side. Also, the blind child could speak up with a reminder from time to time. Avoid the extremes of (a) letting him stand by sadly while others grab the swing each time it is free, or (b) always giving him a turn immediately, even if others have been waiting.

EXAMPLE 3: *INCREASING INDEPENDENCE*

In the fall, before school opens and as school proceeds, review what has already been learned, and see that the child increases independence rapidly.

"You know how to find the jungle gym by yourself. Do you know where the little bouncing ponies are? Which is farther from the building?...Yes, the ponies are farther away. Show me if you know where they are..."

[In this example, assume that the child approaches the ponies, but misses them by staying too far away from the sidewalk.]

"Good! You were close, and almost found them. I'm standing by them—come over and I'll show you this time.... Now, let's go back to the jungle gym and I'll show you how to find the ponies...."

"If you're at the jungle gym, here, remember where the building is and where the sidewalk is. Let's point to the building...point to the sidewalk.... Now, walk away from the building, but get closer to the sidewalk. Pass the overhead bars. Make a wide arc with your cane. And if other children are playing, you may hear them bouncing.... If you get all the way to the other grass, then you've gone too far, and should turn around and come back."

Practice finding the ponies from the school door.

Continue practice as much as time allows in relation to other priorities. Often the student will learn where things are through playing with other children. Correlate your lessons with what the other children, teachers, and aides may show the child. Guide them in giving the right kind of help, and the right amount—not too much or too little.

Insist that the blind child play on various pieces of equipment, rather than getting "stuck" playing in one certain place.

Practice walking with various terrain underfoot—grass, gravel, sand, etc.

Work on finding various pieces of equipment, in relation to each other as well as in relation to the school. It is not productive, however, to spend great amounts of time practicing paths which are hard to define and hard to learn. It is acceptable for the student to have help from other students in finding some things.

EXAMPLE 4: *LINING UP*

Build independence in lining up with the class after recess.

Usually a given class will line up at essentially the same place every time. If it is in a clearly-defined location (as, the second line from the left, at the bottom of the steps), the student should learn that easily.

In this example, various classes line up three abreast facing the building, near the playground teacher as she stands on the sidewalk by the playground. The youngest classes assemble closest to her (closest to the building). The teacher does not always stand in exactly the same spot, although the general area and arrangements are consistent.

The blind child easily learns to recognize the "line-up" signal: one long whistle, as distinguished from short whistles which are meant to stop misbehavior. He follows the other children running to assemble.

When he arrives on the sidewalk, he asks where his group is, and others guide him by voice or physically. (Other students soon learn to anticipate this and become *too* eager to help. Teachers remind them to help only if clearly needed.)

The blind student soon becomes familiar with the overall pattern: the first graders are closest to the whistle, and his class is in the middle of the walk as he faces the teacher. If he finds another class, he knows which direction to go.

Coach the child about standing in line appropriately—keeping the cane still, facing the right direction, staying close to the student ahead without pushing, etc. Help him walk in line, with good cane usage. See the Module, "Walking in a Line of People."

EXAMPLE 5: *BOUNDARIES*

Walk around the perimeter of the total area where first graders play. Examine the boundaries.

Often boundaries have tactual characteristics—sidewalk, hedge, fence, etc. If not, help the child to estimate. Remind him, "If you find yourself playing alone, and everybody else seems far away, think about where you are. Walk back toward the group if you aren't sure."

Walk around just outside the perimeter. (Emphasize that this should be done only with an adult.) Examine what is there; often this is very interesting to a child ordinarily not allowed to go there. Discuss where you are in relation to "inside." (See also the Modules, "Outside and Inside the School" and "Outside and Inside the

House.")

Consider whether there are other areas of the school grounds where the student has never been, and which would provide valuable travel practice as well as understanding and interest.

RELATED PRACTICE: Make a tactual map of the playground. Take it outside and practice finding things on the map and in reality.

FOLLOW-UP: Each year the student will probably have a different classroom, and may play in a different area. Practice new routes and relationships as needed:

- A different classroom door (In the same hallway? On the same side? How many doors from the end?)
- A different rest room
- Upstairs or downstairs
- A different outside door
- Lining up in a different place outside
- A wider area in which to play, or a different area altogether
- More classes outside at the same time

The travel teacher may or may not be the one to teach each of these new things. An aide may be directed to help the child learn. An experienced student in a good situation may easily learn them along with his classmates or with help from other children. But the travel teacher must check that the child *does* quickly learn the new aspects, without unnecessary problems. (Example of a problem: The new aide does not realize that the child could walk across an open space. She teaches him to follow the building and the fence in a long, circuitous route to the slide.)

MODULE 43
WHAT'S OUT THERE?
On the School Grounds

Note: This Module deals with features on the school grounds overall. The "Playground" Module deals specifically with play areas.

OBJECTIVE: The student will locate and name [10] major features on the school grounds.

AGE OF STUDENT: Preschool through elementary grades

PRIMARY SKILL EMPHASIS:
Obstacles in path
Landmarks
Compass directions
Correcting a path
General travel (outdoors)
Open space
Moving straight ahead
Orientation overall
Sidewalk
Varied terrain
Responsibility and citizenship

ADDITIONAL SKILL EMPHASIS:
Overhanging objects
Interpreting odors
Weather and temperature
Stowing cane
Right and left
Hills and inclines
Air currents and echoes
Sound direction and meaning
Boundaries
Corners, turns, and angles
Maps
Examining things tactually
Detecting step-downs or drop-offs

SEE ALSO (Other Modules):
    Playground
    Back Yard (Overall)
    Exterior Fire Escape
    Rough Terrain

Walking Independently While Following Someone
Utilities and Trash
Obstacles: Noting Them and Proceeding
Walking Across Open Space
Outside and Inside the School
The Great Outdoors

TEACHER PREPARATION: Learn the names commonly used for prominent features. At Grand School, a deep window well was referred to as "the pit," and a marble bench was called the "Sandow [Memorial] Bench." If the mobility instructor had called them the "window well" and the "marble bench," her five-year-old student would probably not have realized she meant the same things.

Inquire about group activities at the flagpole. An individual lesson there may be unnecessary. However, even if other activities have occurred, the student may never have actually examined the flag and its pulley.

Make an appointment (or help the student make an appointment) with the school custodian to lower and raise the flag. (*Note:* Do *not* attempt to raise or lower the flag yourself without permission and instruction. Flag etiquette is a sensitive matter. Also, operating the pulley is more complex than it may appear.)

CAUTION: Look for hazards, such as a wasp's nest, or a sharp broken branch that could poke the child in the face.

If you accompany the child into places or situations where students are forbidden to go alone, be sure she understands this.

ACTIVITIES:

EXAMPLE 1: *PLAY AREAS*
See the "Playground" Module for detailed suggestions about the area where the student

has recess.

Often, play areas are divided according to age. Sighted children see the places where their class does not go (and anticipate going there later). It is good to let a young blind child play briefly on equipment dedicated to older students, if it is safe. However, when an older child plays on equipment for younger children, an "image" problem is created. The student might *examine* the equipment during school hours, and perhaps play on it after school when the playground is not divided.

EXAMPLE 2: *TREES*
(*Preschool and Kindergarten*)

Locate an area with a number of trees or shrubs, fairly close to one another but not immediately together. Start the child a few steps from a tree.

"There are a lot of nice trees here. Today we're going to look especially at each *trunk*. That's the part that holds up the rest of the tree. Walk forward and find a tree.....How does it sound when your cane taps it?"

The student then feels the bark, and examines the trunk from the ground to as high as she can reach. She hugs the tree and notes whether or not her arms can reach all the way around. Note scents.

Repeat this to find other trees. (The child finds the trunk each time by using her cane, although the teacher indicates which direction to go.) Include at least one large trunk, and another trunk that is slender enough for the child to reach entirely around it.

On other days, repeat this activity but emphasize different characteristics—branches, blossoms, leaves, fruit, etc. Try to find a tree with some exposed roots. Discuss the overall structure of the tree.

Approach an evergreen tree which has branches extending close to the ground. (Check the sharpness of the needles.) "Now you're going to walk toward a very different kind of tree. Your cane will feel something very different from those hard trunks we've been finding." Examine needles (carefully, avoiding scratches). Examine and discuss the structure of the tree. Walk around the tree, noting how it feels to touch these branches with the cane.

Approach a bush. Study it in a manner similar to that with an evergreen. Note the multiple and thin trunks or stems.

Approach a tree which has some branches hanging low enough to touch the child, but not low enough to be easily found with the cane. Discuss this situation. Allow the student to put the free hand up to protect the face; emphasize that this should *not* be done except when there is good reason to expect something overhanging. A cap with a bill is another way to detect such things.

Examine various prominent trees, or groups of trees, around the school grounds. Discuss their characteristics and their use as landmarks.

REMARKS: This activity is described as for a student age 6 or younger, with time available for discussion of different kinds of trees. Even for a young child, the time spent will vary according to needs and opportunities.

With an older student, check understanding of the skills involved. Brief, age-appropriate practice should be provided as needed.

RELATED PRACTICE:

Correlate this activity with a science unit on plants.

Examine and/or construct models of various trees. Make size comparisons with people, buildings, etc. Many blind children have very incomplete concepts of size, shape, and proportion.

Keep a notebook on trees and their characteristics. For each activity, the student composes a Braille description (dictating it for the teacher to write, if the student is not yet able). Mount a specimen (leaf, piece of bark, etc.)

Examine trees and bushes in the child's own yard. Discuss their characteristics and their use as landmarks.

EXAMPLE 3: *FLAGPOLE*

The flagpole is a prominent feature on the grounds of almost every school. Usually it is a landmark near the main entrance–noticeable visually, tactually, and auditorily. The flags and/or ropes flap in the breeze; the pole is distinctive when touched. Furthermore, symbolic significance is high.

Discuss the significance of the flag. Examine the classroom flag and (if available) a tactual picture of the design. Discuss the Pledge of Allegiance.

Note flags inside the school.

If the student does not yet know how to find the outdoor flagpole, give directions for practice. (Example: "Go to the main front entrance. Walk straight ahead on the big sidewalk, but cane the right edge and look for a small sidewalk going to the right. Follow that and find the flagpole. Also, you will probably hear the flag and its rope flapping."

Examine the pole and the rope. Listen to sounds. Review the significance of the flag.

Make an appointment for the custodian to join you at the flag. The custodian should bring the flag down, with the student helping, and explain how the pulley works. The student should examine the flag, noting its size. (Optional: The custodian demonstrates how the flag is removed and folded, then unfolded and replaced.) The student should help run it back up, learning how to tell when it reaches the top.

Discuss flag etiquette, and the symbolism of a flag at half-mast.

RELATED PRACTICE: Correlate with social studies work about citizenship and the flag. Discuss other flags, such as the state flag. (Was the state flag on the same pole, under the U.S. flag?) Is there a school flag? A parochial school may display a religious flag.

Note flagpoles at various public buildings. Some homes display flags, especially at holidays.

Discuss citizenship in general, including alternative methods for voting.

Examine and operate other pulleys. Examine and compare other kinds of poles (including utility poles, etc.)

EXAMPLE 4: *LOOK AROUND*

Each situation is different. One student is very mature and needs only brief explanation of major features at a new building. Another child is very immature and in need of repeated concrete experiences. Generally, the younger the student, the more appropriate it is to examine details of the schoolyard repeatedly. A young child is still learning basic concepts and techniques.

Below is a representative list of features often found on the school grounds. Watch for temporary features (seasonal, construction, etc.), and consider changing plans to take advantage of the opportunity.

- VEGETATION: Trees, shrubs, flower beds, grass, weeds
- UNDERFOOT: Grass, sand, gravel, wood chips, cement, asphalt, weeds, puddles, mud, dead leaves, fallen pine cones or nuts, inclines up or down, steps up or down
- STATIONARY OBJECTS: Trees, flagpoles, people sitting or standing, benches, utility poles, fences, vehicles, trash receptacles, sports and play equipment, walls of buildings, retaining walls, bicycle racks, parked bicycles, sprinklers, lawn care equipment
- MOVING OBJECTS: People running or walking, lawn mowers, buses, cars, trucks (sometimes even on the sidewalk–delivery vehicles may drive up to a door), bicycles, swings, balls, portable play equipment, sprinklers, snow plows
- WEATHER-RELATED, SEASONAL: Piles of snow, snow sculpture, ice, puddles, mud, blown sand or dirt, piles of leaves, holiday decorations
- AREAS: Ditches; hills; streets, driveways, and parking lots; sidewalks; play areas vs. normally forbidden areas
- BUILDING ENTRANCES: An "arcade"

entrance (a roof held up by pillars but without walls) is particularly interesting. Walking under it is a good way to practice listening to the echoes from the cane tip. Young children may be very intrigued by the sound of voices under an arcade.

SAFETY FACTORS: Moving vehicles, swings, boundaries, drop-offs

MODULE 44
EXTERIOR FIRE ESCAPE

OBJECTIVE: During a fire drill, the student will leave the building in the same manner as other students, without holding onto another person.

AGE OF STUDENT: Preschool and up (The Example assumes elementary-school age.)

PRIMARY SKILL EMPHASIS:
Emergency procedures
Communication and instructions
In a crowd or a line
Stairs
Detecting step-downs or drop-offs
Flexibility and confidence

ADDITIONAL SKILL EMPHASIS:
Attitudes toward blindness
Responsibility and citizenship
Doors and doorways

SEE ALSO (Other Modules):
   Fire Drills
   Introducing the Cane
   Description of Basic Techniques
   Walking In a Line of People
   Stairs in Unfamiliar Buildings
   Emergency Exits (In Various Buildings)
   Walking Independently While Following
      Someone
   Outside and Inside the School

STUDENT BACKGROUND: The student should have experience with regular stairs before walking on a fire escape. If possible, she might be introduced beforehand to other stairs without risers, as in a basement.

General fire safety and drill procedures should be discussed.

TEACHER PREPARATION:
Determine which classes ordinarily use the exterior fire escape. If the student's own class uses it, practice should have high priority. If not, the student should practice before she reaches the grade level that does use it.

Check with the principal to make arrangements for practicing.

If access is through a classroom, find the least disruptive time to practice – probably when students are at lunch or recess.

Women and girls will prefer to avoid wearing high heels or full skirts for this practice, if possible.

An advanced student should be introduced to this experience even if her school has no exterior fire escape. Seek one out. (See the Module, "Emergency Exits – In Various Buildings.")

REMARKS: If others of the same age use the exterior stairs, the blind child should also. If an alternative arrangement is considered, it should be only temporary while the student is learning. (This assumes the student does not have an additional physical disability which by itself would prevent use of the fire escape.)

Practice on the fire escape is a valuable experience even if the student never expects to use it (e.g., she is in sixth grade and only the primary grades use it). An unusual situation, such as an errand, could place her in that location. Also, she might encounter one elsewhere.

ACTIVITIES:

EXAMPLE 1: *PRIMARY GRADES*
(This Example assumes that next year, in fourth grade, the student will be in a classroom near the fire escape.)

Review procedures for fire drills.

Explain that one of the new and interesting experiences in fourth grade will be the outside fire escape. Examine the fire escape from the bottom. Discuss its structure and how it is supported.

Consider the student's general confidence. Some people (sighted or blind) are quite fearful of iron fire escapes. Others find them exciting and fun.

It may be desirable to go *up* first, since that may be easier for a nervous student. (Caution: be sure you can get in the door at the top in case you decide not to walk back down immediately. It is likely to be locked from the outside.) Note that the stairs have no risers. Everyone should hold the handrail.

Go down the stairs at moderate speed. Note that the cane tends to get caught in the iron steps; it may need to be tapped extra-gently. (It would *not* be right to conclude that the cane should not touch the steps at all. As always, the cane verifies that the step is safe.)

With practice, the student should be able to go down at a brisk speed appropriate for a regular drill.

From inside the building, practice finding the exit. It may be helpful to sit down and simulate "reading class," then announce "Fire drill!"

Simulate a group by walking immediately in front of the student in one instance, immediately in back at another time.

RELATED PRACTICE: Discuss various kinds of fire escapes. Mention that some have an extra-large step at the bottom. Describe the type where the last few steps fold up and have a counterweight.

Years ago, many schools had a tubular "chute" (slide) as an escape. These are now rare.

If any unusual exits might be used by the student in the near future, provide practice.

FOLLOW-UP: Be sure that the student actually goes down the outside stairs at least every few months, so that this remains a familiar skill.

MODULE 45
OUTSIDE AND INSIDE THE SCHOOL

OBJECTIVE: At six locations along the exterior wall of a building, the student will: (a) while outside, state what room is inside; (b) while inside, state one or more landmarks which are outside.

AGE OF STUDENT: Preschool through early elementary grades

REMARKS: Beyond the early grades, some of the activities described would make the student appear odd. If this work is done with an older student, it is wise to have an easily-observed purpose (apart from general orientation) and work on it conspicuously. For example, notes could be written (using a Braille slate and a clipboard) about building construction.

PRIMARY SKILL EMPHASIS:
Structure of buildings
Floor plans
Orientation overall
Maps
Corners, turns, and angles
Landmarks
Compass directions

ADDITIONAL SKILL EMPHASIS:
Varied terrain
Doors and doorways
Right and left
Boundaries
Hills and inclines

SEE ALSO (Other Modules):
Outside and Inside the House
Alternate Routes Within a Building
Doors Closed or Open
Fire Drills
Utilities and Trash
What's Out There? (On the School Grounds)

FIGURE(S):
FIGURE 45-1: Outside and Inside

TEACHER PREPARATION: Walking close to the building, especially if the windows are touched, is very distracting to students inside. If possible, make arrangements to talk to someone through certain windows at a convenient time. Elsewhere, move along as inconspicuously as possible. In this example, consider walking by the upper-grade rooms when those students are out at recess.

It is sometimes wise to mention your plans to all teachers beforehand.

STUDENT BACKGROUND: This activity is usually most effective after the student is already somewhat familiar with the building and grounds. It is a good way to integrate learning in a unified manner, and it adds variety and interest.

REMARKS: This description assumes it is realistic to go around the entire building in one session. If that is not appropriate, a part of the building may be used. Often it is good to do this with each of several parts of the building, and then later go around the whole way quickly.

ACTIVITIES:

EXAMPLE 1: *VIEW FROM THE OUTSIDE*
(See Figure 45-1)
This Example assumes an L-shaped building which is easily analyzed. If there are hallways at various distances from the outside walls, walk as close to the perimeter as practical.

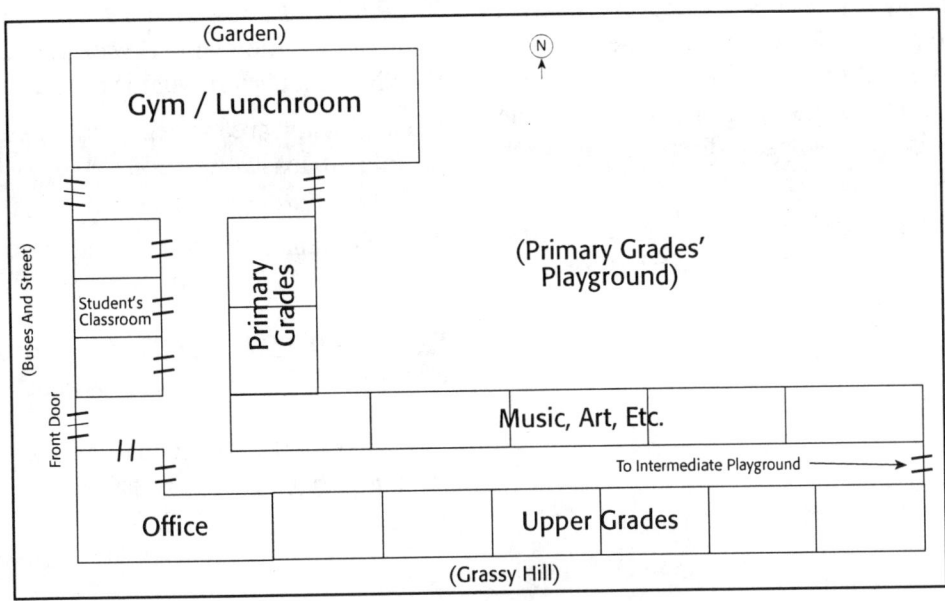

**Figure 45-1
Outside and Inside**

Review the inside:
Walk around the inside of the building. Quickly review important aspects of various parts of the building. In this Example, the vertical "leg" of the "L" extends north and south: the gym/lunchroom is at the north end, and lower-grade classrooms extend along that hallway. The upper grades are in the hallway which goes east to form the horizontal leg of the L shape; the exit at the far end faces east toward the Intermediate playground. The principal's office is at the southwest corner, with the main front door nearby (facing west).

Proceed outside:
Explain that today you will walk around the outside of the building – right along the wall. You will examine the wall in some detail, and discuss where you are in relation to the rooms inside.

Go out the far east door, near the Intermediate playground. Walk back along the south outside wall, going west. Examine some of the windows as you go by. Note that they are the windows of upper-grade rooms, and that you are walking parallel to the east-west hallway. Note the building construction – bricks, metal siding, etc.

The student touches the building with the cane frequently as she walks along, and notes when the southwest corner is reached. What room is at this corner? Help her understand that this is the office. Knock gently on the window, as prearranged, and talk with the secretary through the window. (Students often find this hilariously funny.)

Around the corner, continue to the front door. Walk inside a short way to verify location. Say hello to the secretary again inside the building.

Go back out the front door and continue north. Note that you are now walking parallel to the north-south hallway, and the windows are those of the lower-grade rooms. As arranged, knock gently on the window of the student's own classroom. Talk briefly with classmates and teacher through the window. Look around near this window: what is out here? What view do classmates see through the window? Describe things that are far away or not easily examined by touch.

Continue all the way around the building. Continually discuss what rooms are being passed, at least in a general way. Discuss also what parts of the school grounds you are passing. Emphasize the Primary playground and the door leading to it.

When a particularly familiar room or landmark is passed, note any special characteristics. (For example, the gym windows are especially large; also, the siding is different because the gym was built after the rest of the building.) Whenever a main door is found, go in briefly and verify the location. Discuss compass directions at each corner.

End by returning inside at the same place you started – the east door near the upper grades.

EXAMPLE 2: *VIEW FROM THE INSIDE*
In a comparable manner, walk around inside the building and discuss what is outside.

In each major area which borders the perimeter, go into at least one room. Go to the window and discuss what is outside.

At each main door, step outside and verify what is there (e.g., kindergarten play yard).

RELATED PRACTICE: Make or study a tactual map of the building and grounds.

FOLLOW-UP: Work in a similar way with a building which has a very different shape.

IN THE COMMUNITY – OUTDOORS
BASIC

MODULE 46
WALKING INDEPENDENTLY
WHILE FOLLOWING SOMEONE

OBJECTIVE: The student will use his or her cane and walk independently over varied terrain, while following someone else by means of sound and verbal explanation.

AGE OF STUDENT: Preschool and up (see examples)

PRIMARY SKILL EMPHASIS:
Walking in company with others
In a crowd or a line
Sound direction and meaning
Varied terrain
Correcting a path
General travel

ADDITIONAL SKILL EMPHASIS:
Finding a person
Human guide
Stairs
Sidewalk
Obstacles in path
Communication and instructions
Carrying things
Attitudes toward blindness

SEE ALSO (Other Modules):
   Human Guide
   Carrying Things
   Walking Toward a Sound
   Auditorium or Theater
   Walking in a Line of People
   Visiting a Blind Adult at His/Her
      Workplace

FIGURE(S):

FIGURE 46-1: Following Independently

TEACHER PREPARATION: Find a location where the child can practice in a manner appropriate to his skill level. Select an interesting object or activity to approach.

REMARKS: Avoid referring to "following a sighted person." The leader could be a competent blind person. Instead, speak of "following someone."

ACTIVITIES:

EXAMPLE 1: *PRESCHOOL AND KINDERGARTEN*

"Here we are in Mr. Kopecky's yard. We're going to swing on his big porch swing. Follow me, now – you know your cane will tell you if there's anything in the way, and it will tell you what is under your feet. I'll keep talking as we walk along."

(Deliberately walk across both grass and sidewalk, and in a path where the child will probably encounter some small trees. Keep talking.)

"Now I'm on the *porch*. Did you hear how my footsteps sounded when I was walking up the steps? You'll be finding your way up here too."

Stand at the top of the steps and keep talking. The child finds the steps and comes up. Sit down in the swing and invite the child to join you. Enjoy swinging for a short while.

Repeat this three times. Each time, the child follows you down the steps and across the yard for some distance, then back to the swing again. Note the sound of the cane on the wooden porch.

On the third trip, the child is allowed to swing for a longer time as the lesson ends.

EXAMPLE 2: *PRESCHOOL THROUGH ELEMENTARY GRADES*

"Here we are on the sidewalk. I'm going to walk along the sidewalk, and I'd like you to follow me. I'll talk some, but mostly you will listen to my footsteps. I made sure not to wear soft shoes today; you can really hear my footsteps! We will stay on the sidewalk all the time, and your cane can help you find it...."

"I'll go straight ahead for awhile. Then you'll hear me turn, and you follow. Remember to sweep your cane to help you stay on the sidewalk, and to check in case anything is in the way."

Walk along briskly, making sure your footsteps are clearly audible although not unnatural. After awhile, turn onto a branch sidewalk.

Continue in the same vein, with the length and complexity of the activity depending on the child's ability and experience.

REMARKS: It is important for a blind traveler to be able to follow a sound while walking independently. However, as the child matures, it should not be necessary to hear a *constant* sound. The example below brings this out.

EXAMPLE 3: *ELEMENTARY GRADES*

"Today you're going to practice following me when you can't hear my footsteps well, and when I am not talking *all* the time. I'll talk a lot, but not every second. And I'm wearing tennis shoes, which are very quiet.

"I need to put a lot of things in my car, and I'd like you to help me. We'll each carry a load.

"Now, first we'll go out the south door and turn right, along the sidewalk.... [keep walking, but deliberately pause in your speech]... Now, here, turn left across the teachers' parking lot [pause in speech].... Yes, this way, straight ahead [pause].... that's right, keep coming this way [pause].... Here's my car. Thank you! Set things down here, please."

Thus, the leader alternates between speaking aloud or making some other sound; giving specific directions; and continuing briefly without being heard. This is a realistic life situation that works well. The leader should not need to talk constantly except for a beginner or a very complex situation.

Depending on the route, the follower may be behind or beside the leader from time to time, just as anyone would do. This practice is excellent preparation for following along with a group.

REMARKS: If this kind of practice is never done, some students become very dependent upon constantly hearing or touching the companion, and become frightened when they cannot.

FOLLOW-UP:
ALL AGES

Deliberately plan for the student to follow a person (with sound clues) from time to time. Urge parents to do this routinely.

An experienced student can follow comfortably almost anywhere, and need not necessarily take someone's arm. However, in a crowded and/or noisy situation, it may be simplest to take someone's arm in order to stay together easily. But the blind person should continue to use his or her cane.

DON'T LET THIS HAPPEN: A ninth-grade student followed me across a large parking lot to my car. "What's this?!" he exclaimed each time as his cane encountered a low concrete barrier, a grassy traffic island, and then a utility pole. He had expected to walk around parked cars, but was genuinely surprised to find any of these other things in a parking lot. His parents had always guided him completely around them. They had also encouraged him to surrender responsibility for direction. Despite the straightforward path to my car, this student had no idea how to return to the school building.

Don't let this happen to your students.

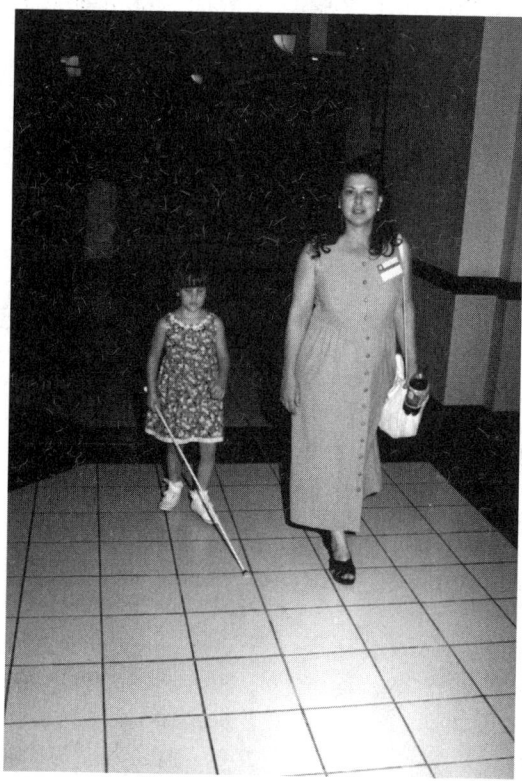

**Figure 46-1
Following Independently**

MODULE 47
SIDEWALKS

OBJECTIVE: The student will walk on a typical sidewalk at a normal speed. He/she will locate a branch sidewalk going right or left, turn onto it, and proceed.

AGE OF STUDENT: Preschool and up (see Examples)

PRIMARY SKILL EMPHASIS:
Sidewalk
Right and left
Compass directions
Moving straight ahead
Posture, grip, gait, and arc
Corners, turns, and angles

ADDITIONAL SKILL EMPHASIS:
Obstacles in path
Hills and inclines

SEE ALSO (Other Modules):
Sidewalk Flawed or Obstructed
Walking at Curbside
Recognizing the Curb
Around the Block
Walking Across Open Space
Right and Left
Compass Directions
Posture, Gait, and Arc
Description of Basic Techniques

FIGURE(S):
FIGURE 47-1: Avoid Following the Edge

ACTIVITIES:

EXAMPLE 1: *STRAIGHT, EASY WALKING*

A long, straight stretch of normal sidewalk is one of the best places to practice basic stance and stride. Help the student move ahead briskly.

Strenuously avoid teaching your student to cane the edge of the sidewalk, the wall, etc., with each and every arc. Instead teach her to move ahead and simply *notice* whenever she naturally encounters an edge or barrier. If she continually runs into the grass on her right, then she should keep a bit more to the left. If she bounces back and forth from one side to the other, she is correcting too much.

A beginner may practice walking from one end of the block to the other, turning around when she comes to the curb/street at each end.

Beginners under 8: With a very young or hesitant beginner, you may need to give extra guidance at first. Some students hesitate so much at first, with great uncertainty about what they are finding, that they move only a few steps at a time. It may be unrealistic to expect independence immediately. To help the young child get the idea, place your hand gently on her shoulder and move her along—at first most of the time; later, when she hesitates at an edge; then only occasionally.

EXAMPLE 2: *SIDEWALKS BRANCHING OFF*

The beginner can quickly learn to examine one side or the other to find another sidewalk branching off. She should arc the cane as usual, but extend the arc a little farther to one side to contact the edge of the sidewalk or the grass. The touch on the opposite side should be in the usual place.

It will be necessary to walk close to the side. (Note that when one is *not* looking for a perpendicular sidewalk or a doorway, one should *not* hug the edge of the grass or the wall.)

This is a good chance to work on right and left and/or compass directions. (However, with a young student who is still learning these concepts, avoid discussing too many terms at once.)

With younger beginners, don't expect too much too soon. With a young student, help her through this process one or more times—with physical assistance as necessary—before expecting her to proceed independently.

With a five-year-old you might say, "OK, keep caning the left side here, because we're looking for the little sidewalk that goes to Bill's door. On the left you're finding grass...grass...more grass...aha! What did you find on the left now?... Yes, you feel hard cement now over there. So we've found where we can turn left and be on another sidewalk. Go ahead, turn...now we have turned left. We're going along on the little sidewalk, and soon we will find the steps to Bill's house...."

Concepts and vocabulary: The beginner may need help to realize that she *is turning*. Even an experienced traveler, when faced with a gradual turn or many complications, may not always realize that she has turned a corner.

With an older student, mention various common terms for a right angle: 90 degrees; perpendicular; sharp turn; as well as simply "turn right" or "turn left."

Arrange experiences also with branches going at other angles, and discuss terms commonly used for that: off angle; partial turn; curving somewhat; angle to the right/left; etc.

Concentrated practice: Perform a door-to-door delivery project (actual or simulated) – i.e., proceed along the main walk for a given distance, walking up each branch sidewalk to each front stoop in turn.

EXAMPLE 3: *SIDEWALK IRREGULAR, BROKEN, OR ABSENT*

(NOTE: The Module, "Sidewalk Flawed or Obstructed" deals with this subject in detail.)

The student needs to realize that a sidewalk may not be perfectly regular, and that alert cane usage must continue. See that she sometimes encounters a broken or uneven surface; toys or bicycles left on the walk; a tree root pushing up a segment; etc.

Soon after beginning, provide experiences with walks that become wider or narrower, bend, or even disappear. Emphasize the student's overall understanding of where she is, proceeding in the desired direction regardless of distractions.

Emphasize overall orientation and the use of various clues. Traffic is a superb guide. Be aware of what is found if the traveler wanders too far to the side (on one side, a curb and the street; on the other side, yards or buildings).

If the walk widens, the student should not passively wander. Among other things, it may "widen" into a large parking lot. This illustrates the importance of *not* following an edge as a guide ("shorelining"). See Figure 47-1.

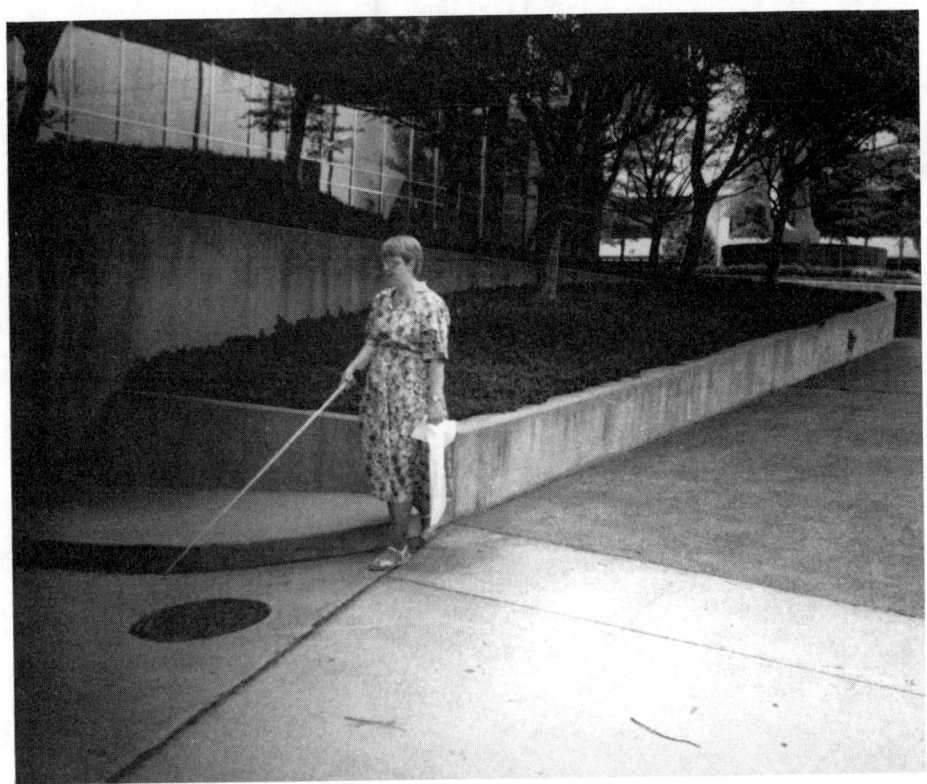

**Figure 47-1
Avoid Following the Edge**

Sliding the cane rather than tapping it is sometimes helpful when traveling next to a parking lot. There may be a substantial crack or ridge between the sidewalk and the parking lot. The cane may be slid across from one side to the other until it encounters the crack or ridge. This technique is of limited value, however, since a crack or ridge may not be detected easily.

If the walk narrows, the student may believe it has ended. She may assume that she is going the wrong direction. Help her to make a quick check to look for the walk, keeping track of the desired direction, and then proceed regardless. Emphasize (and practice) the possibility of walking on without a sidewalk – either on the grass or at the edge of the street. This may be preferable to a lengthy, confusing search for an elusive sidewalk.

Refer to "Sidewalk Flawed or Obstructed" for detailed suggestions.

EXAMPLE 4: *EXAMPLES IN DAILY LIFE*

Usually, in the course of instruction, some practice occurs in places where the student will frequently walk. Especially with a younger child, seek out such places and urge follow-through on the use of her skill. For example, can the first grader walk down to the third neighboring house, alone, and ask if her friend can play?

MODULE 48
AROUND THE BLOCK

OBJECTIVE: The student will walk around a familiar city block and recognize when he/she returns to the starting point.

AGE OF STUDENT: Four years and up (See Examples and Remarks)

PRIMARY SKILL EMPHASIS:
General travel (outdoors)
Compass directions
Right and left
Corners, turns, and angles
Communication and instructions

ADDITIONAL SKILL EMPHASIS:
Street crossing
Addresses
Maps
Orientation overall
Parallel and perpendicular
Street patterns
Sound direction and meaning
Traffic movement
Sidewalk

SEE ALSO (Other Modules):
  Right and Left
  Compass Directions
  Street Crossing with Little Traffic
  Street Crossing with Lights (Basic Skills)
  Non-Square "Blocks"
  Asking Directions And Figuring It Out
  Driveways, Alleys, and Streets

FIGURE(S):

FIGURE 48-1: Around the Block

REMARKS: A student of preschool age may not yet understand the concept of a city block. A somewhat older student in a very rural environment, or in a development with very irregular streets, may not understand the concept well either. However, an older student in an area with regular blocks should already understand the concept, even if he has not had experience in walking independently.

Be attuned to the student's age and experience. Try to give just the right amount of explanation about the definition of a block, the names of the streets, the definition of a "corner," etc.

ACTIVITIES:

EXAMPLE 1: *INTRODUCTION*
(See Figure 48-1. A square block is shown, bounded as follows: Maple Street on the south side, Fifth Street on the west side, Elm Street on the north side, and Fourth Street on the east side. The student's home is in the middle of the block on the Fourth Street – east – side.)

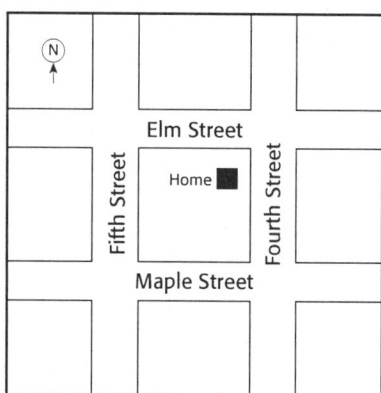

Figure 48-1
Around the Block

Go to the corner of Fourth and Elm. Discuss how you know you are at a corner – traffic sounds (if present), the curb, changes in surface, etc. Face north and imagine crossing Elm. Face east and imagine crossing Fourth Street.

Name the four streets surrounding the block.

To the extent appropriate for the student's experience, discuss compass directions. With a newly-blinded eighth grader, you might say, "We are at the northeast corner of the block. Now let's walk west... We are walking along Elm Street.... We are walking along the north side of the block...."

Note the sound and direction of traffic, if any. Occasionally ask the student to point toward the street itself and then toward the buildings on your own side of the street. Discuss what buildings are being passed. If this is the student's home block, mention familiar neighbors' names.

Note how driveways and/or alleys differ from the street. How do you know when you arrive at the corner of Fifth Street?

Proceed in a similar manner to note each corner and analyze each side of the block. When the corner of Fourth and Elm is reached again, be sure the student understands that you have returned to the same place.

EXAMPLE 2: *CONCEPT DEVELOPMENT*
(Fourth grade and up)

From the beginning, emphasize the compass direction which the traveler is facing as he goes around the block, together with his own left and right. If he is heading west and turns left, then he is going south; if he is heading south and turns left, then he is going east; etc.

Also stress that a person can go around a block by turning the same direction at each corner until he is back at the start.

The teacher may say, "Go west from this corner, to the next street; turn left or south and go to the next street; turn left or east and go to the end of the block there; turn left or north to the end of the block; and you will then be back here where we started." Even though the student may not fully understand and remember all of this description at first, it becomes familiar eventually if it is said enough times. With a reference point at the start, compass directions are correlated with turning left in this instance. From time to time, quiz the student about which compass direction he is changing to as he turns.

Before too long, proceed in a similar manner around a block by making four *right* turns.

In time, routes should often be assigned by describing only the compass directions, so that the student must understand and rely on the compass directions to complete the route.

Ask the student to repeat the directions before beginning the route. This helps you to find out how well the student understands, and to resolve problems beforehand. Students who cannot verbalize where they are going are unlikely to be able to get there. The requirement to repeat also causes the student to pay attention to directions more carefully.

It is interesting and helpful to equate directions with a map of the United States. ("You need to go toward Mexico.") Also, talk about the sun rising in the east, moving along in the southern sky, and setting in the west.

EXAMPLE 3: *CONCEPT DEVELOPMENT*
(Primary grades and below)

With younger children, avoid discussing too many aspects of directions at once. If the student is still learning such concepts, he will probably be confused by discussing all of these on the same day:

- Northeast corner of the block
- Walking west
- Turning left
- Walking on the south side of Elm Street
- North side of the block
- Traffic moving east on Elm
- The street is to our right; buildings are on our left

To avoid confusion, select one (or a few) of these concepts to be discussed at a particular time. Gradually help the maturing student to integrate them so that he can discuss all of them at the same time.

EXAMPLE 4: *STARTING IN THE MIDDLE OF THE BLOCK*

Go around the block in a manner similar to the first example. However, start at a clearly-defined location that is *not* a corner.

In this example, the student's home is on Fourth, between Maple and Elm.

After returning, a young student may not immediately understand that he has covered the entire Fourth Street side, but in two segments — i.e., he walked from his home to Elm, and then later walked from Maple to his home.

EXAMPLE 5: *IRREGULAR BLOCKS*

Discuss any irregularities in the block, as compared to a perfect square. Are two sides longer than the other two? Are the corners perfectly square?

Walk around some other "blocks" that have noticeable deviations from a perfect square. Note that some areas do not have "blocks" in this sense at all.

Once a student is familiar with the idea of a city block, the concept can be used in giving directions even when the blocks are not perfect. For example, one might say,

> "From the bus stop to my home it's the distance of about three blocks, but only one cross street goes through."
>
> "Our house is back-to-back with the Smiths'; we have a fence in common. But if we want to go around the block to their front door, we can only go north. If you try to go around to the south, there's the creek."

See also the Modules, "Non-Square 'Blocks'" and "Irregular Streets."

EXAMPLE 6: *THE OTHER SIDE OF THE STREET*

Go to the corner of Fourth and Elm. Cross Elm. Proceed around the four sides of the home block, but on the *other* side of each street. Discuss as above examples.

REMARKS: If a student lives where there are no regular blocks, introduce the concept by the early elementary grades.

RELATED PRACTICE: A tactual map can be helpful and interesting, especially with a less mature student. This may be simple or detailed, as:

- Examine a square of thick cardboard and compare it to the city block.
- Glue a square of thick cardboard onto a background. Place a Braille label for each of the four surrounding streets.
- Examine (or make) a detailed map showing many city blocks. It may be the student's own city, or another city.

MODULE 49
STREET CROSSING WITH LITTLE TRAFFIC

OBJECTIVE: The student will cross an uncomplicated intersection which has little traffic.

AGE OF STUDENT: Preschool and up (see examples)

PRIMARY SKILL EMPHASIS:
Street crossing
Moving straight ahead
Correcting a path
Detecting step-downs or drop-offs
Sound direction and meaning
Traffic movement

ADDITIONAL SKILL EMPHASIS:
Compass directions
Right and left
Parallel and perpendicular
Right and left
Sidewalk

SEE ALSO (Other Modules):
   From House to Curb
   Recognizing the Curb
   Walking at Curbside
   Around the Block
   Street Crossing With Lights (Basic Skills)
   Stop Signs
   Driveways, Alleys, and Streets
   Rural Environment

FIGURE(S):

FIGURE 49-1: Desired Path, Crossing Fourth Street

FIGURE 49-2: Desired Path and Other Paths

TEACHER PREPARATION: When working near a school, inquire whether there are special crossing guards. Inquire as to when they are present, so that lessons can be scheduled with and without them. (See the last Example.)

STUDENT BACKGROUND: With a child of kindergarten age or below, often it is wise to provide considerable practice elsewhere before working on street crossings. Depending on circumstances, however, street crossings may start very soon – as soon as the second lesson. If the adult is right with a young child (even holding onto him), crossing a quiet street with help should not be difficult or frightening.

An older student may find crossing uncomplicated intersections to be easy and confidence-building.

In any event, the student should begin to cross streets with the cane within a few weeks of the first lesson. The youngest student can begin to listen to traffic and use his cane, even if an adult always holds his hand when near a street. If delay is too long, the student will form habits which are inefficient and exclude the cane.

REMARKS: A significant amount of traffic *helps* a student to know how the streets are aligned and to cross efficiently. It should *not* be assumed that a street with little traffic is innately easier to cross. This module should be used in conjunction with modules which include more traffic. With a very young child who would not yet cross busy streets if he were sighted, readiness-level practice with traffic is desirable (i.e., independence is not expected at this time, but the child becomes accustomed to crossing a busy street in an aware and alert manner.)

REMARKS: When a child begins to move around the yard and the neighborhood, parents sometimes ask the city to erect a warning sign saying "BLIND CHILD." However, a special sign tells everyone that blind children cannot manage as well as others of comparable age. An ordinary "CHILDREN AT PLAY" sign is adequate and avoids many disadvantages. Teach appropriate boundary cues, cane usage, and other skills as the child grows more mobile. See also the Modules, "Back Yard Boundaries" and "Back Yard (Overall)."

ACTIVITIES:

EXAMPLE 1: *PRESCHOOL OR KINDERGARTEN*

See Figure 49-1.

"You're doing a fine job of walking on the sidewalk with your cane. Today we're going to go a little farther. You'll walk along the sidewalk here on Elm Street, just like last time. But when we get near the corner I won't tell you to turn around. This time we will go on across the street. I'll keep hold of your hand while we are at the street, because you're just starting to learn. But I will talk about what we are finding, and you can start to learn how to cross the street.... We're going to cross Fourth Street....."

"Now, pretty soon your cane will feel a step down. There will be just one step, and that will be the curb at the edge of the street.... There! Did you notice your cane going down? We'll stop here a minute. I'll help you move your cane up and down a couple of times and feel that curb. Also, let's tap the sidewalk here, and then the street ahead of us...it sounds a little different. The sidewalk is very hard cement, and the street is 'blacktop,' a little softer."

"Now, listen carefully, please. Do you hear any cars?...No, we don't hear any cars or trucks or buses or anything. So we can go. Let's walk across together. Tell me when your cane finds the curb on the other side...."

"Yes, now we're stepping up on the curb. Your cane found it before your feet did. Keep your cane sweeping—there might be something in the way. Now we will keep walking for awhile here, on the other side of Fourth Street. That's the name of the street we just walked across: Fourth Street. We're still walking *beside* Elm Street. Point to Elm Street, beside us. It's on our right. On our left are some more houses. Now point back to Fourth Street, behind us, where we crossed...."

"Now we'll stop and turn around....Point to Elm Street beside us. We turned around, so it's on our left now. Point to Fourth Street—it's in front of us now, because we turned around."

"We will go on back now, and cross Fourth Street again. You tell me when there are no cars, so we can go ahead and cross—and then tell me when your cane finds the curb and we step up on the other side."

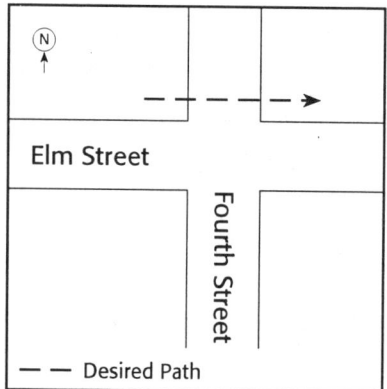

**Figure 49-1
Desired Path
Crossing Fourth Street**

REMARKS: With a beginner of kindergarten or preschool age, it is best to start with the concept, "We cross the street when no traffic is coming—we can't hear any traffic nearby." That is the the concept usually taught to very young sighted children—"Cross when there are no cars coming." A very young child is likely to grasp this idea before he learns to wait for a particular set of traffic to stop.

EXAMPLE 2: *ALL AGES*

The above example describes a typical first lesson for a very young child who has not been crossing streets independently. In proceeding through more lessons with a very young or immature child, avoid emphasizing too many concepts at once. For example, at first you might concentrate only on crossing the street and noticing the curbs, and not comment on directionality or street names. Later, you might emphasize left/right during some lessons, and begin to introduce compass directions during other lessons.

For a more mature student, much less help would be given, concepts would be developed quickly, and explanations would be in mature language.

The progression in regard to independence is as below, with each level encompassing anywhere from a few minutes to many weeks.

Preparation
An adult holds onto the child (or remains extremely close) at all times, while directing and explaining the activity.

Beginning
The adult holds onto the student less and less, but remains nearby. The child is guided to increase independence.

Independence With Guidance
The student crosses without physical or verbal assistance. (For as long as necessary, or as required by school policy, an adult continues to watch from a distance. The adult helps if there is a problem, and provides feedback to the student later.)

Flexibility and Competence
As the student becomes independent, he learns to handle more details and complications.

HINTS AND SUGGESTIONS:

(1) Some corners do not have a clearly defined curb. Instead, one can note a slight slope into the gutter (both from the sidewalk and from the street); a change in surface; and (if present) the sound of traffic. The student should experience corners with poorly defined curbs and with wheelchair cuts.

(2) If there is no traffic, the student may start to cross the street without realizing he is doing so. He may even arrive at the opposite curb before realizing he is crossing. Explain that this is not necessarily a problem, *if* the student remains alert at all times, and *if* he would not have proceeded upon hearing traffic. An experienced traveler does not necessarily *stop* at the curb; instead he may only hesitate slightly as he decides to proceed across.

(3) Sometimes one may step off the curb and *then* hear a vehicle approaching. If one has barely stepped off the curb, going back may be prudent. But if a person has walked more than a step or two into the street, going back is not only inadvisable but dangerous. The approaching driver assumes that a pedestrian will proceed in a consistent path, and steers his vehicle accordingly. If the pedestrian reverses his path suddenly, he is more likely to be hit.

(4) Walking straight across will require continued work. The student who walks briskly has a momentum which helps in walking relatively straight. Practice, with as much help as is appropriate, builds confidence and accuracy.

(5) One possible problem is veering into the street which is beside the traveler, and walking along in that street. In our Example, this results in walking *in* Elm Street — as in dotted line #1 in Figure 49-2 — instead of on the sidewalk beside it. To avoid this, one should deliberately angle very slightly away from Elm Street. A miscalculation in the other direction is not dangerous (going a little too far from Elm Street, as in dotted line #2 in Figure 49-2).

(6) Extreme overcompensation, however, could result in turning much too sharply. (See the two variations of dotted line #3 in Figure 49-2.) The traveler may walk along in the cross street (Fourth, in this instance), as in path 3a. Or, he may continue a curved path and return to the same curb from which he started, as in path 3b.

(7) A student may find himself walking along in the street, and be unsure which (if any) of the above errors he has made. Suggest the following correction:

Walk two more steps to be sure of walking far enough. Then turn 90 degrees and walk to the curb. The direction of the 90-degree turn depends on the position of the parallel street when the crossing was begun. If the parallel street was on the right (Elm Street in this example), turn left. Note that this will help regardless of which error occurred.

Similarly, if the parallel street was on the left at the beginning, the 90-degree turn should be to the right.

(8) When stepping up onto the opposite curb, it is important to sweep the area with the cane to check for obstacles such as poles. At the same time, however, impress upon the student that it is dangerous to remain in the street. Any exploring on the other side, such as looking for the sidewalk, should be done *after* stepping out of the street.

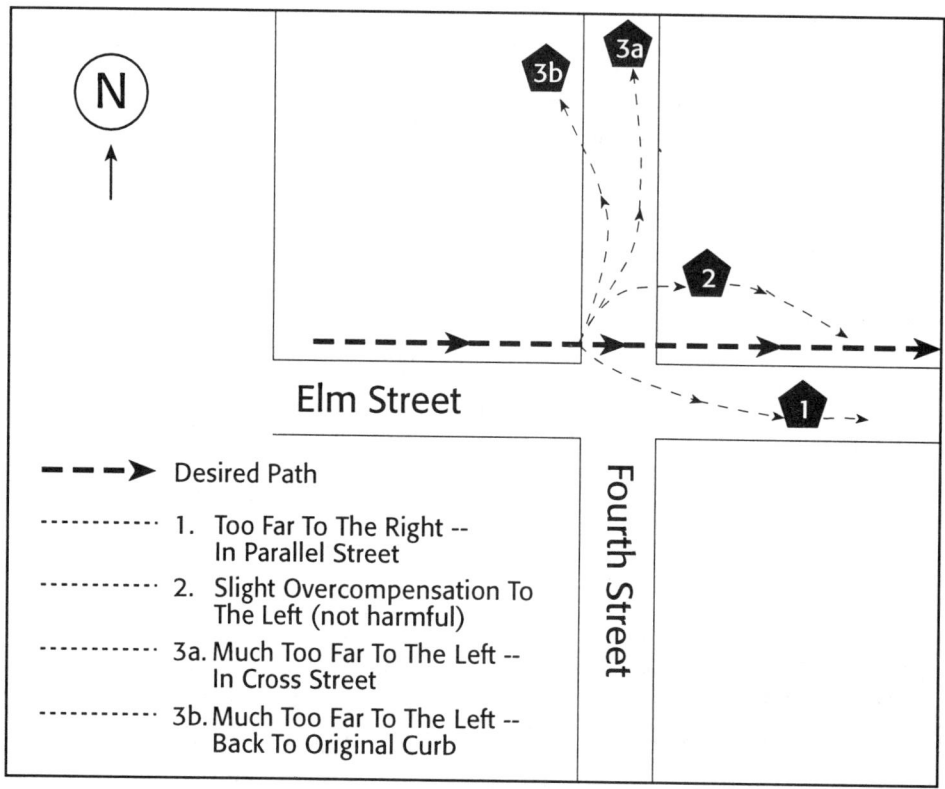

**Figure 49-2
Desired Path
And Other Paths**

EXAMPLE 3: *WITH SCHOOL PATROL GUARD*

Busy crossings near schools often have special guards while students are coming or going. They may be adults or selected students.

The blind youngster should have experience both with the guard's help and without it. However, it is very confusing to try to practice independent crossings while the guards are present. Instead, practice using their help while they are present, and practice crossing alone when they are not present.

After consultation with the principal, talk with the guards about the blind student's methods. If any special help is needed at first, explain it. If the student needs no special help, ask them to treat him normally. Watch the guards at work so that you understand their locations and procedures.

With a beginner, explain in detail. Conduct a practice session with yourself acting out the part of the guard (extending your arms, saying "Wait, don't go yet," etc.) Then practice with the regular guards.

With an older student, go over roles and schedules.

REMARKS: A relatively mature student may easily learn the basic crossing technique in one lesson. Continued practice, moving into more complex and varied situations, is important.

Avoid working for a long time on crossing streets with very little traffic. (A possible exception is a very immature child of preschool age.) The sound of traffic is an excellent directional guide, and helps greatly with the problem of walking straight across. Also, working for a long time on very quiet streets encourages the incorrect belief that crossing with traffic is extremely difficult.

MODULE 50
DISTINCTIVE SOUNDS

NOTE: This Module deals with recognizing and interpreting environmental sounds. The Module, "Walking Toward a Sound," complements this one.

OBJECTIVE: The student will identify [10] common sounds in the outdoor environment, and [10] common sounds in the indoor environment.

AGE OF STUDENT: Preschool and up

PRIMARY SKILL EMPHASIS:
Sound direction and meaning
General travel
Landmarks

ADDITIONAL SKILL EMPHASIS:
Air currents and echoes
Orientation overall
Weather and temperature

SEE ALSO (Other Modules):
　　Walking Toward a Sound
　　Distinctive Odors
　　Echoes and Air Currents
　　Meeting a Car
　　Rural Environment
　　Various "Street Crossing" Modules

TEACHER PREPARATION:
Note where distinctive sounds may be heard.

Be aware of the child's maturity level. Inquire about experience with particular sounds (e.g., dogs barking) and their associated experiences.

REMARKS: Usually a child will have had experience with environmental sounds while with her family. The teacher needs to give attention to this as well, however. A particular child may not have experience with a given sound because of individual circumstances or overprotection. Also, the teacher coordinates other skills with awareness of sounds.

Incomplete knowledge may foster unnecessary fear. A child who has been cautioned, "The lawn mower might run over you!" needs to realize that the mower will not collide with someone on the sidewalk. Similarly, well-planned practice overcomes fear of busy streets.

Usually, explanation and experience overcome fear. Children of kindergarten age and younger, however, sometimes develop irrational fears that cannot easily be removed. At that age, sometimes it is best to avoid a given situation as much as possible for awhile, and approach it again later. Sometimes, on the other hand, kindly firmness is necessary. Consult an early-childhood expert if a child seems extremely fearful.

ACTIVITIES:

EXAMPLE 1: *OUTDOORS: WALKING PAST A BARKING DOG*
(*Preschool*)
Note a location where a dog is confined but can be heard barking as a person passes by.

If the child tends to be fearful, approach this carefully and gradually. Walk on the other side of the street at first.

Walk along the sidewalk with the child. When the dog is heard, comment, "There's an animal inside the fence [or house]. It can't come out here. What animal is it?" Be matter-of-fact. If the child is fearful, be reassuring. Consider holding the child's hand for reassurance – a good illustration of the student's continued use of the cane while holding someone's hand for personal reasons.

Discuss how a person knows that the dog is restrained. Note city laws.

Arrange for students to meet and pat friendly animals. Examine a particularly calm dog all over, to understand body structure.

Discuss why it is generally unwise to pet a strange dog. If maturity permits, discuss what to do if a strange dog follows you.

EXAMPLE 2: *OUTDOORS: OTHER SOUNDS*

Call attention to common and less common sounds in the course of various activities. When appropriate, structure a lesson to emphasize a particular sound. Sometimes, as in the "dog" example, the emphasis is on identifying the sound and preventing confusion or fright. In other instances, the sound gives specific information for orientation. (Examples: the familiar bark of the neighbor's dog verifies that home is near; heavy traffic shows where Main Street is.) Certain sounds demand healthy respect and care to avoid hazard.

Below is a representative list:

- Lawn mower
- Street repair (jackhammer, pump, etc.)
- Traffic
- Trash collection
- Shoveling snow (with shovel or with snow blower)
- Hedge trimmer
- Chain saw
- Garden tractor
- Children playing in a yard
- Large group of children playing in a schoolyard. (The sound of a large group at recess can often be heard several blocks away. A preschool child can understand this, and can learn that the playground is silent when class is in session.)
- Flagpole with flag and cable
- Trees and other things blowing in the wind
- People walking, running, talking, shouting
- Car doors slamming
- Autumn leaves (being walked on, raked, jumped in)
- Bicycles, tricycles, wagons
- Lawn sprinkler
- Portable radio
- A truck backing up
- Birds
- Dogs barking
- In a very rural area, sounds would include various animals, a tractor, other farm equipment, etc.

EXAMPLE 3: *INDOORS: GYM CLASS*
(*Kindergarten and primary grades*)

When a young student is learning her way around the school building, distinct sounds from certain rooms aid in orientation. A good example is the sound of bouncing balls and shouting from the gym.

In this example, the first grade student is standing in front of her classroom door, listening to the travel teacher.

"Now I'd like you to walk to the third grade playground. When we get there, you may go outside and play on their equipment for a few minutes.

"Let's think which way to turn as we start walking. Remember which rooms we walk past to get to the third grade playground. There's one room that often has very loud sounds – I think I hear them now....

"Yes, that's correct – we will go past the gym. Do you hear those bouncing balls? And there's Mr. Inland's whistle.

"So which way do we turn?...Yes, you're turning left and going toward the gym....tell me when we pass the gym.

"Hmmm...we just passed the gym. I think you didn't say anything because it's quiet now. Let's stand still and listen carefully, and maybe we can hear Mr. Inland talking. The boys and girls are sitting down and listening while he explains the next game....We know we are near the gym, because it's at this corner. We can smell it a little bit, too – gyms have a special smell.

"The sound of the bouncing balls helped us for awhile, but we don't hear that *all* the time....We pay attention to a lot of different things to help us know where we are....

"Now, go on to the third grade playground and find the monkey bars."

EXAMPLE 4: *INDOORS: OTHER SOUNDS*

Below is a representative list of common sounds heard inside a school building.

Emphasize that most sounds are heard only intermittently and should not be relied upon as the *only* clue for finding something. A good example is a refrigerated drinking fountain which buzzes when the motor is on.

Also note that some sounds may be heard in more than one place (e.g., various clocks), and others may move around (e.g., the voice of a teacher who is not in his/her own room).

- Drinking fountain
- People walking in various directions
- Music (vocal, instrumental, radio)
- Computer and printer
- Gym class
- Voices of teachers and other staff
- Voices of children
- Rattling dishes in the kitchen
- Furnace, fan, etc.
- Clocks that click or buzz (continually or on the hour)
- Fluorescent lights that buzz faintly
- Rain, sleet, or wind on the roof or windows
- Doors being opened or closed

FOLLOW-UP: With an experienced student, continue to call attention to various sounds and how they help with orientation.

Certain sound patterns (notably traffic) are complex and varied, requiring ongoing study.

MODULE 51
DISTINCTIVE ODORS

OBJECTIVE: The student will correctly name [5] distinctive odors as they are found in the environment. He/she will demonstrate making use of odors as a clue in orientation.

AGE OF STUDENT: Preschool and up (see Examples)

PRIMARY SKILL EMPHASIS:
Interpreting odors
General travel (outdoors)
Landmarks

ADDITIONAL SKILL EMPHASIS:
Purchase or transaction
Orientation overall
Doors and doorways
Sidewalk
Daily living skills
Finding a person

SEE ALSO (Other Modules):
   Distinctive Sounds
   Lunchroom and Kitchen
   Grocery Store
   Restaurant
   Service Station
   Doctor's Office
   Malls
   Swimming Pool or Beach
   Utilities and Trash

TEACHER PREPARATION: Look for locations with a strong, localized, distinctive odor.

ACTIVITIES:

EXAMPLE 1: *PRESCHOOL*
The student walks on the sidewalk in the block that has the bakery. She is using her cane, but an adult is walking along. Discuss the scent and what it means. Help the child find the door, open the door, and walk in. Observe what items are for sale. Note the scent indoors. The child assists in making a purchase. A treat is enjoyed.

EXAMPLE 2: *PRIMARY GRADES*
The student walks independently along the sidewalk, noting the scent of the bakery. She finds the appropriate door with her cane, using scent as one of many clues to the location. She enters and purchases a small treat.

EXAMPLE 3: *FOURTH GRADE AND UP*
Walk around a shopping mall, discussing its overall layout and characteristics. Note scents such as:

   Popcorn stand
   Fresh-ground coffee
   Fudge
   Cafeteria
   Ethnic food
   Shoe store
   Bookstore
   Decorative pool or plantings

Attention to scents should be integrated with general travel skills; avoid over-emphasis on any one type of clue.

RELATED PRACTICE: Emphasize that similar scents may be noticed in more than one place – e.g., another bakery in the next block. Do not be misled by over-relying on scent and disregarding other information.

Note odors inside various buildings. Include the less obvious scents, such as tools in a hardware store, books in a library, and shoes in a shoe store. Also, the basic construction of a given building, together with the materials used in cleaning it, often provide a distinctive odor.

Note other odors around town and neighborhood, pleasant and unpleasant. Include seasonal ones such as lilacs. Over how wide an area is each scent noticeable?

How do wind and weather affect odors? In Cedar Rapids, Iowa, one can smell the cereal factory in certain parts of town and the syrup factory in another area. This varies with wind and weather. Some people complain about the odors. However, many say they are pleasant (or at least neutral) and make a person feel at home.

MODULE 52
ECHOES AND AIR CURRENTS
(Including "Facial Vision")

OBJECTIVE: In [3] appropriate situations, the student will explain how he/she is using echoes and air currents as one clue during travel.

AGE OF STUDENT: Preschool and up (See Remarks)

TEACHER PREPARATION: Look for locations where air currents and echoes are particularly noticeable.

PRIMARY SKILL EMPHASIS:
Air currents and echoes
General travel
Sound direction and meaning
Flexibility and confidence
Obstacles in path

ADDITIONAL SKILL EMPHASIS:
Corners, turns, and angles
Landmarks
Weather and temperature

SEE ALSO (Other Modules):
> Obstacles (Noting Them and Proceeding)
> Distinctive Sounds
> Apartment House or Condominium
> Unfinished Basement, "Crawl Space," or Attic
> Routes for New Buildings and New Classrooms
> Malls
> Rural Environment

REMARKS: Each activity described will vary in difficulty according to the air motion, the characteristics of the particular buildings, other sounds present, etc. It may not be the same from day to day. Try to find a particularly obvious and consistent example for a beginner. Help the advanced student continue to develop his sensitivity to echoes and air currents.

ACTIVITIES:

EXAMPLE 1: *PASSING A BUILDING*
The student walks past a building, close to it but *not* caning the wall. He notes the rush of air as he passes the end of the building. Also, the sound of the tapping cane (when on a hard surface) echoes off the building and results in a change of sound when the building has been passed.

Walk back and forth several times so that the student confidently notices the change. Practice passing two or more separate buildings in sequence and noting these effects as each is passed.

EXAMPLE 2: *UNDER A ROOF*
Approach a building entrance where there is an arcade (i.e., a low roof over an area outside the door, so that passengers can keep dry while getting out of cars in inclement weather). Call attention to the "closed-in" effect felt as the cane tip and footsteps echo under the arcade. Repeat and have the student tell you when he steps under the arcade.

EXAMPLE 3: *HALLWAY WIDENS*
Inside a building, walk along a hallway which leads to a more open area—e.g., a large lobby or a much wider hallway. Call attention to the change in echoes or air patterns. Repeat and ask the student to detect the change without caning a wall. He should learn to discern this with and without other people present.

EXAMPLE 4: *PASSING A SIDE HALLWAY*
Walk down a hallway and go past the place where another hall branches off. Help the student detect changes in echoes or air currents, indicating where the side hall is. Walk back and forth, as the student practices noticing the side hall without caning a wall. This should

particularly be practiced when there are not many other people present; if the student hears others turning the corner, he has another clue that obscures the one he is practicing.

REMARKS: The first two Examples (passing a building, and walking under an arcade) should not be hard even for beginners. The two indoor Examples may be too advanced for a young child who has just begun; however, they should not be difficult with experience.

The student might tap his cane a bit more loudly than usual while analyzing differences in a hallway. Do *not*, however, allow him to stamp his feet or make various sounds with his mouth or hands. Many blind persons, including those with partial sight, develop bizarre-looking habits to detect echoes. A cane, tapped appropriately, is sufficient. (NOTE, however, the importance of a metal tip.) Early training with the cane is important in preventing the unnecessary and unattractive habit of stamping the feet or making noises.

If a student has great difficulty hearing echoes in many different situations, consider the possibility of a hearing problem. However, if a student is already known to have a hearing impairment, do not assume he cannot make any use of echoes.

This Module tends to speak of "air currents" and "echoes" together or interchangeably. In a clear-cut situation such as passing a building while the wind is blowing, it is easy to tell just what is being noticed. Often, however, a person may not know whether he is actually hearing a sound or feeling a change in air pressure.

A popular myth suggests that blind people innately have a sixth sense to make up for the lack of sight. Some people do have a sense which is sometimes called "facial vision." It is the ability to sense objects, and is believed to be due to changes in sounds or air pressure. It can be useful, but is not necessary for good travel. It also can be inaccurate; thus some students will need to be told to ignore it. It is not mysterious or wonderful. A sighted person wearing sleep shades may have this sense, and some blind people do not possess it at all. It cannot be taught, but those who possess it may find it convenient in locating landmarks.

Usually it is not important to analyze all of this in detail. It is important, however, to develop the kinds of skills described in this Module.

MODULE 53
WALKING AT CURBSIDE

OBJECTIVE: The student will walk along beside a street, with or without a sidewalk.

AGE OF STUDENT: Preschool and up

PRIMARY SKILL EMPHASIS:
Obstacles in path
Parallel and perpendicular
Street crossing
Detecting step-downs or drop-offs
Sound direction and meaning
Sidewalk

ADDITIONAL SKILL EMPHASIS:
Right and left
Landmarks
Traffic movement
Varied terrain
Correcting a path
Street patterns

SEE ALSO (Other Modules):
　From House to Curb
　Sidewalk Flawed or Obstructed
　Recognizing the Curb
　Street Crossing With Little Traffic
　Street Crossing With Lights (Basic Skills)
　Rural Environment

TEACHER PREPARATION: Locate an area where the sidewalk (if any) is set back somewhat from the curb, and where there are a number of utility poles, signs, etc., near the curb. Also locate an area where there is no sidewalk but where pedestrians can walk safely in the street or on the grass.

ACTIVITIES:

EXAMPLE 1: *WHAT DO WE FIND?*
"Walk along on the grass (close to the street), for a block. Cane the curb or the street now and then to stay close, but be sure to make your cane sweep to both sides each time. The things you will find here help to show why it's important to make a full sweep with your cane."

The student finds utility poles, signs, etc., with her cane. She walks a block (or more) at a brisk pace without stopping. Then she walks along the same area, but stops to talk about each obstacle.

Examine each item; can the student tell anything about it? (For example, she should be able to identify a fire hydrant; recognize a sign as such, though she may not know what it says; recognize a utility pole.) Explain further as needed. Discuss the meaning of traffic signs. With utility poles, examine the guy wires (if any) also.

Note that it is indeed possible to walk without using a sidewalk. Why would a person do this? (If no sidewalk exists, or it is hard to find; if the sidewalk is being repaired or otherwise is blocked; etc.)

If there is a sidewalk, walk back and forth between it and the curb. In many areas, a strip of grass (often called the "parking" strip) exists between the sidewalk and the curb.

Traffic, if present, makes it easy to walk essentially parallel to the curb.

When crossing a street in this area, note: (a) It is always important to sweep the curb area with the cane when stepping out of the street; there may be poles or other obstacles. (b) It is *not* necessary or desirable to remain in the street while trying to find the sidewalk. There may be no sidewalk; and even if there is, walking on the grass is safer than standing in the street.

(Note: For an inexperienced student, reverse the overall procedure above. First, walk slowly and discuss each item in the way. Then ask the student to walk along the same route quickly.)

EXAMPLE 2: *WHERE TO WALK*
Walk in an area where there is no sidewalk. Walk for at least two blocks, with street crossings. Is there a curb?

Walk for awhile on the grass beside the street. Note how to stay near the street if there is no sidewalk:

> Listen to traffic.
> Cane the curb or street frequently if there is little traffic.
> Realize that if you veer far from the street, you will probably find gardens and houses.

Walk for awhile *in* the street (in a location where this is not dangerous). Keeping left is recommended for safety. To avoid walking in the middle of the street:

> Listen to traffic.
> Cane the curb or verge continually.
> Note subtle changes in the street surface as you move toward or away from the curb. The gutter area may have a different surface than the rest of the street. There is a downward slope toward the curb for drainage.

Discuss when you might choose to walk in the street or road, and when it would not be desirable.

CAUTION: With a young child who has little judgment, it is usually unwise to allow her to walk independently in the street. However, in some neighborhoods there are no sidewalks and everyone walks in the street. Consider the child's maturity in conjunction with the traffic patterns.

MODULE 54
STREET CROSSING
WITH LIGHTS
Basic Skills

OBJECTIVE: (*Preschool and kindergarten*) The student will indicate the direction in which a nearby car is going, and begin to tell whether a light is red or green.

OBJECTIVE: (*Elementary grades*) The student will cross an uncomplicated intersection having red/green lights and moderate traffic.

AGE OF STUDENT: Preschool: readiness and limited independence.
Elementary school and up: increasing independence as appropriate for age.

PRIMARY SKILL EMPHASIS:
Street crossing
Street patterns
Traffic movement
Sound direction and meaning
Parallel and perpendicular
Right and left
Corners, turns, and angles
Moving straight ahead
Correcting a path

ADDITIONAL SKILL EMPHASIS:
Compass directions
Communication and instructions

SEE ALSO (Other Modules):
   Around the Block
   Uncontrolled Intersection
   Street Crossing With Little Traffic
   Street Crossing – Developing Flexibility and Competence
   Complicated Street Crossings
   Street Crossing With Obstruction

FIGURE(S):
FIGURE 54-1: Crossing Fourth Street

CAUTION: Although a competent blind traveler is no less safe than a competent sighted traveler, everyone should exercise appropriate caution in traffic.

Assist young children and beginners as necessary for safety, with independence increasing as skills grow.

REMARKS: Talk with parents and other teachers about how much independence will be allowed outside of the lesson.

After school hours it is the parents, not you, who have authority to permit a youngster to cross a given street. Invite them to watch a lesson or demonstration, as preparation for their granting added privileges.

ACTIVITIES:

EXAMPLE 1: *READINESS*
(*Preschool*)
The youngest student can begin to listen to traffic and use her cane, even if an adult always holds her hand when in or near a street. The parent or teacher should talk with the child, explaining what is happening and gradually helping her to interpret traffic independently.

Sometimes, explain in full detail: "OK, now we are waiting to cross. We can't go, because cars are going back and forth in front of us." [Take the child's hand – the hand that is not holding the cane – and move her hand back and forth from side to side to imitate the motion of the perpendicular traffic.] "Our light is red now...."

"Listen – they are stopping.... Now we hear the cars beside us going." [Move her hand again, forward and backward to indicate motion of parallel traffic.] "Here we go; our light is green...."

Note: Wait until parallel traffic actually moves – an instant *after* the light turns green.

The child can then hear the change of directionality, understand what is going on, and start walking with the timing she will use when crossing alone.

Later, start asking the child herself to state when to cross. Just as very young sighted children do, she can call out "Green, go!" long before she is old enough to be allowed to cross alone.

(Note: A common misunderstanding occurs when parents think the child is "late" in recognizing the green light, when actually she is correctly noting when the traffic actually moves. When teaching a young child to understand what she hears, the adult should also call it "green" only when the traffic actually *starts:* an instant after the light itself changes. Otherwise the child and the helper will never quite agree, and the child will be confused.)

Provide prompting: "OK, now we are at the corner. Is our light red or green?... Yes, it is red, because the cars are going back and forth in front of us...."

"Keep listening....Yes, now it's green. Here we go. Listen to the cars going along beside us...."

EXAMPLE 2: *VOCABULARY*
(*Preschool and elementary grades*)
Children of preschool age may not know the word "traffic." It is best to say "cars" at first. Later, if desired, teach the term "traffic."

Similarly, younger children will not know the terms "parallel" and "perpendicular." (The youngest ones cannot even pronounce them!)

At first, speak of "cars going across in front of us" and "cars beside us." Supplement with physical demonstration, as with the hand motion described above.

Preschoolers may even be unclear about the meaning of "beside."

Practice with toys and stuffed animals may be helpful. Also note examples of role-playing, below.

EXAMPLE 3: *DIRECTIONAL CONCEPTS*
As with vocabulary in general, consider the child's age in relation to directional concepts.

A preschool child is still learning about right and left, and may have no idea of compass directions. She does not have the maturity to learn these in their entirety at the present time. This does not mean that she cannot start to cross streets. But it does mean that vocabulary must be simplified, and independence will be only partial at first.

The Example in this Module on "Pacing of Instruction" gives steps for gradually increasing independence. The teacher can use more and more sophisticated language as time goes on, and the student can do the same.

See the Modules "Right and Left" and "Compass Directions" for detailed suggestions for activities, many of which relate directly to street crossings.

EXAMPLE 4: *LISTENING*
Tell the student to listen closely and line up as straight as she can by listening to the parallel traffic flow. If she is wrong, correct her before she starts to cross. Then ask her to listen again to determine the parallel and perpendicular traffic. (When facing the wrong direction, the student may verbalize, "The traffic is running at an angle," without realizing *she* is the one who is crooked.)

If a beginner has trouble comprehending traffic movements at the intersection, move to the middle of the block and listen. A half block from a light, there will be notable stops and starts in the flow of traffic. With some practice in noting this change (in two directions instead of four), the student can more easily grasp the various directions found at the intersection.

EXAMPLE 5: *BASIC CROSSING*
Standing at the edge of the street, the student listens carefully. If she hears the traffic moving across in front of her, she knows her own light is red. If she hears traffic moving parallel to the path she plans to take, she has the green light. However, if she arrives in the middle of a green light, she should wait through a cycle until the light turns green again. (See Example below,

"Stale Green.")

In Figure 54-1, the student stands on the northwest corner of the intersection. She plans to cross Fourth Street, which runs north and south. When she hears the traffic on Fourth slow and stop, and the cars on Elm start to move east and west, the student begins to cross.

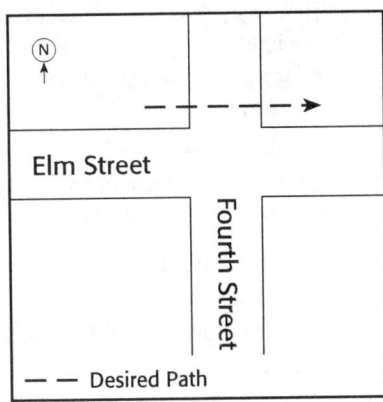

**Figure 54-1
Crossing Fourth Street**

She should move briskly and assertively. If she is very hesitant, drivers may genuinely doubt that she is really going to cross.

To cross correctly, the student listens carefully to determine direction, proceeds parallel to the traffic which is moving *beside* her, and continues to listen to the vehicles (including idling motors of stopped cars on Fourth) at all times. She walks as fast as possible, because she will get across faster and walk in a straighter path.

(Listening to the footsteps of other pedestrians is *not* a reliable guide. Many people cross at odd angles or against the light.)

Upon reaching the opposite curb, it is important to sweep the area with the cane to check for obstacles such as utility poles. At the same time, however, note that it is dangerous to remain in the street. Any exploring on the other side, such as looking for the sidewalk, should be done *after* stepping out of the street.

EXAMPLE 6: *DIFFERENCES FROM SIGHTED TECHNIQUES*

Explain to students and others that a blind pedestrian will not always cross in exactly the same way as a sighted person, and that this is all right. For example, people may worry if the blind traveler is not *exactly* on the marked crosswalk. Actually, as long as she is crossing in essentially the right area, it is not necessary that she walk precisely on the painted lines. However, by listening to where the idling cars are, the student can have a good understanding of the location of the crosswalk.

Similarly, the blind person's crossing may not precisely coincide with the timing of the "walk" light (if present), and this too is all right. The cane gives her the right to cross at a reasonable time. However, she must realize that she cannot count on immunity from danger solely because she is using a cane; it is necessary to pay attention to traffic and proceed carefully.

If there is so little traffic that she cannot determine whether the lights are red or green, she should simply cross as though there were no controls. Otherwise she might stand there forever.

EXAMPLE 7: *PHYSICAL STRUCTURE AND ARRANGEMENT*

Do not assume that a student – even one with considerable useful sight – understands all about the physical structure of an intersection. A tactual map or model is very helpful. Examine the map. Walk through the actual intersection and analyze various aspects. Ask questions to probe the student's understanding. Encourage the student to ask questions, making it clear that you will not belittle any question.

Does she understand where the crosswalk is in relation to the corner, and that lines are painted on the street? Explain that she need not be exactly on the lines, but should be in the right general area.

Does she understand about traffic lanes, again with lines painted on the street?

We speak of "the traffic light" at a particular corner. In fact, however, there are lights facing four different directions. Moreover, at a busy corner there are usually several complete fixtures, all operating together. Explain this, and examine things physically when possible.

Kindergarten classes often have model traffic signals which are low and accessible.

Examine the control box; discuss normal operation and possible malfunction. Note the clicking sound which can often be heard. The student should understand what this is, and realize that sometimes it can be an added clue to the changing lights. Emphasize, however, that this is only supplementary. It varies with different systems, may be heard on only one of the corners, and cannot be heard over loud ambient noise. Traffic, as always, is what the student should mainly attend to. (One instructor said, "Listen to the traffic—not the stoplight. No one ever got run over by a stoplight.")

EXAMPLE 8: *PARALLEL AND PERPENDICULAR*

Age 8 and Below

Most younger students (and some who are older) need considerable explanation and demonstration of parallel and perpendicular traffic.

Explain: "The *cross* traffic goes across in front of you—back and forth, like this.... *Perpendicular* is another name for the *cross* traffic. When that traffic is moving, it has the green light; therefore, your light is red and you do not move.

"The *parallel* traffic moves beside you, like this.... When it moves, you and the traffic both have the same green light, so you can move."

Listen to actual traffic. Examine tactual maps. Move model "traffic" around (using toy cars or other small objects, or simply tracing paths with the fingers.)

With a first grader we recently did some role playing:

> "Kari will pretend to be the cars going north and south on Fourth Street. Jim will be the cars going east and west on Elm. You [Gunar, the beginning student] will be the light; I'll stand with you and help you know what to do.
>
> "OK, now, your head is the traffic light... Yes, that's quite a silly idea, isn't it? Yes, pretty funny.
>
> "Your face is the green light facing north, and we also pretend you have a green light on the back of your head facing south. So when you're facing north, like now, the lights are green for Kari.
>
> "Go ahead, Kari. Show us the cars going north and south.... [Kari "drives" back and forth, north and south, making suitable traffic noises]
>
> "OK, Traffic Light, now you are changing colors. Your lights are yellow, and you are going to be facing the other way. [Kari screeches to a stop.]...
>
> "The green lights are east and west now, for Elm Street." [Jim "drives" back and forth, with suitable sound effects]....

This kind of demonstration is fun and very graphic. As necessary or desired, the person playing the light can operate with much or little help; roles can be exchanged; etc.

Over Age 8

Older students may benefit from a brief, age-appropriate version of role-playing. For example, I asked an 11-year-old to face north while I walked back and forth saying, "I'm the north-south traffic." Then she faced west while I walked back and forth saying, "I'm the east-west traffic."

EXAMPLE 9: *WALKING STRAIGHT ACROSS*

Detailed suggestions for walking straight across appear in the Module, "Street Crossing with Little Traffic."

The traveler must avoid two opposite errors—veering too *close* to the parallel traffic (i.e., walking *in* the parallel street instead of beside it) or too far *away* from it (i.e., wandering along in the cross street).

The presence of traffic actually makes it easier to cross straight. However, a student accustomed to quiet streets needs to learn to include additional information. She must pay close attention both to moving cars and to idling motors, so as to walk in the clear path between the parallel traffic and the stopped traffic.

EXAMPLE 10: *CAR IN CROSSWALK*

Provide experience with a car stopped *in* the crosswalk. Help the student to recognize this and to be careful without being frightened. If at all possible, it is much better to go around the front of the car, to maximize being seen by the driver. But if crossing in front would put the traveler into a busy stream of parallel traffic, it may be necessary to go behind.

The Module, "Street Crossing With Obstruction," has more detail on this subject.

EXAMPLE 11: *"STALE GREEN"*

After some experience, a traveler may walk toward an intersection and realize (before stopping) that the light is green. Discuss whether it is wise to simply continue without stopping.

My instructor called this a "stale green," and said that it was worse than stale bread. If the traveler starts to cross after the light has been green awhile, it will probably change to red long before she reaches the opposite curb. Therefore, tell your student to stop until the light turns red and then green again. Then she can step out just after the traffic first begins to move, on a light that is not "stale."

A short-timed light may still change to yellow before she finishes crossing, but she should be able to cross basically within the intended time.

A good rule is, "If you aren't sure about when to go, then don't go." There is no fire. There is no danger in waiting. Also, many beginners need extra time to line up straight by listening to the traffic patterns. The most important things to do before crossing are to listen carefully and line up straight.

An exception: An experienced traveler, approaching a familiar intersection and hearing the change to green as she approaches, may indeed correctly gauge whether enough time is left. But usually the rule, especially for beginners, should be "Never cross on a stale green light."

Position While Waiting: When the traveler is standing and listening at length, she should pull the cane up vertically to indicate she is not crossing. When she is ready to cross, however, she must not suddenly step out without warning. When the traveler is expecting to cross soon, the cane should be at the normal angle well *before* she starts to move, as a signal to motorists.

EXAMPLE 12: *SCHOOL PATROL*
(*Elementary grades*)

Elementary schools often have a "School Patrol." At busy crossings near the school, an older student (or an adult) stands at each curb, directing the children when to cross. (Typically, the guard holds his arms out to the side when the light is red. When the light is green, he steps aside, or may walk part way across with the children.)

Discuss the Patrol with your young student, possibly demonstrating with role playing.

You may decide to talk with Patrol members about the blind child's ability. Urge them to say something aloud when they release students to cross. Explain that the student can cross with as much independence as others.

EXAMPLE 13: *AROUND ALL FOUR WAYS*

Have the student go all the way around an intersection. Ask what color the light is at each point; insist that the student only cross at the beginning of a green light.

Ask her to describe the traffic pattern, including where cars are coming from and whether they turned or went straight. Emphasize compass directions, as, "That car was going north on Fourth and turned east on Elm."

Go around at least once clockwise, and at least once counterclockwise.

EXAMPLE 14: *TURNING TRAFFIC*

The student must understand that a turning car does *not* safely indicate when and where she should cross.

Readiness:

Help beginners recognize whether a car is turning or proceeding straight ahead. Stand at the corner (with cane pulled up vertically, to indicate that one is not crossing) and listen through several cycles. Discuss the direction of various vehicles. Help the student move her hand to indicate motion, including turning—this is particularly graphic and helps you know how well she understands.

Such practice helps to prevent the beginner's following a car's path around a corner, instead of proceeding in the straight path desired.

When to step out:
When the traveler hears the parallel traffic beside her start up, she should not actually step out until the first car has gone far enough to make it clear that it is going straight. Otherwise, the vehicle might be making "right turn on red," in which case pedestrians do not have a green light either.

She should step out when the majority of traffic moves, or the straight traffic, rather than when she hears a single car start up. She must listen to *all* of the traffic, not just a single car which may be about to turn.

Emphasize that the movements of other pedestrians are *not* a reliable guide.

EXAMPLE 15: *PACING OF INSTRUCTION*

Pacing is an important responsibility of the teacher.

One student may be thrilled at emerging independence and eager to cross many times during the first lesson. Another may be very fearful and reluctant. Most are somewhere in between.

Observe the student to see what she does when things do not go right; watch for signs of fear or poor judgment. Provide coaching and physical assistance as needed.

Younger students, especially, often cannot grasp all aspects at once. But this is no excuse for putting off instruction altogether. Instead, provide help with one or more aspects while expecting the student to handle others. Following is a good sequence for gradually increasing independence.

This sequence may be completed in a lesson or two for a mature student. A preschool student will probably not achieve full independence at that age; but proceeding part way through the sequence provides a basis for fast progress later.

The Module, "Street Crossing with Little Traffic" has many suggestions also relevant here.

Sequence for Increasing Independence
- The student takes your arm (using the human-guide technique), and walks across with you while you explain traffic movements.
- The student helps to decide when to start across. While walking across with you, the student explains traffic movements.
- The student decides when to start across, and does not take your arm. However, you walk behind with your hand on her shoulder, gently guiding her path and encouraging appropriate speed of walking.
- As in the previous stage, you walk behind the student and guide her as needed. However, you place your hand on her shoulder less and less. If there are turning vehicles or other complications which the student does not yet understand, you tell her what to do.
- You walk close to the student, but no longer provide physical guidance. You continue to explain traffic patterns she does not understand.
- The student crosses an uncomplicated lighted intersection independently. She understands turning traffic.

NOTE: At all times the teacher expects to intervene if the student (a) is placing herself in danger which she is not prepared to handle, or (b) is having difficulty which is beyond her skill or maturity.

FOLLOW-UP: Incorporate lighted crossings into ongoing practice. Do not let your student become "rusty."

MODULE 55
STOP SIGNS

OBJECTIVE: The student will cross an intersection which has stop signs in one or more directions (with his/her own path protected).

AGE OF STUDENT:
Preschool and kindergarten: easy, familiar situations
Primary grades and up: Varied situations

PRIMARY SKILL EMPHASIS:
Street crossing
Traffic movement
Sound direction and meaning
Parallel and perpendicular
Street patterns

ADDITIONAL SKILL EMPHASIS:
Compass directions
Right and left
Correcting a path
Maps

SEE ALSO (Other Modules):
> Around the Block
> Uncontrolled Intersection
> Street Crossing With Little Traffic
> Street Crossing With Lights – Basic Skills
> Street Crossing – Developing Flexibility and
>   Competence
> Driveways, Alleys, and Streets
> Rural Environment

FIGURE(S):
FIGURE 55-1: Four-Way Stop
FIGURE 55-2: Series of Two-Way Stops

ACTIVITIES:

EXAMPLE 1: *COMPARISON WITH LIGHTED CROSSING*
At a light-controlled intersection with considerable traffic, there is a clear-cut flow in one direction and then a clear-cut change. Listening to this pattern helps a student to understand the pattern of an intersection with a stop sign. You might say, "With a light, several cars move in one direction, then several in another direction. It's like that with a stop sign, except that only *one* car goes at a time."

Comparison with lights is helpful even if that kind of crossing is not yet on the program for the child to learn. The student can walk through a light-controlled intersection for readiness and observation – i.e., listen, discuss, and cross with the teacher.

EXAMPLE 2: *FOUR-WAY STOP*
Explain that *every* approach to this intersection has a stop sign. Traffic in each direction is stop-and-go, in a seemingly random pattern. (See Figure 55-1.)

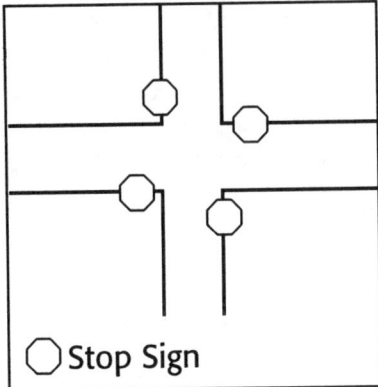

Figure 55-1
Four-Way Stop

Walk through one or more crossings with the student, discussing what is heard. Stand at the curb and listen for awhile. (Note, however, that motorists will tend to wait, expecting you and the student to cross. You may wish to wave them on.)

For independent crossing, the student listens to traffic in the relevant direction and makes sure the vehicle really is slowing to a stop. He listens to the idling motor and uses other clues to make a smooth crossing to the opposite curb. (See the Module, "Street Crossing With Lights – Basic

Skills.")

With a four-way stop, no traffic should be moving fast. The student should realize, however, that a car from another direction may come toward his crosswalk. Clearly, such a vehicle *should* yield the right-of-way to a pedestrian already in the crosswalk. However, the student should realize the possibility of stopping in the middle if necessary.

Note that the sequence of movement is not consistent in the manner of a lighted crossing. If there is no car in a particular position, cars in other positions go ahead (as opposed to waiting for a green light).

Remind the student that if there is no traffic at all in the relevant direction, he should simply go ahead.

EXAMPLE 3: *TWO-WAY STOP*

Often a pedestrian will proceed for several blocks along a "through" street, with each of the side streets controlled by a stop sign. At each intersection he notes the "through" traffic moving beside him, listens for the traffic on the side street to stop (or verifies that there is none), and goes on to the next block. (See Figure 55-2.)

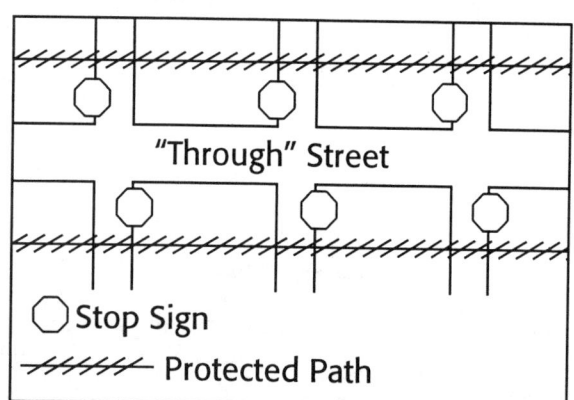

**Figure 55-2
Series of Two-Way Stops**

A two-way stop such as this can be quite easy even for a beginner. (See the Module, "Street Crossing With Lights – Basic Skills" for details on making a smooth crossing without excessive veering.) If the side street forms a "T" intersection, the principle is the same.

Since the traffic on the "through" street may be moving fast, turning traffic is a potential danger. Although he has the right-of-way, the student in the crosswalk should be prepared to stop or hesitate if he hears a car turning in front of him.

Use a simple tactual map to show a series of two-way stops. Explain that if you are walking along the busy, "through" street, the stop signs protect you and help you be assured of a smooth, undisturbed walk. (This is shown as a "Protected Path" in Figure 55-2.) But if you are walking along a side street (one of the less busy streets, where drivers stop for a stop sign) and desire to cross the "through" street, you need to be especially careful. Drivers on the "through" street have the right-of-way and are not expecting to slow down.

See the Module, "Uncontrolled Intersection," for discussion of crossing a "through" street.

EXAMPLE 4: *IS THE INTERSECTION CONTROLLED OR NOT?*

At first, the instructor will tell the student what kind of crossing to expect (lights, stop signs, uncontrolled, etc.) But a maturing student needs to learn to assess this for himself.

Listen with the student at a light-controlled intersection and then at one with stop signs. Contrast the patterns of movement.

As the student approaches an intersection, help him assess its characteristics while approaching. He may be well advised to stand and listen at the corner for a few moments, but he should have heard and learned quite a bit while still walking toward it.

Sometimes, give the progressing student partial information. You might say, "The corner is controlled in all four directions. But I am not telling you whether it has lights or stop signs. After you cross, tell me which it is."

The mature traveler should not need more detailed directions than would be given to anyone. For example, when getting directions in a strange city, a person might be told, "Turn left at the next corner, which is Forest. After about four blocks you'll cross Aurora – it's a very busy boulevard. The theater will be on your left in the next block after Aurora."

EXAMPLE 5: *ONE FAMILIAR, EASY CROSSING*
(*Preschool/kindergarten*)

With a very young child, it often is appropriate to work with one or two particular intersections near the home or school. In this situation, the teacher should emphasize the characteristics of that particular crossing. Too much information about crossing in general may confuse a very young beginner. At this age, it may not even be necessary for the child to understand the entire intersection (all four approaches), but only the specific crossing which he himself makes.

FOLLOW-UP: Discuss traffic laws and the concept of right-of-way. Discuss "Yield" signs and other variations. Provide continuing practice in many situations.

IN THE COMMUNITY
OUTDOORS
INCREASING SKILLS

MODULE 56
SIDEWALK FLAWED OR OBSTRUCTED

OBJECTIVE: The student will detect an obstacle in his/her path, proceed around it, and continue in the desired direction.

AGE OF STUDENT: Preschool and up

PRIMARY SKILL EMPHASIS:
Sidewalk
Varied terrain
Obstacles in path
Orientation overall
Correcting a path

ADDITIONAL SKILL EMPHASIS:
Weather and temperature
Hills and inclines
Air currents and echoes
Flexibility and confidence

SEE ALSO (Other Modules):
  Sidewalks
  Obstacles – Noting Them and Proceeding
  Rough Terrain
  Street Crossing With Obstruction
  Inclement Weather
  Rural Environment

FIGURE(S):

FIGURE 56-1: The Unexpected

STUDENT BACKGROUND: The very first lesson(s) on a sidewalk should be with a fairly regular surface, relatively free of obstructions or major flaws.

However, if the logical place for starting outdoor instruction (e.g., the sidewalk in front of a four-year-old's home) has an unusual surface, it may be logical to start there and deal with the flaw immediately.

Once the child gains some skill in easy situations, he/she should become accustomed to irregularities.

REMARKS: Often it is not necessary to plan specifically for these experiences. Flaws and obstacles are encountered in the normal course of things.

However, especially for a younger student, it is well to do some conscious planning. It is all too easy to arrange practice in "ideal" locations and avoid places that are messy or inconvenient.

Also, with a very young student the lessons may all occur within a limited area – e.g., the modern school building and the fine new sidewalks near it. Parents may lead the child around construction areas without comment.

If too much time passes without the student's meeting unexpected flaws, it becomes harder and harder to develop flexibility.

ACTIVITIES: As soon as the student has some experience with sidewalks, talk about flaws and obstacles. Recall any that have already been encountered. See that the student has experiences such as the following.

EXAMPLE 1: *HOLES, CRACKS, ETC.*
The student needs to detect holes, breaks, etc., well enough to avoid falling or otherwise having real difficulty. Any pedestrian may trip slightly on a piece of broken cement, or walk more slowly on a very uneven surface. The blind pedestrian should not have significantly more trouble than others. At times, sliding the cane from side to side may be preferred rather than lifting the tip during the arc.

Note various reasons for flaws. The cement may be old and cracked; a tree root may raise the walk and break it; construction may cause temporary obstacles or permanent changes.

Walk on a sidewalk/surface with overall flaws or irregularities. Examples include a very old, uneven walk; cracks with grass growing through; cobblestones.

EXAMPLE 2: *OBJECTS IN THE WAY*

Recognize that unexpected objects may exist at any time. Stepping on the object, or running into it, may harm the object and/or the pedestrian. For example, stepping on a skateboard can cause a painful fall.

If obstacles are never encountered, set some out occasionally on purpose. (Caution: Avoid inconveniencing other people, and always remove items promptly afterward.) Explain to the student that you would not place her in a situation for which she was not prepared, but that you would not be teaching properly if you never exposed her to obstructions.

Sometimes, ask the student to point in the direction where she is headed—before, during, and/or after going around an obstruction. (She should point in the conventional manner with the free hand, *not* with the cane.) If necessary, hold onto her hand as she walks along, keeping her finger pointing in the correct direction. ("This finger is your compass pointer. I will help keep it on target.")

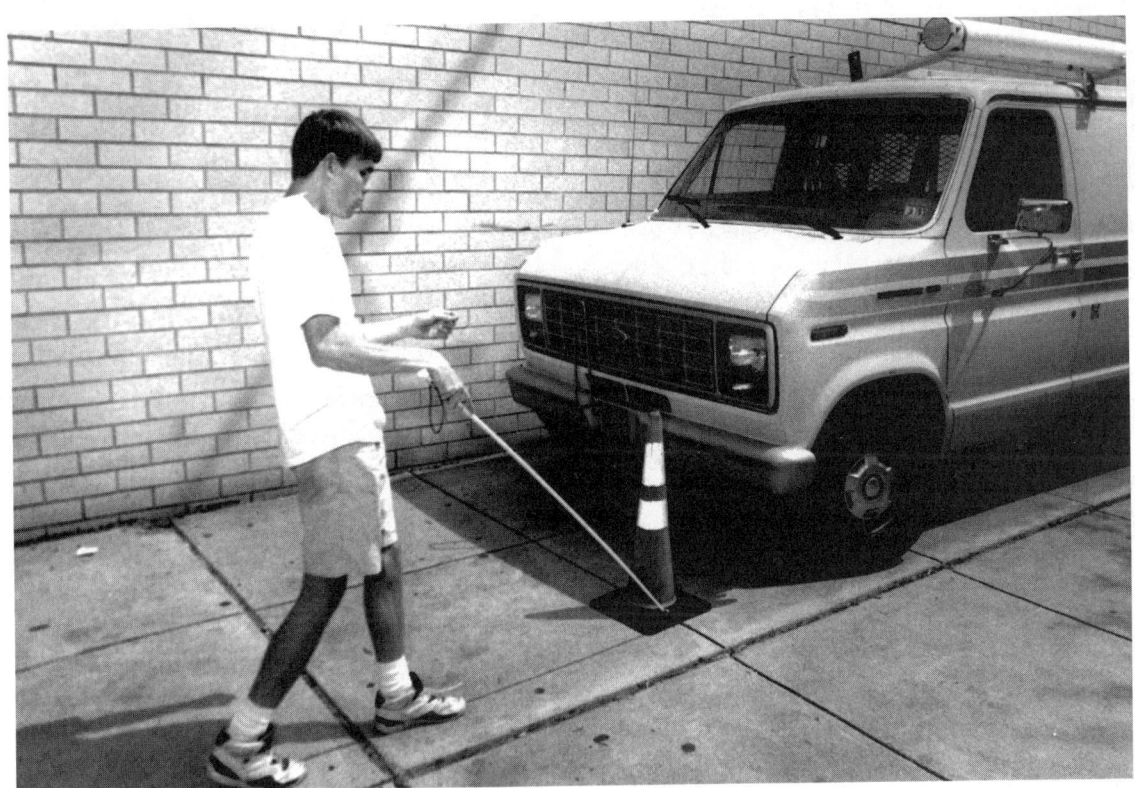

Figure 56-1
The Unexpected

EXAMPLE 3: *SIDEWALK WIDENS OR NARROWS*

(Or appears to do so)

The student must develop the ability to walk in a particular direction, reasonably straight. She should walk with adequate speed, not wobbling and wavering. She must *not* be dependent on following a sideline, such as the edge of the walk or the side of a building (sometimes called "shorelining").

Although following an edge can be one clue, it should *not* be the main guide for determining the direction of travel. If a person does become dependent on following a sideline (such as the edge of a sidewalk), there are many undesirable results. The edge may curve off in a non-desired direction, but the traveler will not notice if she is only attending to the edge itself. Also, there are many situations where there is no edge to follow. Students develop a false sense of security if encouraged to follow a wall or edge routinely.

Then, where there is no wall or edge, they feel frightened or at least unsure of themselves.

The sound of traffic is the best guide to direction.

Practice in Varied Situations
Go to a location where the sidewalk becomes narrower. For example, one building is much closer to the curb than the previous building is, and the walk suddenly narrows. The student begins where the sidewalk is wider, and proceeds past the change of width. She realizes that the width may change, and is able to continue in the desired direction regardless.

Go to a location where the sidewalk becomes wider, or appears to do so. The student realizes that this may occur, and that the apparent widening may actually be a parking lot or driveway. She continues in the desired direction without mindlessly following the edge.

The student remains alert to various clues to her location. For example, if she wandered into a parking lot, the surface might be different; there would be unexpected parked cars; she would be farther away from traffic. If she should wander up a driveway, she would come to a garage or yard. If she wandered down a driveway, she would notice a slope and then would find herself in the street.

EXAMPLE 4: *BARRICADES*
Recognize that if the sidewalk is blocked, it is usually possible to walk on one side of it. Practice walking on the grass. Walk briefly in the street when traffic is not extremely heavy, keeping close to the curb.

Occasionally (especially in commercial areas) construction may totally prohibit walking on the sidewalk or in the street beside it. One must walk on the other side of the street or take a different route. Advanced students should, if possible, examine such a location and note how it may be recognized. The approach to the sidewalk will be completely blocked, perhaps along with part of the street itself; there may be barricades some distance away to deter people from crossing toward the affected area. Sometimes a covered boardwalk is provided when a much-used sidewalk is blocked.

Take time to discuss how a traveler learns that there is construction:

- A fence or barricade
- Rope or tape around the area
- A hole or major irregularity
- Rough ground where the sidewalk should be
- Policemen or others giving directions
- Noise of jackhammers, etc.

Also discuss how to find the best alternative path, including the choice of crossing the street when there is no way through.

- Walk to the left and/or to the right to look for a way around
- Estimate the size and nature of the situation (e.g., slightly broken sidewalk vs. many large barricades)
- Ask construction workers
- Accept assistance from construction workers if it seems the best solution

A rope or tape is often strung right over the edge of the hole itself. This means that the cane tip will drop over the edge of the hole *before* the traveler actually encounters the rope or tape. Again, the importance of good cane technique is underscored.

EXAMPLE 5: *NO SIDEWALK*
In some places there are no sidewalks. Also, if a sidewalk is hard to find or extremely flawed, a person may choose not to walk on it for a time. Provide practice in walking on the grass near the curb. Emphasize that this is acceptable, and much preferable to lengthy efforts hunting for a sidewalk.

In some neighborhoods there are no sidewalks, but the streets have little traffic. The student can readily walk along in the street at the edge (preferably on the left if possible), keeping track of the curb with the cane. She should cane the curb continually to avoid drifting out into the middle of the street.

MODULE 57
VISUALLY CONFUSING APPEARANCE

OBJECTIVE: The student will discuss situations where alternative techniques are more effective than attempts to rely on inadequate vision. He/she will travel effectively with and without sleep shades in locations where the environment is visually confusing.

AGE OF STUDENT: Elementary grades and up

REMARKS: This is a special lesson which is sometimes helpful for a student with partial sight. The value varies greatly with the individual. Most students understand this concept as soon as they learn to travel confidently with sleep shades, and need no special demonstrations or practice. For most students, an occasional *discussion* about visually-confusing appearance will suffice. Daily life outside of lessons provides an abundance of situations where the cane will be used without the eyes being covered.

The activity below is irrelevant for a student who is totally blind or nearly so. You may, however, choose to discuss it with a totally blind student, especially if he has friends with partial sight.

FIGURE(S):
FIGURE 57-1: Visually Confusing Surface

PRIMARY SKILL EMPHASIS:
Detecting step-downs or drop-offs
Varied terrain
Attitudes toward blindness
Flexibility and confidence
Understanding vision and partial vision

ADDITIONAL SKILL EMPHASIS:
Posture, grip, gait, and arc
Moving straight ahead
General travel
Open space
Obstacles in path
Stairs

SEE ALSO (Other Modules):
Posture, Gait, and Arc
Sleep shades
Poor Lighting Conditions
Rough Terrain
Walking Independently While Following Someone
Unexpected Drop-Off or Step-Down
Swimming Pool or Beach

TEACHER PREPARATION: Look for places where the visual appearance of the surface underfoot is likely to be visually confusing, especially to someone with partial sight. Examples:

Decorative tile in a mall or lobby – conspicuous, contrasting colors in broad, irregular patterns
Sharp shadows on a sidewalk
A place where carpeting ends with strong contrast to the bare floor, and there might appear to be a step-down

This lesson as described works best when the area is not crowded with people. (Other variations, however, may be more effective when the area is crowded.)

STUDENT BACKGROUND: See Remarks

REMARKS: Many other lessons in this curriculum, and many situations in daily life, demonstrate "an obstacle or step-down which would not be seen reliably with partial sight."

This lesson illustrates the opposite: "a place where, with partial sight, there would appear to be obstacles or step-downs where actually there are none."

An *occasional* lesson like this (perhaps one lesson out of 20 or more) is sometimes helpful in (a) demonstrating the value of the cane, and (b) helping the student learn to *rely* on the cane in daily life (outside of lessons), when the eyes are not covered, and (c) contrasting efficient and easy travel relying on the cane vs. confusing and slow travel relying on partial sight.

Normally, during lessons a partially sighted student should wear "sleep shades" to cover the eyes, so that he positively will learn what the cane can do. However, an *occasional* planned demonstration or practice without shades is helpful to some students, especially younger ones. (See the Module, "Sleep shades," and the *Handbook*, pp. 182-184.)

ACTIVITIES:

REMARKS: Make a clear separation between this kind of practice and the regular lessons in which sleep shades are always used. You might label the combination work as "extra practice," and carry it out in a different location or at a special time.

EXAMPLE 1: At the South Mall, the floor tile has a striking black-and-white pattern. The colors alternate approximately every two feet, in irregular patterns. Here and there, a large circle appears in red. The student is not familiar with this mall.

Say to the student, who is wearing sleep shades: "Today we're going to have a different kind of lesson. We're going to do several things here at the mall. First I'd like you to walk straight ahead to the east end of the mall. I'll talk to you there."

At the east end, say to the student (who is still wearing sleep shades): "Tell me about what you found underfoot ... a plain floor made of tile, yes ... Anything in your way?... One pillar, yes.... Any steps up or down?...No...A very easy path to the end of the hall... You walked quickly; very good..."

Next, ask the student to cross the wide hallway and turn around to go back. Say, "Now, in a moment I will ask you to walk back in the other direction. You're on the other side of the wide mall hallway, and remember it may not be the same over here. You may find almost anything in a mall – steps up or down, pushcarts, pillars, fountains, all sorts of things – and of course, people. Today for awhile I'd like you to have an 'extra practice' session with your sleep shades off. Take them off, please, and walk to the west end of the mall."

As the student walks, observe whether he walks as quickly and easily as before, or whether he continually hesitates when he sees a color contrast in the floor.

At the end of the hall, if the student has proceeded briskly and easily, compliment him on relying on the cane to check the underfoot surface.

If he was hesitant, say, "OK, tell me about what you found underfoot this time...Yes, it looked like a lot of things to your eyes, but what did the cane find?...A plain level floor, yes. Again, a couple of pillars...No steps up or down, not even one...It turned out to be a very easy path, just like the other side. So this helps to show that your eyes won't tell you reliably what's underfoot.

"You know that when there actually is a step, you often can't be sure of it with your eyes. Well, here's the opposite – sometimes it will *look* like a step or something, but really will be just a color change. So the best thing to do is let your *cane* tell you what is really there.

"You walked about three times as fast with your shades on as you did without them, and you also went much straighter. Go back to the east end once more, please. Walk quickly, and rely on what your cane is telling you. Then put your shades back on, and we'll do some shopping."

EXAMPLE 2: Demonstrate the opposite situation, where there actually is an obstacle or step-down, but it is not reliably seen with partial sight.

REFERENCE(S):

Willoughby and Duffy. *Handbook for Itinerant and Resource Teachers of Blind and Visually Impaired Students*, pp. 182-184.

Richard Mettler. *Cognitive Learning Theory and Cane Travel Instruction: A New Paradigm*, pp. 66-106.

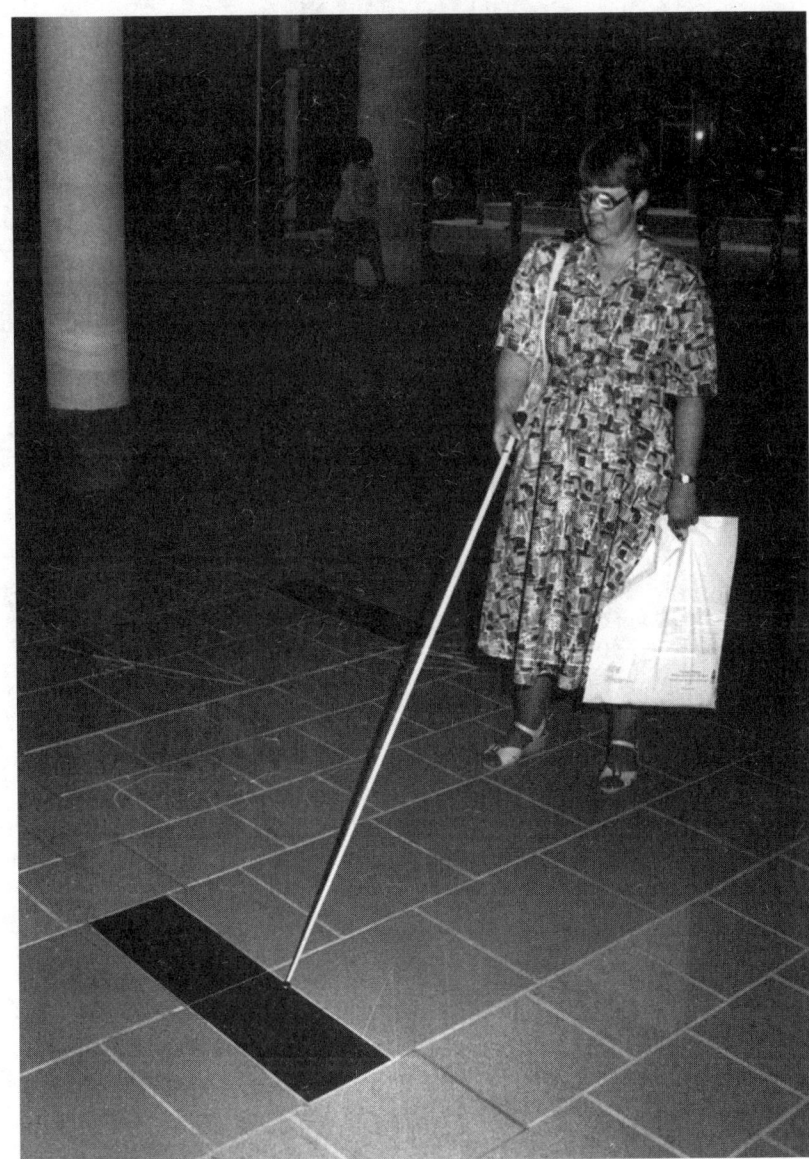

**Figure 57-1
Visually Confusing Surface**

MODULE 58
INCLEMENT WEATHER
Including Ice Underfoot

OBJECTIVE: The student will travel in inclement weather conditions, wearing suitable clothing. This includes walking on snow and ice [if applicable in local climate].

AGE OF STUDENT: Preschool and up (NOTE: Most of these Examples assume the student has learned to cross streets. However, experiencing inclement weather is important for very young students also. Most principles apply to any outdoor location. Also, walking beside a street, or crossing a street with someone else, provides readiness for future independence.)

PRIMARY SKILL EMPHASIS:
Weather and temperature
Varied terrain
Sound direction and meaning
Street crossing
Flexibility and confidence
Posture, grip, gait, and arc
Sidewalk

ADDITIONAL SKILL EMPHASIS:
Carrying things
Correcting a path
Air currents and echoes
Interpreting odors
Daily living skills
General travel (outdoors)
Hills and inclines
Obstacles in path

SEE ALSO (Other Modules):
   Rough Terrain
   The Great Outdoors
   Rural Environment
   Obstacles (Noting Them and Proceeding)
   Poor Lighting Conditions
   Carrying Things
   Sidewalk Flawed or Obstructed
   Echoes and Air Currents

TEACHER PREPARATION: Think about skills which the student has learned but may never have practiced significantly in inclement weather. Have plans in mind, ready to take advantage of weather conditions when they occur.

CAUTION: Be aware of any special health concerns – e.g., special sensitivity to cold; tubes in ears (water could enter the ear); etc. Be aware of general safety factors.

REMARKS: Consider discussing plans with parents and/or administrators, to prevent misunderstanding about why lessons are sometimes carried on in inclement weather.

It is easy for a blind youngster to fall into a pattern of avoiding all inclement weather. The stereotype of the "frail" blind person lurks unconsciously. A blind child may stay in while his playmates run through the rain or snow; a blind adult may be picked up at the door while others walk to the car. Help your student and his parents avoid such harmful overprotection.

STUDENT BACKGROUND: Appropriate clothing and other protection (umbrella, book bag, etc.)

ACTIVITIES:

EXAMPLE 1: *RAIN*
Find a time when it is raining significantly, but there is no dangerous lightning or hail. Suitably dressed, the student walks at least two blocks and crosses at least two streets with some traffic.

Points for discussion:

– How can you carry an umbrella (if desired) and still use the cane? It can be done. However, many people prefer to wear a raincoat and rain hat instead of using an umbrella, partly because it makes it easier to carry other things.

Help your student develop a personal preference.
- Sounds are somewhat altered by rain, often seeming louder. Vehicles tend to sound closer. Practice may be needed to avoid disorientation.
- If possible, step back slightly when waiting at the curb; vehicles may splash you.
- We may or may not enjoy walking in the rain, but it is often necessary.
- Study safety precautions for thunderstorms. For example, avoid taking shelter under a lone tree.
- Be extra careful around traffic. Drivers may see poorly and have less traction.

EXAMPLE 2: *WIND*

Select a time when there is significant wind. It may or may not be accompanied by rain or snow, but should not include dangerous lightning or hail.

The student walks at least two blocks and crosses at least one street with traffic. Practice turning left, turning right, and walking straight. Walk on the grass (or snow) as well as on the sidewalk. Go into and out of the school building.

Bring out these points:

- Wind can alter sounds. Traffic and other sounds may seem slightly different.
- The wind can "catch" a door and bang it against you or the wall. Be careful; grasp the door handle firmly.
- Young and inexperienced children may be nervous and need reassurance. (If appropriate, discuss how we identify and deal with a truly dangerous wind such as a hurricane.)
- Children with physical handicaps or very poor coordination may have considerable difficulty. Seek advice from a physical therapist or other expert.
- The wind may blow you enough to cause confusion in making a precise turn or an exact motion. It can blow you slightly off your planned path. Practice recovering.
- When carrying anything, hold on tightly. Try to wrap or contain things, especially loose papers.
- Watch clothing. Is a cap likely to blow off? Will a skirt blow upward at the street corner?

EXAMPLE 3: *FOG*

Fog may alter perception of sounds and odors. Sounds tend to be muffled. Industrial odors may be trapped. A temperature inversion may bring similar effects.

If waterways are nearby, listen to the foghorn. Students in other areas will enjoy learning about foghorns.

Explain the nature of fog. ("A cloud is made up of tiny drops of water floating in the air. A fog is a cloud which is down on the ground.") Discuss local characteristics of fog, such as typical timing.

Walk representative routes while fog is present. Take extra care because drivers cannot see well.

Discuss how a blind person can determine that fog is present. (Other people's comments; radio or TV; foghorn. Sounds and odors may change. Heavy fog may be directly perceptible.)

EXAMPLE 4: *SNOW*

Make a point of continuing outdoor lessons during the winter months. If necessary, make outdoor lessons very short, but do not omit them. Include the following:

- Walking on a shoveled sidewalk: How does the cane find the difference between the sidewalk and the snow on either side?
- A sidewalk that has not been shoveled: If the path is not well-trodden, the cane can probably detect the sidewalk through the snow. If the path is well-trodden, the cane will detect the relatively hard surface of snow or ice in comparison to the soft snow at the side. Remember that if the sidewalk cannot be found easily, you can walk by the curbside.

- Crossing the street: Snow may be piled up at the street; there may be a path through, or you may need to climb over. The curb itself may be buried. Slush in the street may alter the sounds of traffic and feel different underfoot. Traffic sounds may be generally muffled, especially in fresh snow. Emphasize the "whole picture" rather than over-relying on any particular clue.
- Holding and using the cane feels somewhat different while wearing gloves or mittens. Gloves permit more precise use of the fingers. Mittens, however, are warmer. Help your student develop a personal preference.
- Walking in snow or sleet that is still coming down: See "Rain" and "Wind," above.
- Remember that drivers have less traction and control.

Related suggestions about uneven terrain are found in the Modules, "The Great Outdoors," "Rural Environment," and "Rough Terrain."

EXAMPLE 5: *ICY SURFACE UNDERFOOT*

REMARKS: Parents should include walking on icy areas naturally and continually from the time the child learns to walk. As with any child, offer some support when the child is young, but expect that falls are not ordinarily harmful. As the child gets older, expect him to walk on slippery surfaces as others do.

TEACHER PREPARATION: As winter approaches, watch for places where ice is likely. Inquire about the student's previous experience with walking on ice. Plan to include specific practice on ice when the opportunity arises.

ACTIVITIES: Direct the student to walk through an area where an icy surface is present. With an inexperienced child, give help and reassurance as appropriate; hold the child's hand at first if needed.

Discuss how to get along on ice. Anticipate when and where it is likely to be present, and be alert. The cane can usually help warn of ice; there is a different sound and feel than with a non-icy surface, and soft snow is quite different. (Note that hard-packed snow is essentially like ice.)

Talk about how *all* persons tend to take smaller steps on ice, walk more slowly, and bend the knees slightly. Another thing to keep in mind is to put your foot down with weight centered on it. However, all of this should not result in overly-cautious and unnecessarily slow walking.

Practice walking in various slippery locations – sidewalks, street crossings, driveways, etc. Note that sidewalks may be very slippery without actual "ice," (as with a light dusting of wet snow – or even rain – under some conditions). Sprinkle sand and see how it adds traction.

If a sidewalk is very slippery, a person may prefer to walk *beside* it, with better traction on the snow or snowy grass. (A wide arc with the cane can keep track of where the sidewalk is, and check for improvement in the surface.)

RELATED PRACTICE: There are many enjoyable things which are not strictly "travel lessons," but which add to ability to move in a snowy or icy environment. For example:

- Ice skating
- Sledding and tobogganing
- Skiing (both downhill and cross-country)
- Sliding for fun without skates – on the level or on a slight hill. (Check before allowing this on a school playground – it may be forbidden.)
- Wading through deep snow
- Climbing on a snow "mountain"
- Making a snowman, snow fort, snowballs, etc. (Note: snowballs are generally forbidden on school playgrounds.)

In climates where freezing weather is rare, describe it. (When discussing it with a young child, offer ice cubes to feel as a comparison.) Is there an ice-skating or ice-hockey rink that might be visited?

MODULE 59
UNEXPECTED DROP-OFF
OR STEP-DOWN

OBJECTIVE: The student will detect step-downs and drop-offs with the cane, and proceed appropriately.

AGE OF STUDENT: Preschool and up (see comments in Examples)

PRIMARY SKILL EMPHASIS:
Detecting step-downs or drop-offs
Posture, grip, gait, and arc
Flexibility and confidence

ADDITIONAL SKILL EMPHASIS:
Varied terrain
Street crossing
Hills and inclines
Addresses
Communication and instructions
Doors and doorways
Stairs
Sidewalk

SEE ALSO (Other Modules):
> Posture, Gait, and Arc
> Description of Basic Techniques (Including Stairway Technique)
> Recognizing the Curb
> The Great Outdoors
> Rural Environment
> Bridges and Overpasses
> Swimming Pool or Beach

TEACHER PREPARATION: Look for places where there is a sharp drop-off or steep downward slope. Examples include: a steep hill beside a sidewalk; a parking lot three feet higher than the sidewalk; steps which interrupt the sidewalk and lead down to a basement office; etc.

If you plan to go to a place where the public does not ordinarily go, ask permission beforehand. (Example: the loading dock described below)

Consider the student's experience and confidence level in comparison to the surprise factor.

ACTIVITIES:

EXAMPLE 1: *STEEP SLOPE OR BANK*
Scene: A long sidewalk has grass on each side. For part of the way, there is a steep downward slope on one side.

Direct the student to walk south on the sidewalk to the end of the block. If he happens to cane the slope and remarks about it, immediately proceed with the activity below. Otherwise, at the end of the block have the student turn around to walk north, and give him directions according to his ability:

> (For a kindergartner or a nervous older beginner): "On the right is a hill. Find it and tell me if it slopes up or down."
> (For a student beyond kindergarten, with some experience): "There's something interesting on your right. Find it and tell me what it is."
> (For an older, advanced student): "Now turn right and walk across the grass. Stop when you find a driveway."
> [CAUTION: Before giving a student directions with a significant omission, as in the last instance, it is wise to make it clear that you may do so from time to time. Previous instructors may always have warned of "unusual" things.]

Have the student walk down the slope, using his cane, and proceed some distance at the bottom. Then direct him to turn around, walk back up, find the sidewalk, and proceed south to the end of the block. Then he should turn around, go north again, and look for the slope – i.e., cane past the edge of the sidewalk. When the slope is found, the student goes down to the bottom and back up again.

EXAMPLE 2: *LOADING DOCK*

Scene: The back door of a grocery store leads to a loading dock which is 18" above ground level. There are no steps.

Direct the student to walk out the back door, proceed to the alley, turn right, and go to Eighth Street. The alley will be easily recognized because it has a gravel surface. As you direct the student, include the degree of warning appropriate to his experience:

- (For a child below 7 years of age): This would be a "readiness" experience for which independence would not be expected. Stay right with the child and give close guidance at all times. A child of this age would not be at a loading dock unless closely supervised.
- (For a student in the early grades, or an older beginner): "Outside the door is a very large step-down. Find it with your cane and stop to talk about it."
- (For a student with considerable experience): "When you get outside the door you'll find something unusual. Be careful."
- (For an advanced and competent student, age 12 or older): Do not warn of the drop-off. However, be sure that he knows you might not warn him of such things. See comments above.

With an advanced student, say nothing until he arrives at Eighth Street. Then compliment him on handling the drop-off confidently.

With a less experienced student, stop and talk when the drop-off is found.

The student bends over as necessary, extending the cane to touch the ground. He sweeps the ground briefly to be sure it is safe to step down. (If desired, he also may walk around the dock to look for steps or a lower place to step down.)

"Is it safe to step down?" If the child is very small or multiply handicapped, the conclusion may be "no." (Go back in and go to the alley by another way.)

A child with little experience may need help and reassurance in climbing/stepping off. Practice getting on and off the dock several times.

An experienced person may anticipate that there might be a loading dock behind a store. However, the above example illustrates that the cane can find even dramatic and unexpected things. One need not be restricted to walking in "regular, normal" places.

EXAMPLE 3: *VERY HIGH DROP-OFF*

Find a drop-off where the cane *cannot* reach the ground. Recognize that climbing off is *not* safe. (Caution: if it is possible to fall off, hold onto a young child during this experience.)

EXAMPLE 4: *BASEMENT STAIRS, OUTSIDE*

Scene: The sidewalk in the downtown area is adjacent to the buildings, and usually is continuous and wide. But occasionally it is interrupted by steps going down to a basement. In walking near the building, the traveler suddenly encounters a stairway going down.

Direct the student, "Imagine, please, that you have asked directions to the drugstore. You were told, 'It's the first door from the corner.' Show me where the drugstore is."

[As in the Examples above, give the student an appropriate degree of warning–or no warning–that he is about to encounter an unusual step-down.]

When the student finds the steps, compliment him on recognizing them without stumbling. Walk down to the basement; observe that there is trash accumulated on the stairs, and the door is locked. The imaginary person giving directions was not counting this unused entrance when he said "the first door from the corner." Go up the steps and proceed to the first ground-level door, which is the drugstore.

(Alternate procedure: allow the student to proceed to the drugstore without interruption. Then return to the steps to discuss and examine them.)

Walk some distance back, and practice approaching the steps again.

Discussion:
- This is an excellent illustration of why it is important to keep arcing the cane well and paying attention.
- Sometimes a below-ground entrance is in current use. A person giving directions would probably mention that the entrance is downstairs.

VARIATION(S): Other examples of "unexpected drop-offs" include:
- Swimming pool
- Extra-high step or curb
- Edge of stage or platform
- Orchestra pit
- Tiered classroom or theater (including outdoor amphitheater)
- Approach to an apartment house via a small footbridge: if the traveler does not find the bridge, he abruptly finds a steep embankment
- Retaining wall

FOLLOW-UP: As the student gains experience, incorporate unexpected drop-offs in lessons from time to time. The competent traveler remains alert to this possibility. Even in a "familiar" environment, a person may encounter a step-down without expecting it. Distractions or obstacles may cause him to approach a step from a different angle or at a different time than he had expected.

REFERENCE(S):

Richard Mettler. *Cognitive Learning Theory and Cane Travel Instruction: A New Paradigm*, pp. 66-106, 116-117.

MODULE 60
WALKING ACROSS OPEN SPACE

OBJECTIVE: The student will walk across an open area for at least [20] feet, maintaining a reasonably straight path. He/she will use appropriate techniques to maintain orientation at the end of the open space.

AGE OF STUDENT: Preschool and up (See examples)

PRIMARY SKILL EMPHASIS:
Open space
Orientation overall
Boundaries
Correcting a path
Flexibility and confidence
Moving straight ahead
Orientation within a room

ADDITIONAL SKILL EMPHASIS:
Right and left
Corners, turns, and angles
Doors and doorways
Landmarks
Varied terrain

SEE ALSO (Other Modules):
> The Great Outdoors
> Rural Environment
> From House to Curb
> Back Yard Boundaries
> Back Yard (Overall)
> Orientation Inside New Classroom
> Playground
> Rough Terrain
> Swimming Pool or Beach
> Malls

FIGURE(S):
FIGURE 60-1: In a Large Room
FIGURE 60-2: Across a Parking Lot
FIGURE 60-3: Across a Grassy Area

TEACHER PREPARATION: Find one or more locations where a person might want to walk across a sizeable open space with few landmarks. A ball field or an empty parking lot is a good example for an older child. For the very young child, it may be a space of just a few steps.

STUDENT BACKGROUND: From the time a child starts to walk, she should learn to walk across open spaces of increasing size. The toddler can walk a few steps toward a person's voice, without expecting to touch things on the way. The preschool child should walk confidently across the middle of a familiar room and across the middle of the back yard.

ACTIVITIES:

EXAMPLE 1: *ACROSS THE ROOM*
(*Preschool*)
(See Figure 60-1)

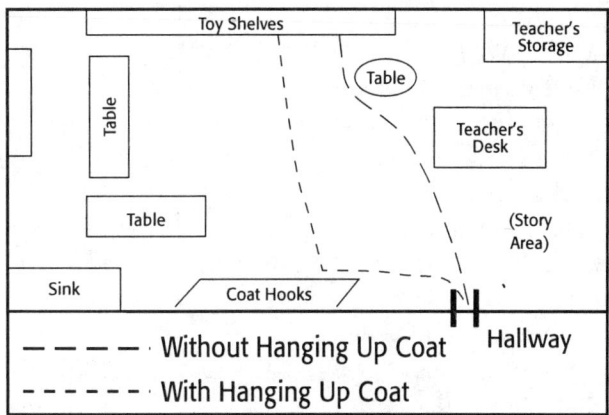

Figure 60-1
In a Large Room

This description assumes that a four-year-old is being introduced to her new preschool classroom before class begins. In a previous session, she has walked around the room, met the classroom teacher, and begun to learn what is in the room.

The cane travel teacher has decided to emphasize finding the toy shelves first. The child remembers enjoying them. Also, children are usually allowed to get a toy when first arriving at preschool.

The toys are along the wall which is opposite the door. If the child walks straight ahead from the door, however, she will encounter the teacher's desk. (The toy shelves are slightly to the left, along the wall.)

Today's session proceeds:

The child walks in from the car, holding someone's hand but also using her cane. As she approaches the preschool door, she canes the wall and finds the door.

"This is Mrs. Carey's door. Today I'm going to help you start finding some interesting things by yourself. Do you remember the toy shelf?....What were some things you played with last time?....

"Now I'm going to walk with you to the toy shelf. I'll hold your hand this time. We're going through the door....kind of straight ahead, but we keep just a little bit to the left. We keep on going....and what have we found? Yes, it's the toy shelf. Look at a toy and tell me what it is....Now, we'll do that again, and when we get back here you may stay awhile and play with a toy.

"Can you point back toward the door? I'll walk there with you. We'll go out and come in again."

The second time you enter, ask the child to walk to the toy shelf by herself. Instead of holding her hand, walk behind her and gently guide her by placing a hand on her shoulder occasionally. She continues to use her cane as she goes around a small table and then finds the toy shelves. She plays with a toy briefly.

Repeat once more, giving even less assistance. If the child goes the wrong direction, allow her to proceed until she reaches something substantial. Then help her understand where she is in relation to the toy shelf—for example: "OK, we're getting closer. You've found Mrs. Carey's desk. When you find her desk, you know that you're almost there, but you need to keep more to the *left* [touch the child on the left arm]. We'll go around the desk, on the left... find the wall... go some more to the left....and here's the toy shelf."

The child is allowed to play with the toys for a short while. Then she is briefly introduced to a slightly different relationship:

"Here we are at the door again. We're going to look at one more thing. We'll turn left as soon as we come in, this time, and go along this wall.... What are these?....Yes, these are the coat hooks where you and the other girls and boys will hang your coats. If you have a coat on, you'll need to hang it up here before you go over to the toys. Can you point toward the toys?.... [Correct the direction, as needed.] Since we already went to the left to get to the hooks, we are straight across from the toy shelf. Again now, we need to walk *across* the room to get there. If we find a table, we'll go around it. I'll walk behind you and give you a little help if you need it."

The above practice is a good introduction, but a child of this age will probably need much more practice before she can find the shelves reliably. Also, she needs to understand where other things are. After the class begins, everyone helps the child to grasp the overall arrangement of the room. They do not let her form a habit of always walking around the perimeter.

For awhile, she may receive help for part of the way across the room each time and then proceed by herself.

The cane travel teacher continues to give concentrated, planned lessons such as the one above.

EXAMPLE 2: *ACROSS THE PARKING LOT*
(*Intermediate grades and up*)
(See Figure 60-2)

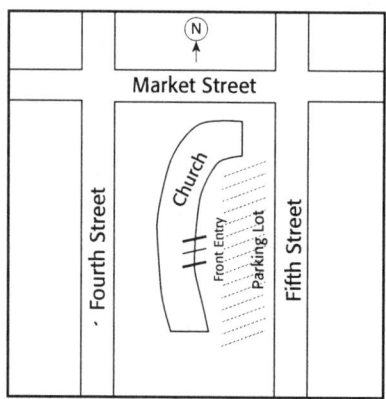

Figure 60-2
Across a Parking Lot

This example is described as for a fourth grader. It assumes the student has had experience in walking along a street and crossing streets.

"Here we are, leaving your church. As we stand in front of this door, we are facing east toward Fifth Street, in the middle of the block. There's a parking lot here, between you and Fifth Street. It's pretty empty today – hardly any cars parked.

"You will walk straight ahead from this door. When you find Fifth Street, turn left on the sidewalk and walk north. Go on north to the corner of Market Street. Turn west and walk on along Market. I will meet you at Fourth Street."

Emphasize walking briskly, arcing evenly, and maintaining good posture. If there is any traffic on Fifth Street, use it as a clue. (Extensive traffic would make this an easy task: simply walk toward the traffic. That is valuable practice, but the student should also practice crossing an open space when there is no consistent sound to walk toward.)

EXAMPLE 3: *ACROSS THE GRASS*
(*Preschool and up*)
(See Figure 60-3)

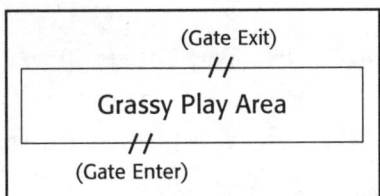

Figure 60-3
Across a Grassy Area

The student wishes to cross a grassy play area, exit through a gate on the far side, and continue on a short cut to her home. She has learned to enter at the first gate and walk toward the exit gate at approximately the correct angle. However, when she reaches the opposite fence she has difficulty finding the gate. Her parents consult you about helping her walk directly to the gate. They also ask whether following around the perimeter would be better even though it is farther.

A blind traveler should not expect to walk "straight as an arrow" across an open space toward a precise point such as the gate. Some correction should be expected. In this case, if the student reaches the opposite fence and does not immediately find the gate, she should follow the fence for a few feet to the left or right, and then try the opposite direction if necessary.

It *is* reasonable for the blind traveler to learn to walk in a fairly straight line so that the correction is relatively minor. Walking quickly and confidently is important; the slow and hesitant traveler wobbles and has no clear direction.

In some instances the student might choose to go around the perimeter if it is really more efficient. However, that should not be the only option considered. With practice, the student should be able to cross an open space of moderate size with little difficulty.

REFERENCE(S):

Richard Mettler. *Cognitive Learning Theory and Cane Travel Instruction: A New Paradigm*, pp. 107-120, 140-144.

MODULE 61
STREET CROSSING
Developing Flexibility and Competence

OBJECTIVE: The student will cross at least four different controlled intersections, each of which has considerable traffic, including vehicles turning in various directions.

AGE OF STUDENT: Elementary school and up (with increasing independence as appropriate for age)

PRIMARY SKILL EMPHASIS:
Street crossing
Corners, turns, and angles
Street patterns
Traffic movement
Correcting a path
Moving straight ahead
Parallel and perpendicular
Flexibility and confidence

ADDITIONAL SKILL EMPHASIS:
Communication and instructions
Sound direction and meaning
Compass directions
Right and left

SEE ALSO (Other Modules):
> Street Crossing With Lights – Basic Skills
> Uncontrolled Intersections
> Complicated Street Crossings
> Non-Square 'Blocks'
> Irregular Streets
> Street Crossing With Obstruction
> Stop Signs
> Compass Directions
> Rural Environment
> Street Crossing With Little Traffic

FIGURE(S):

FIGURE 61-1: Simple Intersection, One-Way Streets

FIGURE 61-2: Several One-Way Streets

FIGURE 61-3: Two-Way Streets, Turning Traffic

FIGURE 61-4: One-Way Streets, Turning Traffic

CAUTION: Although a competent blind traveler is no less safe than a competent sighted traveler, everyone should exercise appropriate caution in traffic. Assist younger children and beginners as necessary for safety, with independence increasing as skills grow.

REMARKS: Talk with parents and other teachers about how much independence will be allowed outside of the lesson. After school hours it is the parents, not the teacher, who have authority to permit a young person to cross a given street. Invite parents to watch a lesson or demonstration, as a preparation to granting added privileges.

ACTIVITIES:

EXAMPLE 1: *BASIC CROSSING WITH LIGHT*
The Module, "Street Crossing with Lights – Basic Skills" contains many suggestions which are applicable even for the most advanced student, but which will not be repeated here because of space limitations. That Module should be regarded as a foundation and a companion piece for this Module. When starting street crossings with a mature beginner, use age-appropriate activities and pacing.

If possible, start with an intersection which has fairly heavy traffic, a consistently timed light cycle, and a regular traffic pattern. However, any crossing where the student would normally cross frequently (e.g., close to home or school) is important to include quickly.

Some students need many lessons on the mechanics of crossing with lights. Use different lights when possible, to help the student generalize principles of crossings, and to eliminate boredom. After two or three lessons at a particular light, assign routes which include that light or a similar one. Always coach as necessary before trusting the student to cross alone in a new situation.

EXAMPLE 2: *DIFFERING CYCLES*

Not all traffic lights have the same kind of cycle.

Lights in large cities are often on a fixed cycle which is determined by the amount of traffic crossing in each direction. The east-west light may always be 20 seconds and the north-south light might always be 40 seconds. Once you have been through a cycle, you can estimate how long this cycle is going to be. A stop watch is not necessary; just count mentally to determine the length of a cycle. (A common method for counting seconds fairly accurately is to say, "one thousand one, one thousand two...")

Some systems vary their timing according to the volume of traffic. For example, lights in Alamogordo, New Mexico, vary from cycle to cycle depending upon the presence or absence of vehicles in turning lanes (as determined by sensors in the pavement), and also whether or not someone has pushed the "walk" button. Any part of the cycle may vary in length – or even be omitted – depending on how much traffic there is. A student should learn to recognize the variations for turning traffic, and should listen to cycles of the light with and without pushing the button.

Even without these sophisticated variations, the timing of cycles will vary from one corner to another.

EXAMPLE 3: *ONE-WAY STREETS*

Readiness

For a beginner – especially a young beginner – a carefully chosen location on a one-way street is an especially easy place to hear traffic start and stop.

Some students will need physical and tactual demonstration of the concept.

Ask, "How do the drivers know they must go only one way?" Examine and describe one-way signs.

Independence

For crossing independently, one-way streets provide less information to the traveler than do two-way streets. In Figure 61-1, the traveler wishes to walk north beside Fifth Street, which is one way southbound.

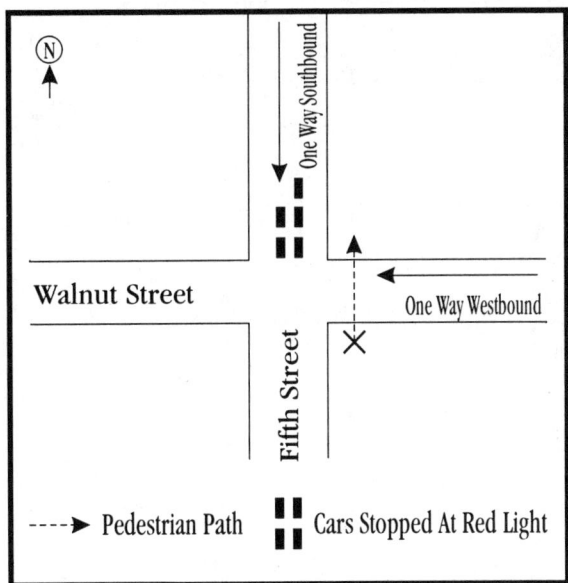

**Figure 61-1
Simple Intersection,
One-Way Streets**

As she waits on the southeast corner of the intersection (ready to cross Walnut), the only parallel traffic is waiting beyond the cross street (i.e., on the north side of Walnut). When the light turns green for Fifth, it is quite some time before that parallel traffic actually passes the pedestrian. A student may need to wait an additional light cycle to be certain that she is starting exactly parallel to that traffic.

Steady traffic in all four directions is the easiest to interpret because of the possible traffic patterns available for determining exact directions.

However, a pattern of one- and two-way streets can be a superb guide to location. Figure 61-2, for example, shows an adapted version of part of downtown Des Moines (a view which includes the intersection shown in the previous Figure). As a person walks north, she crosses the following: Court Avenue eastbound, Walnut westbound, Locust eastbound, Grand westbound, and Keosauqua two-way. If a student walking north desires to turn at Grand, but encounters two-way traffic, she realizes she has gone a block too far and reached Keosauqua.

Figure 61-2 also shows streets which intersect at unusual angles. This situation is discussed in the Module, "Complicated Street Crossings."

The Example, "Turning Traffic," below, includes more detail about one-way streets.

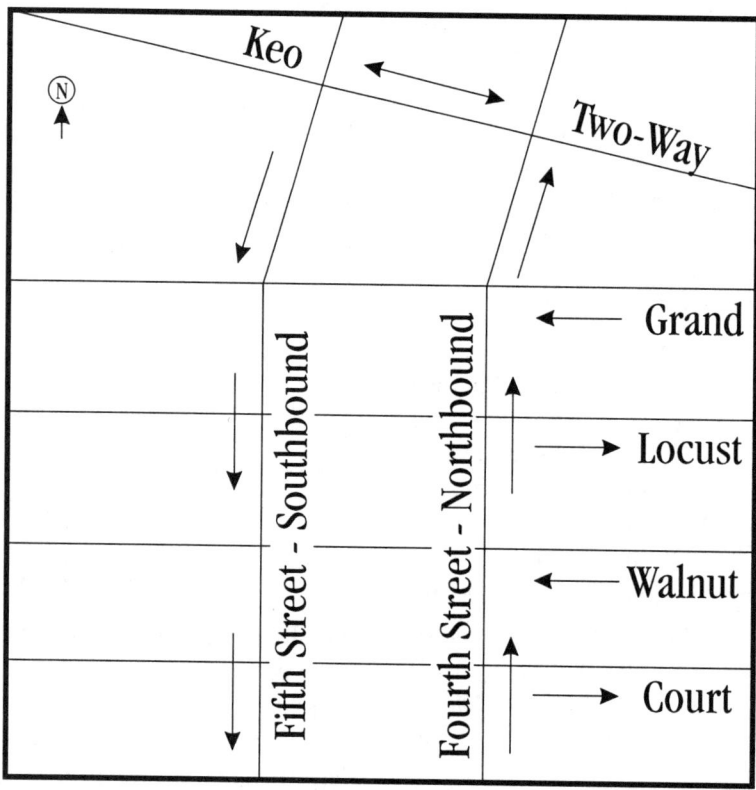

Figure 61-2
Several One-Way Streets

EXAMPLE 4: *"PRESS BUTTON TO CROSS STREET"*

Special school crossing lights

Many schools have a special light at the nearest crosswalk. It is operated by a large pushbutton on the pole. It may work only at certain hours and/or only with the pushbutton.

As with a regular crossing, the blind traveler should rely on traffic movement instead of unreliable clues such as sounds from the control box or from other pedestrians. (Exception: Directions from a School Patrol member should be followed.)

Sometimes a school light is in the middle of the block and relates to traffic on only one street. There is cross traffic only–no traffic parallel to the pedestrian. In this case, it is appropriate simply to wait until the traffic stops and then step out immediately.

Other pedestrian crossings

In some cities, certain poles at busy intersections have signs saying, "Press button to cross [Peach] Street." Pressing the button typically stops traffic and turns on a "walk" light.

This can be helpful to blind pedestrians as to others. However, there are some differences in timing.

The sighted pedestrian waits to see the actual "walk" light before proceeding. The blind traveler's crossing may not precisely coincide with timing of the "walk" light; however, this is all right if it does coincide appropriately with traffic movements. The cane gives the blind pedestrian the right to cross at a reasonable time. However, the traveler must realize that she cannot count on immunity from danger solely because she is using a cane; it is necessary to pay close attention to traffic and proceed carefully.

Also, the traveler should realize that buttons are not always present. Even when present, they may be oddly located and hard to find. Therefore, extensive searching for the button is not desirable. With occasional exceptions, failure to push the button results only in a somewhat longer wait for a favorable light.

EXAMPLE 5: *CURBS ARE VARIABLE*
The curb is *not* reliable as a way to judge what is "straight."

Most newly-constructed corners are rounded, and hence not straight across in front of the pedestrian. Often the curb is "cut" for wheelchair access. These and other factors make the curb an unreliable guide for determining when one has arrived at the street, or for facing in the right direction to cross.

Listening to traffic is the most reliable. If there is little or no traffic, the best guide is to maintain overall directionality (i.e., walking north along Elm Street), pay attention to all information available, and move briskly. A speedy traveler has momentum which maintains the desired directionality; a slow traveler wobbles and wanders.

EXAMPLE 6: *BICYCLES*
Bicycles are very quiet, usually only accompanied by a slight clicking of the gears. They observe traffic laws only slightly more often than the average pedestrian does. Sometimes there may be no traffic coming in any direction – except an almost silent bicycle.

Caution students about this possibility, so they can be listening for bicycles as they cross. Consider arranging for someone to ride by on a bicycle occasionally during a lesson.

Local situations may provide other examples of vehicles with little sound or unusual sounds – electric cars, horse-drawn carts, etc.

EXAMPLE 7: *TURNING TRAFFIC*
A. *Turning traffic is not a guide.*
The student must understand that a turning car is *not* a safe guide for when and where she should cross. As discussed below, a car may make a "Right Turn on Red." With one-way streets, there may be a "Left Turn on Red." Consider also the opposite kind of thing: a driver who has a *green* light, but does *not* proceed because he wants to turn and his path is blocked.

A car in the right-hand lane is always "suspect." Until it actually moves quite some distance, one cannot tell whether it will go straight or turn.

B. *When to step out:*
When the traveler listens to parallel traffic idling beside her, and then hears it start up, she should not actually step out until the first car has gone far enough to make it clear that it is going straight. Otherwise, the vehicle might be making "right turn on red," in which case pedestrians do not have a green light either. She should step out when the majority of traffic moves (or the straight traffic moves), rather than when she hears a single car start up. It is vital to listen to *all* of the traffic, not just a single car which may be about to turn.

Another way of expressing this is, "Let the first turning car go. That is, let a car near you cross. You can't beat him anyway; but go before the light cycle is too far along. If traffic is extremely heavy, it may be wise to wait a cycle and hope for better conditions the next time around."

C. *Which turns would conflict with your path?*
As the pedestrian proceeds in any given direction, certain turns by vehicles would conflict with

her path. Other turns would be compatible or even helpful.

As an example, consider Figure 61-3. Suppose that Fourth Street (running north and south) and Elm (running east and west) are both two-way streets controlled by lights. The pedestrian starts at the southwest corner, as shown, and wishes to walk north across Elm. When Fourth Street has the green light and she would be crossing, the following potential turns would conflict with her path:
- Northbound on Fourth, turning left
- Southbound on Fourth, turning right

At the same time, she realizes that when Elm has a red light, it would be possible for an eastbound vehicle to make a "Right on Red" and thus move through her path.

Thus, three potential paths for turning traffic would conflict with hers. Other potential turns would not conflict.

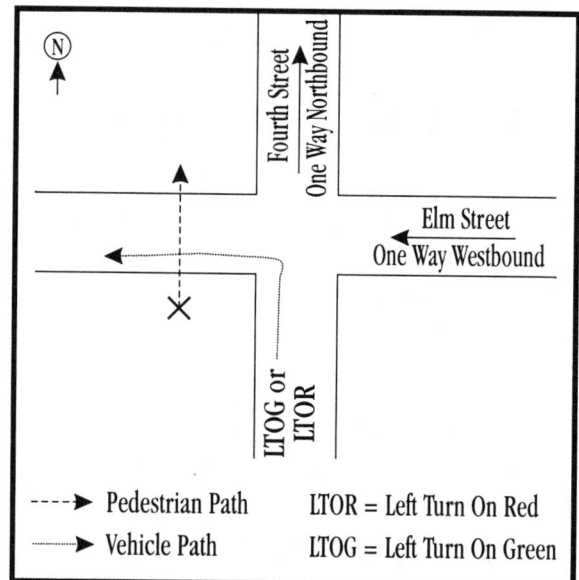

Figure 61-4
One-Way Streets, Turning Traffic

D. *Turning Traffic on One-Way Streets:*
A one-way street provides a simpler (but different) pattern. Suppose that, instead, Elm Street is one-way westbound and Fourth is one-way northbound. (Figure 61-4)

The only possible turns are left from Fourth onto Elm, and right from Elm onto Fourth. The latter would not conflict with this pedestrian.

Her only concern (with legally turning traffic) is vehicles coming north on Fourth and turning west. However, she needs to realize that (a) they will turn from the lane(s) nearest to her, rather than keeping to their right, and (b) they may potentially turn regardless of the light, if "left turn on red" is legal from a one-way street to a one-way street.

EXAMPLE 8: *WHAT ABOUT AUDIBLE SIGNALS?*

Unfortunately, some people believe that street crossings are impossibly difficult, and advocate various special devices to "help the blind." These may include buzzers or bird calls emanating from traffic lights, and various underfoot guidance systems. Such devices actually *cause* difficulty rather than improving opportunities, for a number of reasons.

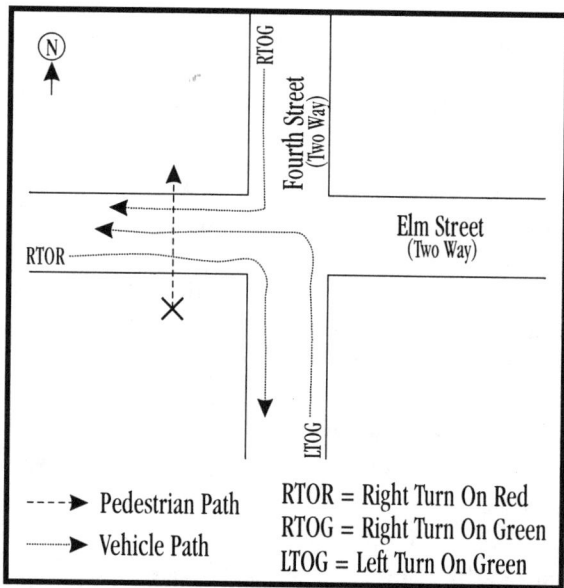

Figure 61-3
Two-Way Streets, Turning Traffic

They promote a false sense of security, discouraging the use of reliable methods for safe crossing. They encourage the idea that it is *not* safe for a blind person to cross at other locations.

If such devices exist in your community, discuss them with your student. If practical, cross at one of them; help your student rely mainly on traffic movements, as usual, rather than mindlessly assuming the signal will solve all problems.

Even when there are no special signals in your area, it is wise to discuss them, since your student will undoubtedly hear about such things. Help her realize they are unnecessary and even harmful.

(Note: The audible signals described here are *not* similar to the slight "click" often heard from regular traffic control boxes. Rather, they are loud buzzers or other unusual sounds.)

EXAMPLE 9: *THE "BIG PICTURE"*

Examples given here are somewhat simplified. Laws differ in various localities. There may be "No Left Turn" signs, lighted turning arrows, or other specialized signals.

At a potentially complicated intersection, it is wise to listen through a complete cycle before crossing. This lets the traveler grasp the overall cycle, orient herself to crossing straight in the desired direction, and decide upon the best time to cross. All the following factors must be taken into account:

- Cross (perpendicular) traffic movement
- Parallel traffic
- Turning traffic, in various directions
- One-way vs. two-way streets
- Light cycles and timing
- Unusual angles or patterns of streets
- Typical speed of vehicles
- Effect of nearby intersections (e.g., if there is a light at every corner, traffic may tend to move in batches and never get very fast)
- Residential vs. business area

Taking all available information into account, the pedestrian steps out at the most advantageous time. Since every kind of information is not always available, it is wise to keep in mind a hierarchy of preference:

Preference list for guidance in crossing

(1) First choice: Parallel traffic going in the same direction as the pedestrian. This is the first choice because this traffic is generally on the same light as the pedestrian.

(2) Second choice: Parallel traffic going in the opposite direction (e.g., traffic coming south when the pedestrian wishes to walk north). This is a second choice because sometimes the traffic may be coming from this direction in order to turn with a turning arrow, or to do something else unusual.

(3) Third choice: Perpendicular traffic stopping. This implies that the pedestrian's light is changing to green.

(4) Fourth choice: No traffic from any direction, and a *large* group of pedestrians starting in the desired direction.

(5) Fifth choice: No traffic and no pedestrians. It is safe to go no matter what color the light is.

Another way of expressing preference is, "Cross when you are least likely to be hit." Without scaring the student unnecessarily, impress upon her the importance of using good principles and being alert to all information.

Also emphasize proceeding in a sensible, predictable way. A good admonition is, "Cars are not trying to run over you, so if you are careful not to do anything they would not anticipate, you will be safe."

Particularly, the traveler must remember:

- DO NOT turn around and run back after crossing an entire lane.
- DO NOT speed up or slow down significantly (unless careful thought determines that this is indeed wise).
- DO NOT do anything unpredictable.

REMARKS: The various Examples above are not necessarily in a particular sequence for instruction. Depending on circumstances, certain situations will be dealt with right away, and others will be left until later.

Watch students carefully for the two extremes of (a) excessive fear and nervousness, and (b) stagnation due to lack of challenge. Pace lessons appropriately according to age, background, and general ability.

FOLLOW-UP: Incorporate various kinds of lighted crossings into ongoing practice. Do not let your student become "rusty."

MODULE 62
STREET CROSSING WITH OBSTRUCTION

OBJECTIVE: The student will detect an obstacle in his/her path, proceed around it, and continue in the desired direction.

[Also see Objectives in other Modules which deal with street crossing.]

AGE OF STUDENT: Preschool and up (see Examples)

PRIMARY SKILL EMPHASIS:
Street crossing
Obstacles in path
Flexibility and confidence
Correcting a path
Traffic movement
Sound direction and meaning

ADDITIONAL SKILL EMPHASIS:
Parallel and perpendicular
Street patterns

SEE ALSO (Other Modules):

Obstacles – Noting Them and Proceeding
Sidewalk Flawed or Obstructed
Street Crossing With Lights
Complicated Street Crossings
Alternate Routes Within a Building

FIGURE(S):

FIGURE 62-1: Parked Cars

FIGURE 62-2: Idling Car Near Crosswalk

FIGURE 62-3: Major Obstruction in Intersection

STUDENT BACKGROUND: When *first* working on a given skill, such as crossing the street, it is best that there be no major obstacles. A few sessions without complications are important in grasping the idea. However, if too much time passes without any unexpected obstructions, it will become harder and harder to develop flexibility.

From the beginning, the student should realize that a desired path is not necessarily without obstruction.

In indoor travel, see that unexpected objects are sometimes in the way. When practicing on the sidewalk, include situations with obstructions, in a manner similar to that below. See that the student deals with real obstructions without undue help. Set up artificial situations occasionally if necessary.

CAUTION: Avoid introducing artificial obstacles where substantial traffic is present. Never leave an artificial obstacle in the street when you are not immediately present. Always keep in mind the safety of the student and yourself, and also the safety and convenience of others.

ACTIVITIES:

EXAMPLE 1: *OBSTRUCTION (NOT IN STREET)*
(*Preschool and up*)
Discuss the concept of unexpected obstructions and why they exist.

Examine a minor hazard such as a pothole or a broken curb. Discuss when a hazard is major enough that the public should be warned. If possible, examine a location with an actual temporary fence or barricades around a hazard. Alternatively, discuss fences with which the student is familiar, and examine a sawhorse as a model of a barricade.

Make it clear that you, the instructor, will from time to time expose the student to an obstruction (or place an artificial obstruction) for learning purposes. You will not place the student in a situation for which she is not prepared; however, you would not be teaching properly if you always warned her of everything.

Practice with Sidewalk Obstruction
If no natural obstacle is available, place a sawhorse or other object, and ask the student to go to a destination beyond it. For an

experienced student, do not warn her. Provide feedback afterward about how well she dealt with the obstacle.

If the student needs extra help, give her warning and explanation as needed. Before and after reaching the obstacle, ask the student to point in the direction where she is headed. (She should point in the conventional manner with the free hand, *not* with the cane.) If this is very hard for the student, walk her around the barricade while you hold onto her free hand, keeping her finger pointing in the correct direction. ("This finger is your compass pointer. I'll help keep it on target.")

Alternatively, practice with an obstacle in a hallway or elsewhere.

The Module, "Sidewalk Flawed or Obstructed," deals with this subject in detail.

EXAMPLE 2: *QUIET STREET*
(*Preschool and up*)
Select a street with little traffic, where the student has the skills to make a routine crossing. Explain that you will simulate a barricade around a hole.

If placing a barricade seems impractical, obstruct the path yourself. Imitate a policeman, telling her to go around you.

EXAMPLE 3: *ACTUAL STREET REPAIRS*
(*Preschool and up*)
Seek out a location with a real barricade. If the situation is too difficult for the student at this time, walk her through it for the experience of a real situation.

Be alert for real obstructions in your community, and see that your student deals with some of them from time to time.

EXAMPLE 4: *PARKED CARS*
(*Preschool and up*)
Figure 62-1 shows Broad Street running east and west, and intersecting with 32nd Street (north-south). (33rd Street also intersects farther west.)

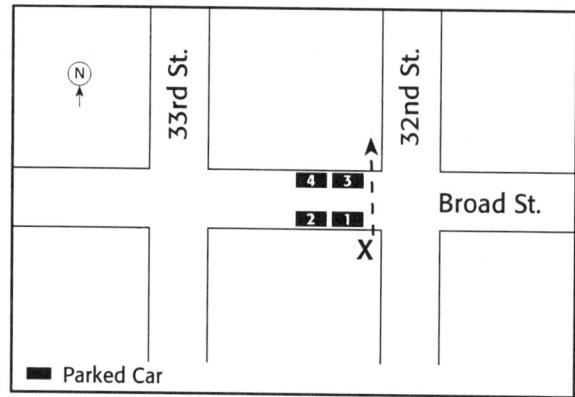

**Figure 62-1
Parked Cars**

At 32nd, a pedestrian wishes to cross from the southwest corner to the northwest corner. Cars are legally parked near the crossing: #1 and #2 on the south side of Broad, and #3 and #4 on the north side.

If the student encounters a parked car on the near side (#1, or perhaps #2), she should regard this as a clue that she is too far from the corner. Since she has not yet actually started to cross, she should move closer to the actual intersection before proceeding. In this example, she should walk to her right until close to 32nd, and then cross Broad in the crosswalk area.

If a parked car is encountered on the *far* side of the street (#3 or #4), priorities are different. It is important to step out of the street quickly. The student should go around the parked car, sweep the curb with the cane and step up, and then make corrections to the path as necessary. In this example, she should realize that she has already inadvertently started west toward 33rd. If she had *wanted* to turn west toward 33rd, she would simply continue west on the sidewalk. If she had instead desired to walk north along 32nd, she would need to go a few steps east.

Practicing with parked cars is easily arranged. It is a simpler task than dealing with idling cars, and can be included at a very young age.

EXAMPLE 5: *IDLING CAR BLOCKING CROSSWALK*
(*Elementary grades and up*)
The most common "obstacle" encountered while

actually crossing the street is an idling car. This can be frightening at first, and the student should have guided practice.

Figure 62-2 is identical to the previous Figure, with the addition of an idling car. Again, the pedestrian wishes to cross from the southwest corner to the northwest corner.

Car #5 is eastbound on Broad, waiting for the light to change at 32nd. It is shown as waiting correctly, just west of the crosswalk. However, this Example also discusses the possibility of its stopping farther forward and blocking the crosswalk.

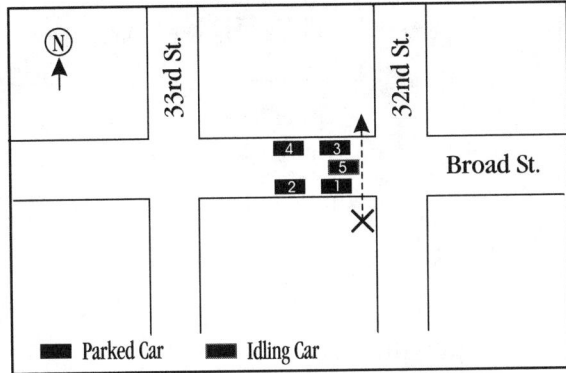

**Figure 62-2
Idling Car Near Crosswalk**

What Have We Here?
If the student starts to cross Broad and veers to the left, she may encounter the near side of Car #5. Help her realize what is happening and continue around the car. Ordinarily this means walking around the front of the car – the pedestrian gets into the normal crosswalk area, and the driver is most able to see her. It is important to keep track of where the car is, rather than wandering vaguely. The traveler must listen to the idling motor, and possibly tap the car gently with the cane as she passes, to keep track of where she is. At the same time, she listens to the moving parallel traffic on 32nd, to be sure she is not being forced too close to it.

If the street is wide, two or more cars may be waiting side by side. The sound of their idling motors is an excellent guide to walking in the correct direction.

No Room In Front?
Sometimes a car actually blocks the crosswalk. In this case, walking in front of it may result in walking into the parallel street and its moving traffic. (In Figure 62-2, if Car #5 were farther forward, it would force the pedestrian to walk in the stream of traffic coming south on 32nd with the green light.)

Walking in front of a stopped car is greatly preferable whenever possible. The driver might decide to back up (knowing he is too far forward). He is less likely to notice a pedestrian who is behind him. However, if going in front is really impossible, and if traffic is truly stopped, going around behind may be acceptable as the best alternative.

The maturing student needs experience with situations such as this. She needs to go through the stage of thinking, "I'm lost in a confused mess of traffic!" while the teacher is there to coach and interpret. Tell her, "Don't panic if you encounter a stopped car," and help her learn how to proceed. Also remind her, "If the noise level changes – the light is probably changing."

EXAMPLE 6: *BUSY INTERSECTION WITH MAJOR OBSTRUCTION*
(Elementary grades and up)
Select a location with traffic, where the student has the skills to make routine crossings. Explain that you will pretend to be a policeman, or a large fence, blocking all access in one direction. The student will need to think of another way to achieve the desired crossing.

For example, Figure 62-3 shows the same location as the previous Figures. Again, a pedestrian stands at the southwest corner of 32nd and Broad, wishing to walk north across Broad and to proceed north on the west side of 32nd. But construction has completely blocked the crosswalk area: anyone trying to go around it would be forced into the traffic of 32nd Street, or forced to cross Broad far west of the intersection.

The pedestrian might choose to face east and go around three sides of the intersection, (the dotted path in Figure 62-3). Another choice would be to walk a block west, cross Broad, and come back on the north side of Broad (the dot-dash path in Figure 62-3). The latter may be wise if the blocked intersection is very messy overall.

Depending on the actual destination, detours in various directions could make sense.

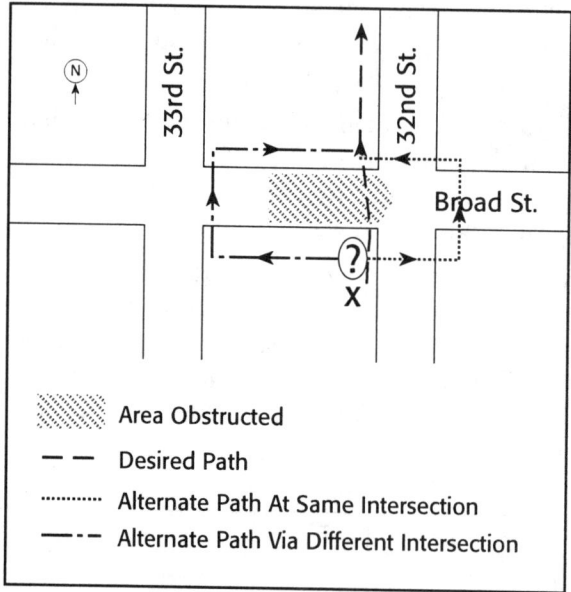

**Figure 62-3
Major Obstruction in Intersection**

MODULE 63
DRIVEWAYS, ALLEYS, AND STREETS

OBJECTIVE: The student will examine typical streets, driveways, and alleys. He/she will describe the usual characteristics of each, and how to distinguish among them.

AGE OF STUDENT: Preschool and up (see Examples)

PRIMARY SKILL EMPHASIS:
Street crossing
Street patterns
Sidewalk
Orientation overall
Corners, turns, and angles

ADDITIONAL SKILL EMPHASIS:
Compass directions
Right and left
Correcting a path
Addresses
Interpreting odors
Sound direction and meaning
Air currents and echoes
Maps
Varied terrain
General travel (outdoors)

SEE ALSO (Other Modules):
> Sidewalks
> From House to Curb
> Street Crossing With Little Traffic
> Street Crossing – Developing Flexibility and Competence
> Echoes and Air Currents
> Walking at Curbside
> Uncontrolled Intersections
> Rural Environment

FIGURE(S):
FIGURE 63-1: Driveways

ACTIVITIES: PRESCHOOL AND PRIMARY GRADES

EXAMPLE 1: *STREET OR DRIVEWAY?*
(*Preschool*)
(Figure 63-1)

"You're getting very good at walking on the sidewalk now. We've practiced going west past the Barbers' and the Perowskys'. Let's do that once more and especially notice their *driveways* when we pass them."

Walk past familiar driveways. Note various characteristics – different surface material, different slope, gravel, etc.

Tap the cane along the edge of the sidewalk and note the change from grass to driveway.

"Now we'll turn around....We'll keep going past your house and walk on east, where I haven't gone with you very often. We will pass some other driveways – you know Mrs. Johnston is next door, and we'll keep going...."

As you pass each home, examine the driveway as before. Emphasize that a driveway leads to *one* particular house.

"OK, here's the last *driveway* on this block. Remember, it goes to just one house. When a car comes in here, the people are coming to *this* house....Now, we are about to get to something different. This is not just a little driveway. Can you tell me what we're coming to?....Yes, the *street*. It's Clemens Street. Notice, we hear lots of cars going by. They are going to lots of different places....

"We will find the curb and listen to the cars a minute.

"How do we know this is not just a driveway?"

While walking back, select one driveway and walk up it to a house. Greet the neighbor, if possible. Examine the width of the driveway and its construction.

Walk back down the driveway and find Beaver Avenue, emphasizing that this too is a *street*.

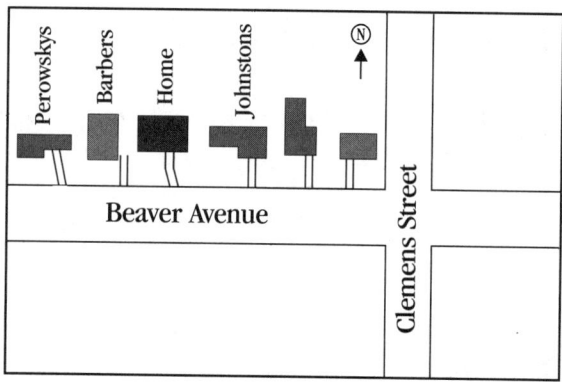

**Figure 63-1
Driveways**

EXAMPLE 2: MORE DRIVEWAYS, MORE STREETS
(*Preschool and primary grades*)

Examine several driveways in a manner similar to the above.

Walk across a street. Note its width and construction.

Go back to a driveway and discuss how it is different from a street.

- A street is much wider than a driveway.
- There are differences in surface.
- Streets (usually) have a clearly-defined curb, while driveways (usually) do not.
- Driveways slope toward the street.
- A driveway leads to one particular location, while a street leads onward to many possible places.
- Cars move slowly in a driveway. On a street they may go fast.
- In a driveway there are only the vehicles for one family (and perhaps guests). In a street there may be a great many vehicles.

Discuss safety in passing driveways. A very young child may be told, "If you hear a car moving in a driveway ahead of you—or even if you hear a car's motor—stop and wait." A somewhat older child can be taught to pause and proceed with caution.

EXAMPLE 3: *EXPLORING A DRIVEWAY*
(*Preschool and primary grades*)

Below are two opposite examples: going too far up a driveway, and going too far down. These experiences usually occur naturally in the course of practice, and they should be discussed and understood.

However, it is often helpful to explore these "detours" on purpose. The student will then understand more readily when he goes there inadvertently.

Encourage the viewpoint that some deviation from the "ideal" path is normal. The goal should not be a "perfect" walk every time, with no deviation from the desired path. Rather, the goal should be to reach the destination with reasonable speed and efficiency.

Down Toward the Street: Walk east along Beaver. Start to cross a driveway, and note how it slopes toward the street. While crossing the driveway, get closer and closer to the street, encouraged by the slope. What happens?

Into the street: If the student has gone all the way to the street, he will find himself walking *in* the street. Although the surface is solid, various characteristics show this is not a sidewalk:

- Traffic imminently close
- A gutter, with drainage from the raised center of the street
- A curb on the left (or on the right, if the student inadvertently crossed Beaver)
- Sewer gratings

Help the student use clues such as these, in order to realize he is in the street and get back on the sidewalk.

Part way toward the street: Sometimes a student may follow the slope of a driveway only part way down to the street. Then, as he tries to "keep walking straight ahead," he finds grass instead of the continued sidewalk.

Help him realize what has happened, continue parallel to the street, and look for the sidewalk. Point out, however, that one should not spend large amounts of time looking for a sidewalk. Sometimes there is none. If the walk is not easily found, simply keep going beside the street. (See the Module, "Walking at Curbside.")

Away From the Street: Walking *up* a driveway (away from the street) is a common experience also. A beginner may tend to follow a solid surface without realizing he is turning. An experienced traveler may be unsure of direction because of curves or other complexities.

The student walks up a driveway, away from the street. Help him note clues such as:

- He has turned, rather than going straight
- Traffic is farther and farther away
- The surface material of the driveway continues and is not replaced by the sidewalk surface
- Bushes, plants, etc. may be found
- Parked cars, bicycles, etc., may be found
- Often the building itself is soon reached, giving a very emphatic clue
- Even if the driveway does not lead to a building, other items typical of a yard are encountered

ACTIVITIES: FOURTH GRADE AND UP

Note: Examples below are described as for a student in the intermediate grades or older. However, if there are alleys in a neighborhood where the student normally travels, they should be explored at any time.

EXAMPLE 4: *ALLEYS, DRIVEWAYS, STREETS*
(*Fourth grade and up*)
(Note: This assumes the student has had experience traveling in residential areas and now is working in the nearby business district. It also assumes the student has not had experience with alleys.)

Review the differences between driveways and streets. Review clues for correction of going too far up or down a driveway. (See examples above.)

Discuss the definition of an *alley:* "It's like a small street going through the middle of the block. The alley goes *behind* the buildings."

Walk with the student as he crosses two alleys and two streets. Note contrasting characteristics. In this example:

- An alley is narrower than a typical street, but wider than most residential driveways.
- An *alley* is shallow and concave (that is, the middle is lower than the sides). A *street* is higher in the center and sloped to drain toward the gutter.
- A street (usually) has clearly-defined curbs, except for wheelchair access cuts. An alley (usually) does not.
- An alley goes behind buildings. One finds back doors, parking areas, loading docks, trash receptacles, etc. There often are distinctive odors. The street, in contrast, goes past the sidewalk and the front doors.

Ask the student to proceed three blocks to the hardware store. He must count the streets without being confused by an alley in the middle of one of the blocks.

REMARKS: Alleys, driveways, and streets all vary in their construction. In a small town, streets may be "blacktop" (tarred surface), alleys may be gravel, and driveways may be any surface. Streets may not have clearly-defined curbs. Note characteristics which apply in your area. As the student matures, expose him to different characteristics.

EXAMPLE 5: *WALKING IN AN ALLEY*
(*Fourth grade and up*)

The previous example assumes the student is crossing a driveway or alley, and does not wish to follow it.

Discuss reasons why a person may choose to walk in an alley:

- A shorter route
- Delivering something to the back door
- An employee entrance in back
- A customer entrance in back
- In some residential areas, alleys are logical routes to neighbors' homes and yards

CAUTION:

Caution that alleys often have little foot traffic. Drivers of vehicles may not expect pedestrians, and may be less careful. There is no sidewalk or clearly-defined path for walking.

In a large city, alleys may be less safe in regard to crime.

Provide suggestions for safety and convenience. As with walking on a roadway, it is usually best to walk on the left. The pedestrian then is facing any oncoming traffic and is more easily seen.

In an Alley, by Choice:

Discuss how to find the back door to Fletcher's Clothing. Many typical clues found at the front may not be available. There may be parking spaces around the door. (A lack of landmarks is another reason why one might prefer to go around by the front, even if it is somewhat farther.)

If a suitable situation is available, direct the student to walk through the alley to a given location. For example, he might proceed until the parking area on the right has ended; pass a fenced-in trash bin; then turn toward the building and find the back door of Fletcher's.

Not by Choice:

Sometimes a traveler intends to turn at a street corner, but instead turns at an alley and begins to walk through there unintentionally. Discuss this possibility. How would your student recognize it if it occurred?

In the alley of a downtown area it may be quiet, cool, and smelly. There is no regular sidewalk, and the terrain generally is not typical of the street front.

Even if an independent lesson in the alley is not planned, walk through with the student so he may experience what it is like.

MODULE 64
NON-SQUARE 'BLOCKS'

NOTE: This Module, "Non-Square 'Blocks,'" emphasizes irregular *patterns* of streets. The Module, "Irregular Streets," emphasizes *individual streets* with unusual characteristics. "Complicated Street Crossings" emphasizes *intersections* with unusual characteristics.

OBJECTIVE: The student will examine street patterns which do not conform to regular, square blocks. He/she will discuss three ways of analyzing irregular street patterns.

AGE OF STUDENT: Elementary grades and up

PRIMARY SKILL EMPHASIS:
Street patterns
Addresses
Street crossing
Orientation overall
Flexibility and confidence

ADDITIONAL SKILL EMPHASIS:
Compass directions
Corners, turns, and angles
Communication and instructions
Landmarks
Maps
Parallel and perpendicular
Right and left
Traffic movement

SEE ALSO (Other Modules):
Around the Block
Irregular Streets
Complicated Street Crossings
Rural Environment
The Great Outdoors
Walking at Curbside

FIGURE(S):
FIGURE 64-1: Benton Circle
FIGURE 64-2: Shady Lane Subdivision

TEACHER PREPARATION: Locate at least two areas which do not have the "standard" square grid pattern. The selections below are examples only.

STUDENT BACKGROUND: Ideally, the student would first become familiar with the "standard" grid pattern, and then work on arrangements which may be harder to analyze. However, the student should become familiar with his own neighborhood immediately, whatever its characteristics.

When the student begins to walk routes of some length, it is important to include some areas with the standard grid arrangement, regardless of how the home neighborhood is laid out. It is also important to encounter irregular arrangements.

ACTIVITIES:

EXAMPLE 1: *STANDARD GRID PATTERN*
See the Module, "Around the Block," and other STREET CROSSING Modules.

EXAMPLE 2: *GRID PATTERN WITH IRREGULARITIES*
See the Module, "Irregular Streets," and other STREET CROSSING Modules.

EXAMPLE 3: *CIRCULAR PATTERNS*
In the Benton Circle development, there is a park in the center, with concentric circles around it–five roughly circular "Streets." (See Figure 64-1.) Eight "Avenues" radiate outward from the park, cutting through the concentric circles. Thus, each "block" is approximately a rounded trapezoid: the two Avenue sides are straight (though not quite parallel), and the two Street sides are somewhat curved.

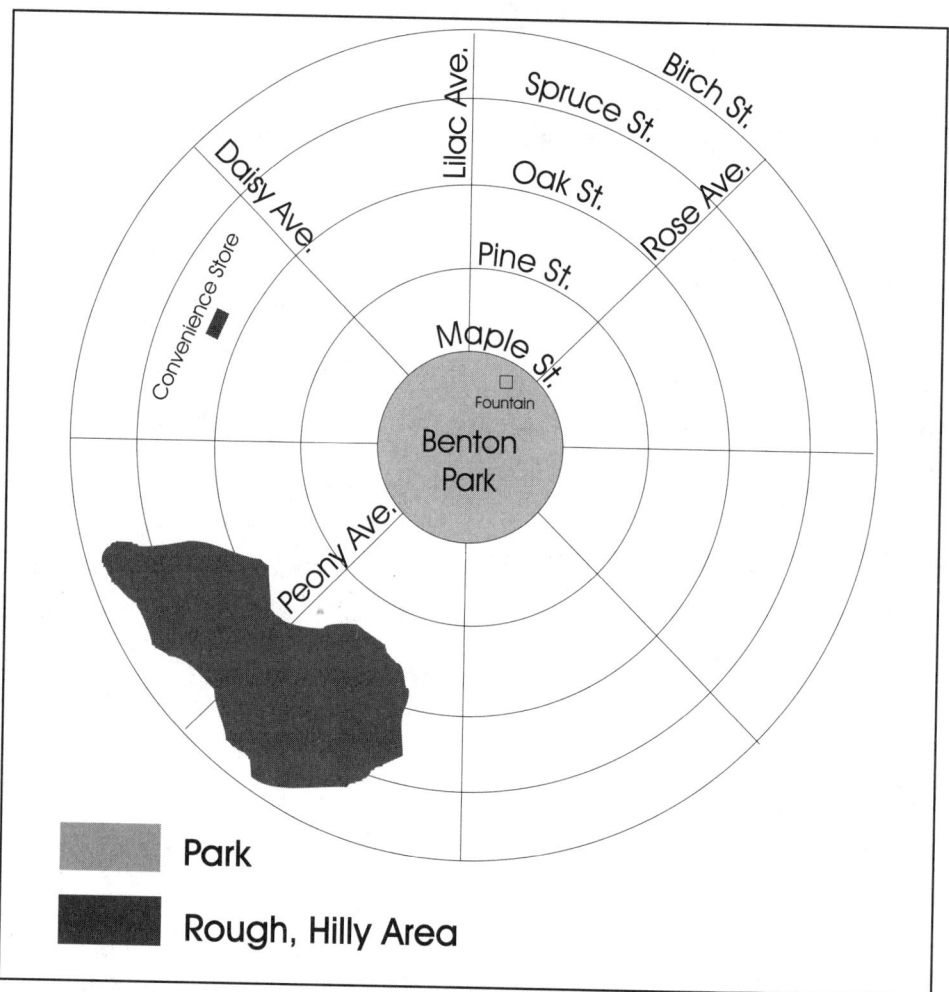

**Figure 64-1
Benton Circle**

Explain this overall pattern. (Use a simple tactual diagram, or take the student's hand to draw an imaginary diagram.) Walking here is similar to walking in an area with square blocks, but with notable differences:

- There is a slight curve on each "street" block, curving outward from the park.
- The two "Avenue" sides of each block are not quite parallel, but fan outward.
- The blocks near the center are much smaller than the outer blocks.
- It is hard to estimate compass directions.

Practice routes which involve both Avenues and Streets.

Route A: Starting at the fountain in the park, walk outward (roughly northeast) on Rose Avenue for two blocks. Turn left at Oak Street and go 2-1/2 blocks. Buy toothpaste at the convenience store in the middle of the block on the "outer" side of Oak Street. Return to the fountain.

Route B: Wear a pedometer. Starting at the fountain, walk all around the innermost Street (Maple) and back to the fountain. Note how far you walked to complete this circle.

[Note: If time and/or endurance make walking the part below inadvisable, it may be covered in a car, noting the odometer.]

Proceed out Rose Avenue, 4 blocks to the outermost circle (Birch Street). Go all the way around on Birch Street. (About halfway around, there will be an extra-long "block." Peony Avenue does not go through to the outer circle.)

Compare the distances around the outer and inner circles.

EXAMPLE 4: *NON-GRID PATTERN*

The Shady Lane subdivision has three main Boulevards, each of which meanders outward from the wide entrance. (See Figure 64-2.) Each main Boulevard has several small branches at irregular intervals.

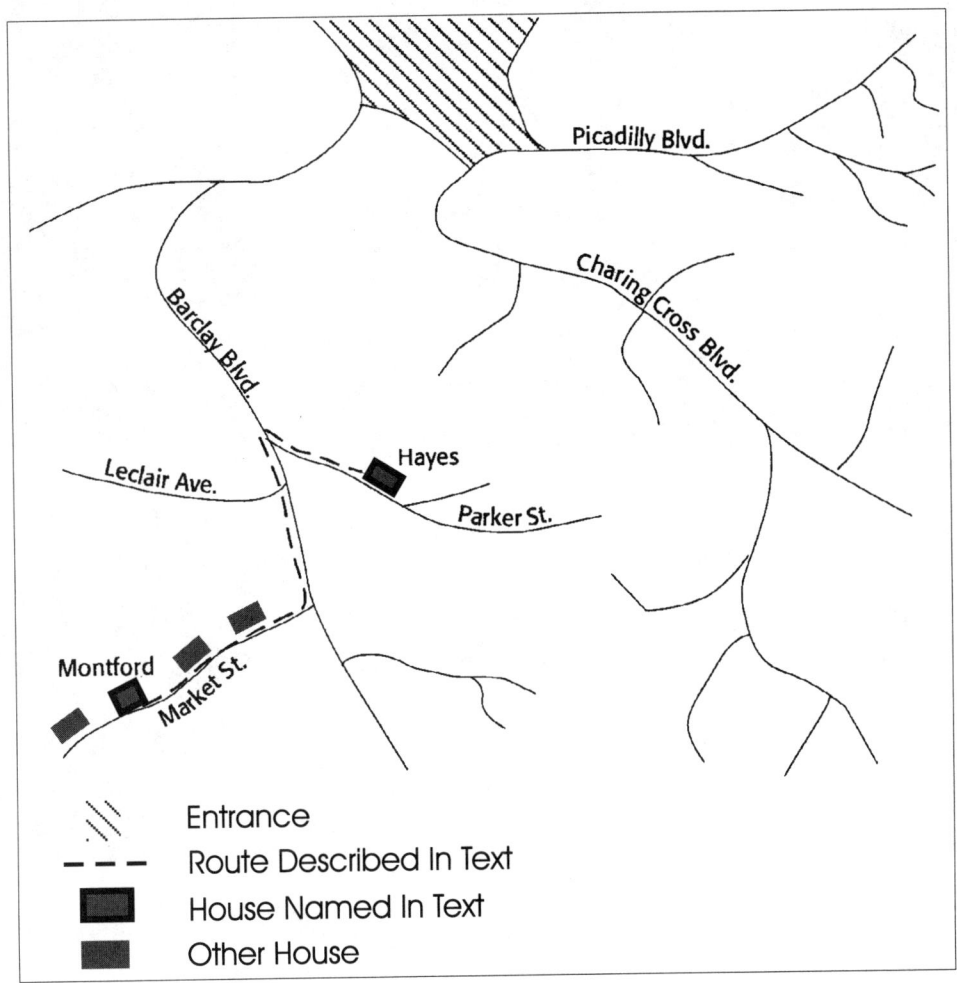

Figure 64-2
Shady Lane Subdivision

Explain that this is not a grid at all. There is, however, a pattern of branches from each Boulevard, though intervals are irregular. Examine an actual tree branch and/or a tactual diagram.

Example of a route: Start from the Hayes' home on the north side of Parker Street, which is a side branch of Barclay Boulevard. Go to Barclay and cross it. Turn left (approximately south) and pass one branch. Turn right at the second branch, which is Market. On the north (right) side of Market, find the third driveway, which is the Montford home.

EXAMPLE 5: *COUNTRY ROADS AND LANES*
See the Modules, "Rural Environment" and "The Great Outdoors."

FOLLOW-UP: When the student has experience with some "non-standard" patterns, then comparisons can be made. For example, there might be a pattern resembling part of a set of concentric circles – e.g., a quarter or half of the Benton Park layout.

RELATED PRACTICE: Tactual maps

MODULE 65
IRREGULAR STREETS

NOTE: The Module, "Non-Square 'Blocks,'" emphasizes irregular *patterns* of streets. This Module, "Irregular Streets," emphasizes *individual streets* with unusual characteristics. "Complicated Street Crossings" emphasizes *intersections* with unusual characteristics.

OBJECTIVE: The student will describe each of the following, and demonstrate at least one technique for traveling where each occurs: "T" intersection; dead-end or cul-de-sac; turning or merging streets; offset intersection.

AGE OF STUDENT: Elementary grades and up (Also note "Student Background," below)

PRIMARY SKILL EMPHASIS:
Street crossing
Street patterns
Corners, turns, and angles
Parallel and perpendicular
Sound direction and meaning
Traffic movement

ADDITIONAL SKILL EMPHASIS:
Maps
Compass directions
Correcting a path
Communication and instructions
Flexibility and confidence
Moving straight ahead
Right and left
Orientation overall

SEE ALSO (Other Modules):
>Street Crossing With Lights – Basic Skills
>Street Crossing – Developing Flexibility and Competence
>Non-Square "Blocks"
>Complicated Street Crossings
>Rural Environment

FIGURE(S):
FIGURE 65-1: 'T' Intersection
FIGURE 65-2: Dead End or Cul-de-Sac
FIGURE 65-3: Street Turns and Name Changes
FIGURE 65-4: Offset or 'Jog'

TEACHER PREPARATION: Select locations where one street ends or is interrupted in some way.

STUDENT BACKGROUND: Some experience with streets is desirable before attempting to discuss this concept abstractly. Preschool-aged children may be unable to understand the concept in general. However, if one of these situations is in a place where the child ordinarily goes, he can learn to find his way, even if full understanding will come later.

ACTIVITIES:

EXAMPLE 1: *GENERAL CONCEPTS*
Discuss: "How long is a *street*? Where does it end?....I'll give you a hint: they're not all the same. Tell me what you know about this, and then I'll help you learn some more."

Name some major streets that are quite long; probably the student is familiar with them. Do they connect with highways going out of the city? Also name some streets (perhaps unfamiliar) that are very short.

Make a tactual map of the areas studied. Discuss the city map as a whole (or examine a tactual map, if available).

EXAMPLE 2: *"T" INTERSECTION*
(Figure 65-1)

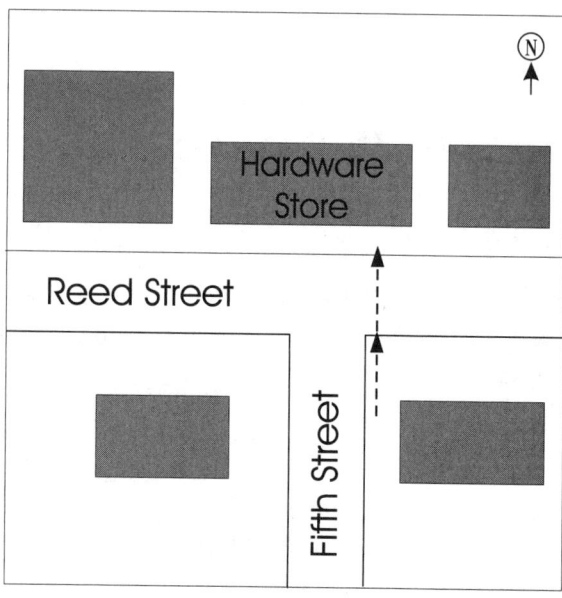

Figure 65-1
"T" Intersection

"Walk north on the sidewalk beside Fifth Street. (Remember, we're on the east side of Fifth.) Cross Reed. On the other side of Reed, the sidewalk does not continue ahead; Fifth Street does not continue."

"If you walk straight ahead anyway, you'll find the hardware store."

(Cross Reed and simulate "trying to go on north." Observe that the hardware store is in your way. Fifth Street does not go through.)

"Turning right or left on Reed is possible. But going north on Fifth is not possible here."

"Suppose you were looking for an address several blocks farther north on Fifth Street. What could you do?" (Recognize that Fifth Street may resume farther on. Try turning left or right on Reed and going around the block. Alternatively, you might ask about this in the hardware store. They may suggest you cut through their store or find a way between buildings. They could probably tell you where Fifth Street will resume.)

Discuss why it is called a "T." Examine the raised print letter.

EXAMPLE 3: *DEAD END OR CUL-DE-SAC*
(Figure 65-2)

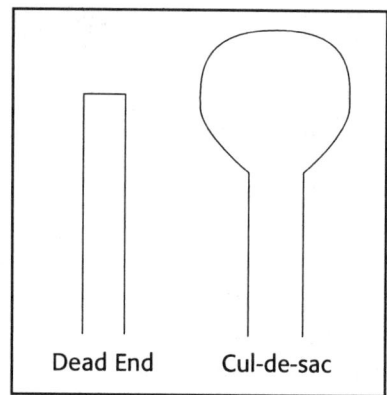

Figure 65-2
Dead End or Cul-de-Sac

"We're coming to a place where Maple Street actually ends. There is no more of it here. It doesn't connect with another street–no 'T' intersection–it just ends. This sign says 'Dead End.' Walk to find the end; then go to the other side and walk back a block on the other side."

Discuss how to tell when you find the end. Was it just an abrupt end, or was it a rounded cul-de-sac?

Note that a dead-end street, like one at a "T" intersection (as discussed in Example 2), may resume farther on with the same name.

Some cities are replacing the expression "Dead End" with "No Outlet," believing that this is a more pleasant expression. The term, "No Outlet," however, may include other configurations besides one street ending straight ahead–e.g., a small "T" intersection leading nowhere.

EXAMPLE 4: *THE STREET TURNS, AND THE NAME CHANGES*
(Figure 65-3)

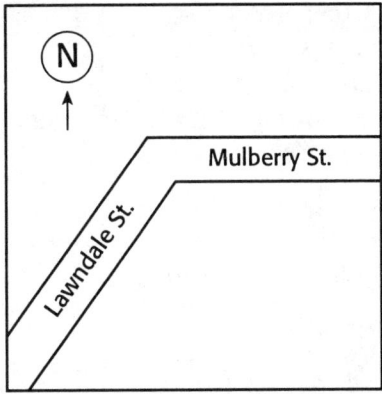

Figure 65-3
Street Turns and Name Changes

"Sometimes a street curves a bit and keeps its same name. But sometimes we find that it has a new name after it curves. This is especially likely if it turns a lot – perhaps a full 90-degree corner.

"Now, here we're going more or less north on Lawndale. The street and the sidewalk turn sharply to the right, here. The street sign says that this is the corner of Lawndale and Mulberry. But there's no other street coming in. We can say that Lawndale *becomes* Mulberry after it turns."

Walk around the turn. Walk some distance on Mulberry. Then cross Mulberry, turn around, and recognize when you are again on Lawndale.

Discuss how it is decided whether a street should keep its same name when it turns. (It is partly a matter of tradition and opinion. But it also depends on the layout of nearby streets and the degree of turning.)

EXAMPLE 5: *NON-SQUARE ANGLES*
See the Modules, "Complicated Street Crossings" and "Non-Square 'Blocks.'"

EXAMPLE 6: *OFFSETS*
(*also called "doglegs" or "jogs"*)
As in Figure 65-4, sometimes a street crosses another and resumes with a slight offset rather than being perfectly in line. These arrangements are called by various names such as "jogs" or "doglegs."

The Module, "Complicated Street Crossings," contains detailed suggestions for crossing such an intersection from various approaches.

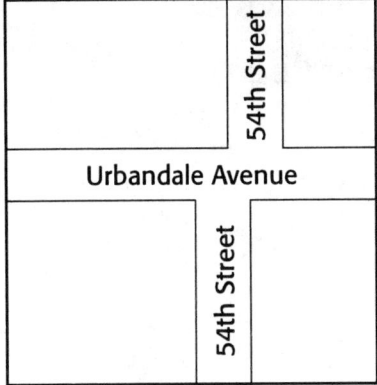

Figure 65-4
Offset or "Jog"

FOLLOW-UP: Incorporate "irregular" situations such as these into routes routinely from time to time.

REFERENCE(S):
Richard Mettler. *Cognitive Learning Theory and Cane Travel Instruction: A New Paradigm*, pp. 136-140.

MODULE 66
COMPLICATED STREET CROSSINGS

NOTE: The Module, "Non-Square 'Blocks'" emphasizes irregular *patterns* of streets. The Module, "Irregular Streets" emphasizes *individual streets* with unusual characteristics.

This Module, "Complicated Street Crossings," emphasizes *intersections* with unusual characteristics.

OBJECTIVE: The student will demonstrate methods for crossing intersections with unusual characteristics, including "T" intersections, offsets, and safety islands.

AGE OF STUDENT:
Specific individual crossings: Preschool and up, as needed.
General learning: Elementary grades and up.

PRIMARY SKILL EMPHASIS:
Street crossing
Street patterns
Traffic movement
Moving straight ahead
Correcting a path
Parallel and perpendicular
Corners, turns, and angles
Compass directions

ADDITIONAL SKILL EMPHASIS:
Sound direction and meaning
Maps
Right and left
Flexibility and confidence

SEE ALSO (Other Modules):
Non-Square 'Blocks'
Irregular Streets
Street Crossing With Lights – Basic Skills
Street Crossing – Developing Flexibility and Competence
Stop Signs
Uncontrolled Intersections
Street Crossing With Obstruction
Rural Environment

FIGURE(S):

FIGURE 66-1: "T" Intersection

FIGURE 66-2A: Offset: Desired Path, East Side of Street

FIGURE 66-2B: Offset: Desired Path, West Side of Street

FIGURE 66-2C: Offset: Mistakenly Walking in the Street

FIGURE 66-2D: Offset: Mistakenly Continuing on Wrong Side of Street

FIGURE 66-3: Unusual Angles

FIGURE 66-4: Traffic "Island"

ACTIVITIES:

EXAMPLE 1: *"T" INTERSECTION*
Discuss or review the concept of a "T" intersection. The Module, "Irregular Streets," includes detailed suggestions for introducing this.

If a young child (even a preschooler) has a "T" intersection nearby, he can easily learn to cross that particular one – provided its other characteristics (such as amount of traffic) are appropriate for his age and skill. In elementary school and above, the teacher should be sure to include various kinds of intersections.

In Figure 66-1, Reed Street runs east and west. Fifth Street comes in from the south to form the leg of the "T."

COMPLICATED STREET CROSSINGS

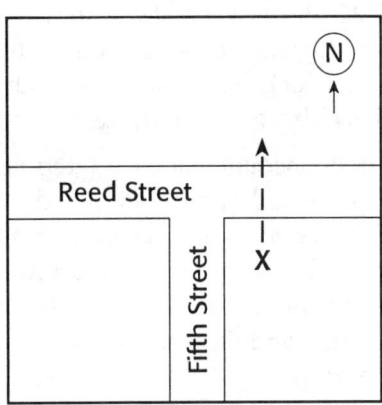

**Figure 66-1
"T" Intersection**

The Module, "Street Crossing–Developing Flexibility and Competence," has detailed suggestions about handling turning traffic. Generally, at a "T" the percentage of turning traffic is especially great. Consider the pedestrian in Figure 66-1, standing on the southeast corner and desiring to cross Reed. He must understand that (a) when his light is green, it is also green for the traffic on Fifth, and much of it will turn east through his desired path; (b) because of that and because of Right Turn on Red, there is likely to be turning traffic on *both* red and green lights.

Help your student listen through a cycle or two to analyze where and when traffic is heaviest. Help him plan to cross when the least and/or slowest traffic is likely to cross his path. The best time to step out may not be immediately after the light changes. Sometimes it is wise to let one car proceed around a turn, and then step out. (This assumes that cars are moving slowly and/or one at a time. Remind the student always to extend the cane before actually stepping out, so that motorists will be warned.)

"Go when you are least likely to be hit" is a good maxim in a complicated situation.

If the traveler in Figure 66-1 wished to cross Fifth Street instead, he would be walking parallel to the ongoing straight traffic on Reed–a helpful guide. He should realize, however, that some of that traffic will turn onto Fifth.

A traveler crossing Reed from the *north* side may find it hard to locate the crosswalk area. There is no intersecting street to define the corner. There may be a curb cut or similar indication. Generally, however, listening must be the main guide. Especially listen to the traffic coming from the "leg" (Fifth Street).

Traffic is a superb source of information and feedback for the traveler. If the first experience with a "T" intersection involves little or no traffic, see that the student soon gets experience with significant traffic.

The maturing student should learn to recognize a "T" without advance explanation.

EXAMPLE 2: *OFFSETS ("DOGLEGS" OR "JOGS")*

Sometimes a street crosses another and resumes with a slight offset rather than being perfectly in line. These arrangements are called by various names such as "jogs" or "doglegs."

The various versions of Figure 66-2 show Urbandale Avenue running straight east and west. 54th Street runs north and south. However, 54th is offset: the segment south of Urbandale is slightly west of the north segment.

In Figure 66-2A a traveler is walking south on the *east* side of 54th and then crossing Urbandale. He would tend to reach the opposite curb a bit east of the connection. To continue south on 54th he would need to walk a few steps west. This is not greatly different from what one might ordinarily do. However, if the offset is large, it may not be easy to find the continuation southward.

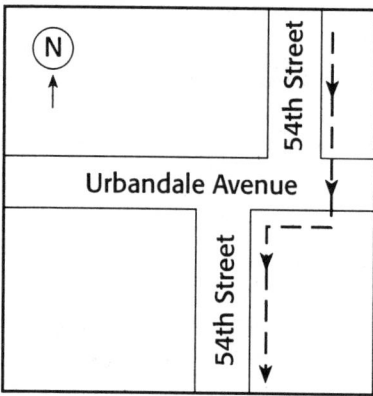

**Figure 66-2A
Offset: Desired Path
East Side of Street**

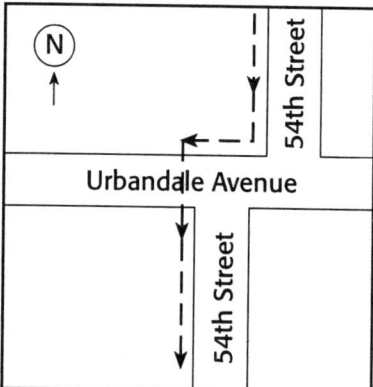

**Figure 66-2B
Offset: Desired Path
West Side of Street**

Figure 66-2B illustrates walking south on the *west* side of 54th. This requires some added understanding and compensation.

Sometimes the traveler will know the situation beforehand. (The area may be familiar; someone else may have told him; or he may recognize the situation while listening to traffic before crossing.) He can then walk a few steps west *before* crossing Urbandale. Or, he may consciously angle westward as he crosses Urbandale.

Figure 66-2C shows a traveler who tries to cross Urbandale (again, walking south from the northwest corner), but continues south *in* 54th instead of arriving at the southwest corner.

His cane may encounter a curb (step-up) to his right or left instead of straight ahead. An inexperienced traveler may conclude that he has found the south side of Urbandale and is simply approaching from the wrong angle. He may step up on the curb and face east or west, believing he is facing south.

If the traveler in Figure 66-2C is out in the middle of 54th, he may not immediately find a curb beside him. An inexperienced traveler may walk on and on, thinking, "Urbandale is a terribly wide street!"

The Module, "Street Crossing with Little Traffic," speaks to the traveler who finds himself walking on and on without encountering the opposite curb. The following advice is offered: Walk two or three more steps to be sure of walking far enough. Then realize that you are probably mistakenly walking *parallel* to a curb. Turn 90 degrees and walk to the curb which is beside you. The direction of the 90-degree turn depends on where you believe you are.

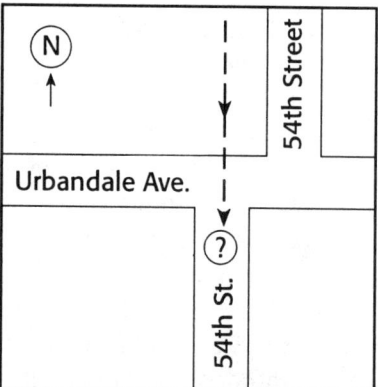

**Figure 66-2C
Offset: Mistakenly Walking
In the Street**

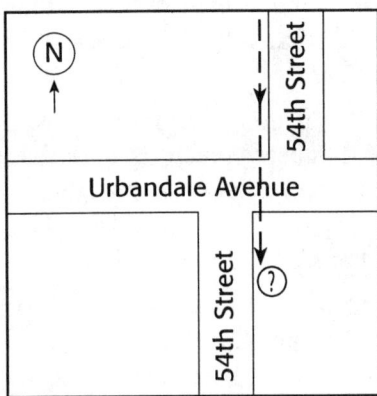

**Figure 66-2D
Offset:
Mistakenly Continuing on
Wrong Side of Street**

In Figure 66-2D (attempting the same desired path, intending to walk on the west side of 54th), the traveler walks south across Urbandale and does indeed find a curb ahead of him. He proceeds south on the sidewalk. However, he has come to the *southeast* corner instead of the southwest corner. He is now walking on the *east* side of 54th instead of the west side.

The alert traveler will soon observe that the street is on his right, when it should have been on his left. He will hear traffic on his right. The curb (step-down) will be on his right.

A beginner, however, may conclude, "I'm supposed to be walking the other way," and mistakenly turn around and walk north. Or, he may go back to the intersection and mistakenly go east in order to put the traffic on his left.

A more experienced traveler will think of several possibilities, including: (a) he walked diagonally across the intersection instead of straight ahead; (b) he made a right-angle turn while crossing, and is now walking along Urbandale; (c) 54th has an offset, as in the diagram. The experienced traveler will listen to traffic, note any other clues, and recall his path during the crossing. He will then make a correction.

Many forms: "Jogs" appear in infinite variations. The offset may be slight or substantial. Streets may be wide or narrow, straight or angled. There may or may not be stoplights, stop signs, traffic islands, etc. The street may or may not keep the same name after the jog. The advanced student should experience many examples.

EXAMPLE 3: *UNUSUAL ANGLES*

Figure 66-3 illustrates streets which come together at an unusual angle – that is, not a 90-degree right angle. These both happen to be one-way streets. Fourth street runs from south to north. Grand runs approximately southeast to northwest.

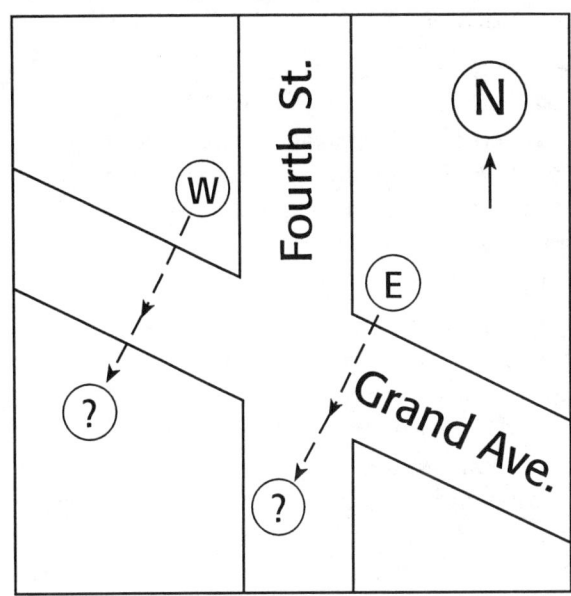

**Figure 66-3
Unusual Angles**

The unfortunate pedestrians in Figure 66-3 (Traveler W on the northwest corner and Traveler E on the northeast corner) both lined up square with the north curb, and square with Grand Avenue. They tried to cross Grand as though the streets were at right angles. Pedestrian W, coming from the northwest corner, reached the south side of Grand considerably west of the intersection. Pedestrian E, coming from the northeast corner, did not encounter the south side of Grand at all; instead, he walked on south *in* Fourth Street, probably encountering the west side of Fourth.

If there is traffic on the street parallel to his path, the alert traveler will use it as a guide to avoid this problem. He should walk beside the traffic which is on Fourth, keeping parallel to it. (Pedestrian W will want to hear the Fourth Street traffic close by on his left; Pedestrian E will want it on his right.)

However, traffic may be intermittent, and may have many turning vehicles. Even an experienced traveler may find that he has proceeded incorrectly as in the illustration.

Pedestrian W will merely need to walk east to find the continuation of Fourth. If there is considerable traffic, this should be easy. (The Example, "Offsets," above, analyzes a comparable situation.)

Pedestrian E, on the other hand, may reach the west curb of *Fourth* Street. Hearing parallel traffic on his left instead of his right, he should realize that something is wrong. He should listen carefully to traffic, note any other clues, and make a correction.

If Pedestrian E does not encounter a curb immediately, he may continue south *in* Fourth Street without realizing it – walking *in* the street which he had wished to walk beside. He should apply the advice for the traveler who finds himself walking on and on without encountering the opposite curb: Walk two or three more steps to be sure of walking far enough. Then realize that you are probably mistakenly walking *parallel* to a curb. Turn 90 degrees and walk to the curb which is beside you. The direction of the 90-degree turn depends on where you believe you are.

Emphasize the importance of a sharp, 90-degree turn. Realizing that something is wrong, a person in this situation is likely to turn slightly from time to time – but this results only in a wavering path down the middle of the street. With a 90-degree turn, however, he will encounter a curb very quickly and get out of the street.

EXAMPLE 4: *FIVE- AND SIX-WAY INTERSECTIONS, "Y" INTERSECTIONS, ETC.*

Occasionally there will be three or more streets coming together, resulting in more than four approaches. "Six Corners" in Chicago is an example.

There is no set pattern for this situation, and often a pedestrian will need to ask other people for information.

One strategy (if there is considerable traffic) is to locate a street which is parallel to your desired path, and cross beside it. Even then, it is wise to check on the other side to be sure you arrived at the place you desired.

A "Y" intersection has some similarities to a "T," but without the helpful square angles. Again, the traveler should analyze traffic patterns and ask directions if necessary.

EXAMPLE 5: *TRAFFIC ISLANDS*

Sometimes the pedestrian's path across a street is interrupted by an "island" – a raised area which divides the street. An island channels the traffic and/or provides a safe place for pedestrians to wait part way across a wide thoroughfare.

Explanation and practice are essential in helping the student anticipate and deal with such interruptions. A beginner may not realize what is happening and become very confused.

Select a situation appropriate for your student's level of experience. Provide a tactual diagram of some kind. (Often it is sufficient to cut a piece of paper in the shape of the island, and to move your student's hand around and over it while discussing the crossing verbally.) Except for a very experienced student, walk through the crossing together and analyze it before expecting him to proceed independently.

Figure 66-4 shows two wide streets intersecting. New York runs east and west; 72nd runs north and south. The northeast corner of the intersection has an island to channel traffic turning north from New York to 72nd. The two sides of the island which are toward the streets are straight; the side facing northeast is somewhat curved.

COMPLICATED STREET CROSSINGS

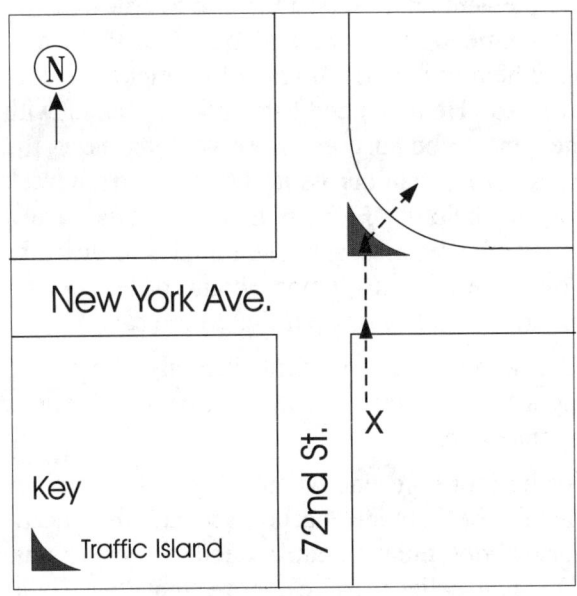

**Figure 66-4
Traffic "Island"**

A pedestrian wishes to cross New York Avenue, going from the southeast corner of the intersection to the northeast corner. For a smooth crossing, he should use the parallel traffic on 72nd as a guide to avoid veering to the right onto New York. (Also, of course, he must not move too far to his left and veer into 72nd Street itself.)

When the traveler reaches the island and is ready to cross the last lane, it is often best to face the curved side of the island and step off perpendicular to that curb, even though this path is not strictly parallel with 72nd. (Note the slight bend in the traveler's path in Figure 66-4.) This is safer because it cuts the risk of walking out into the busy parallel street.

Traffic turning north from New York onto 72nd is likely to make a Right Turn on Red. In fact, it may have only a "yield" sign instead of an actual light. A motorist there may observe that the closest lane on 72nd is free, and proceed at a substantial speed – despite the fact that 72nd Street and the pedestrian have a green light. Realizing this, the student should hesitate on the island and listen, to avoid stepping out in front of a fast-moving car. However, if he stops altogether, a motorist may assume he is not going on. The student should keep the cane extended, indicating he wishes to proceed.

Varied Experiences: Maturing students should realize that islands may be found anywhere, but anticipate where they are most likely to be. They should recognize clues that show they may have found an unexpected island (e.g., more traffic quite close in front, after a step-up has been reached).

Discuss variations and common examples. Provide experience with as many as practical. For example:

- The traffic on the far side of the island may be parallel to the traffic already crossed. Or, as in Figure 66-4, it may be turning or angling somewhat. Or, it may be going in the opposite direction (as on a boulevard with a median).
- On a divided boulevard, typically the median extends for many blocks and is interrupted at each intersection. However, it may or may not be the same at every intersection.
- There may be an island at only one corner of a given intersection (as shown in Figure 66-4). Or, there may be islands at two, three, or four corners.
- Sometimes an island contains a sign post, light pole, or other obstruction. As always, sweep with the cane at all times. A sign or pole may even be in the street without a substantial island.
- There may be more than one island in one's path (as would be true in Figure 66-4 if New York were also a divided boulevard with a median).
- Some intersections have streets going off in more than four directions and/or at unusual angles. These are especially likely to have safety islands.

The best overall approach is to maintain orientation and momentum in the desired direction, while listening to traffic and noting other clues. The mature student does not blithely conclude, "Ah! Here's the curb. Those cars in front of me must be in a parking lot."

EXAMPLE 6: *RAILROAD TRACKS*

The pedestrian may encounter railroad tracks when he is crossing a street or when he is walking along in the middle of the block.

Railroad tracks demand a healthy respect, but they need not cause excessive fear. If a train is coming, its distinctive whistle will be heard. At a controlled crossing, bells will be heard and gates will come down. (Note: Be sure your student knows what the "gates" are like. A small arm-type gate in a parking lot is a good model for demonstration.)

With deft use of the cane, the traveler can note uneven terrain and step over tracks without tripping, while at the same time avoiding getting the cane tip caught.

Sometimes the student finds, after crossing the tracks, that he has drifted somewhat to the left or right in relation to his desired path. He is not quite where he expected to be. A slight correction (by listening to traffic and noting other clues) may be necessary.

Supplementary remarks for young children: In the elementary grades and below, a child may need help to understand how the tracks are constructed. He may need to practice checking with the cane to be sure he is not walking *along* the track rather than across it. (A model train track may be helpful. Explain that the "ties" are a series of short pieces, at right angles to the rails. There are two rails, going on and on. A person should *not* walk along parallel to the rails.)

With a very young student, it is also helpful to use a toy train on a track to illustrate the entire arrangement.

Furthermore, even when a child examines models, he may still harbor serious misconceptions about the size and speed of real trains. (He may believe, for example, that "we could just reach out our hands and stop the train.") If possible, arrange a tour of a real train; examine the cars inside and outside. Emphasize that trains are large and heavy, and that they travel very fast like vehicles on a highway.

MODULE 67
ASKING DIRECTIONS
AND FIGURING IT OUT

By Doris M. Willoughby
And Sharon L. Monthei

OBJECTIVE: The student will ask and follow directions appropriately when needed. On [three occasions per semester] he/she will ask directions from someone at a business or on the street.

OBJECTIVE: Given an appropriate situation where he/she has partial information, the student will figure out where he/she is in relation to the destination, and proceed with little or no assistance.

AGE OF STUDENT: See Examples

PRIMARY SKILL EMPHASIS:
Communication and instructions
Compass directions
Right and left
Corners, turns, and angles
General travel
Meeting the public

ADDITIONAL SKILL EMPHASIS:
Purchase or transaction
Daily living skills
Etiquette
Finding a person
Flexibility and confidence

SEE ALSO (Other Modules):
Compass Directions
Right and Left
IN THE COMMUNITY Modules
PUBLIC BUILDINGS Modules (especially "Malls")
PUBLIC TRANSPORTATION Modules

REMARKS: In most lessons the student should proceed independently, having received age-appropriate directions from the teacher. Continually accepting help from others undermines learning.

Nevertheless, the student also needs to learn how and when to ask directions. Lessons should permit accepting certain kinds of help as appropriate. It is also desirable to have an occasional lesson which *requires* asking directions.

EXAMPLE 1: *GENERAL PRINCIPLES*

Give the student guidance, with changes over time, as to what help he may accept during your various lessons. (Also discuss what help it is wise to accept when he is not working with you.) For example:

Preschool Through Primary Grades

–"If a friend talks to you, you may say hello. But don't let someone else walk with you or keep talking with you. Tell them you're supposed to practice alone."

–"Sometimes when we're on the street, a grownup (someone you don't know) may try to talk to you or touch you. Just ignore him. Or you may say, 'Thank you, but I'm practicing, and my teacher is watching me.' I might say something, too. Remember, I'll always be close by."

–"If I send you into a store to get something, I'll help you know how to find the people who work there. You can hear voices or the sound of a cash register, and I may tell you about some other things. You *should* talk to the people who work there. If the people who work there take your hand to show you something, that's OK too."

Sixth Grade and Above

- "If you meet a friend, and you're sure it's someone you know, you may go ahead and talk *briefly*. Then explain that you're practicing. Don't let a friend walk with you."
- "If you are really having trouble and aren't getting it solved, you may ask directions. Ask for as little help as possible, just to get you back on track. For example, in a department store you might say, 'Could you direct me to the 50th Street door?' Then you may let someone walk a few steps with you, but not far."
- "Remember that someone might make a mistake and give you wrong information. Never rely entirely on what someone tells you. Also, remember that an employee of a business usually will give more reliable information than a member of the general public."
- "If you did receive help, tell me about it afterward. Even though I'm watching you, I want you to tell me; that helps me to understand and to plan future lessons."
- "For each lesson, or part of a lesson, I'll let you know where I will meet you. (As you know, I follow you, but I might be some distance away.) We hope this never happens, but let's talk about what you should do if you can't find me.

"First, be sure you are in the right place. For instance, if I said I would meet you in the camera department at Wal-Mart, ask a clerk whether that is where you are. Then stay there and wait for me.

"If you ever wait a *long* time (more than half an hour) and don't find me as planned, call the school or call your grandmother. I would do the same if I couldn't find you."

REMARKS: The student who is walking routes of several blocks should be building confidence and independence. There is no substitute for practice, and no amount of talking can replace experience. If a student becomes lost, it is his responsibility either to figure out where he is or to seek assistance to determine his location.

The teacher must lay down ground rules about acceptable types of assistance. It is not acceptable for a student to accept a ride, since that is dangerous and does not develop self-confidence. Also, the student should not let someone escort him to a location, but merely should ask whatever questions are necessary to determine present location and how to get back onto the desired route.

EXAMPLE 2: *FINDING A PAY TELEPHONE*
(*Fourth grade and up*)

TEACHER PREPARATION: Look for a location (unfamiliar to the student) where there is a pay telephone, and where the student could logically ask directions. Consider whom the student might call. Provide coins, or arrange for the student to bring them.

STUDENT BACKGROUND: The student should have experience in using a pay telephone. He should also have the maturity and experience to ask and follow the directions required.

ACTIVITIES: Beforehand, explain to the student that he will be practicing two things: (a) asking directions and (b) using a pay phone. Decide whom to call—a family member, the school secretary, etc. Make arrangements with that person if necessary.

Be sure that the needed coins are available.

"In the next block you will find Mama's Pizza, where there is a pay phone. You'll cross Fifth Street, turn left, and walk north about half a block. When your cane finds a parking lot on your right, turn right and go to the building (it's not far from the street). Be sure to listen for moving cars as you cross the lot. Find the door and go in.

"Ask someone where the pay phone is. (If they offer to let you use the restaurant's phone, explain that you are practicing and that you want to use the pay phone.)

"Call your grandmother and visit for a few minutes. Then go back out; ask directions back to the Fifth Street door if you need to. I'll meet you on the corner of Fifth and Elm, before you go back across Fifth."

Provide tips on getting directions efficiently:

- Be alert to the possibility of finding the phone without any help. You might happen to walk by just as someone hangs up, for example. But walking around aimlessly and hunting is not efficient or necessary.
- Usually an employee will give better help than a customer. But it is all right to ask a customer, especially if employees are busy.
- If the person you ask doesn't seem to know, ask someone else. An employee *should* know where the phone is, but a customer may not.
- It is well to *point* in the direction you think the person means for you to go. If they see that you misunderstood, they will correct you.
- If the directions seem complicated or unclear, start off in the direction indicated. Then after awhile, ask someone else. You may want to ask again when you seem to be in the right area but still can't find the actual phone.

REMARKS: In the restaurant, the student gets valuable practice in going around obstacles, finding doorways and walls, etc. He notes that the cane causes people to be especially willing to give directions. It should eliminate sarcasm if he asks about something that would be obvious to the sighted.

EXAMPLE 3: DIRECTIONS TO A PUBLIC BUILDING
(*Sixth grade and up*)

TEACHER PREPARATION: Look for a location where the student should be able to fill in a given gap in information by asking directions of a stranger. The area should be unfamiliar to the student but at the appropriate difficulty level.

STUDENT BACKGROUND: The student should have enough experience to carry out the activity independently, asking only for the missing piece of information. In this example, he also needs one dollar [or, whatever is needed for the chosen transaction].

ACTIVITIES: Explain beforehand that you will direct the student to a given area (or go with him), but will deliberately leave out a necessary piece of information. He is to ask someone for that information.

Explain the task: Find the bank in the mall. Exchange your dollar bill for four quarters. [Alternatively, explain another transaction.]

"All right, here we are at the Northview Mall. Imagine that I am a taxi driver. I'm letting you out, and telling you this is the east door of the mall. I also tell you there is one large hallway in the mall, running north and south. But I don't tell you where the bank is.

"You'll need to ask directions. You may just happen upon a clue, so be alert; but it's probably most efficient to ask directions.

"One good way is to walk into just any business and ask. Many malls do have an 'information' booth. But I'm not telling you whether there is one here; and it would be silly to ask directions to *that*, just to ask more directions when you get there.

"When you get to the bank, locate a teller and exchange the dollar bill for four quarters [or conduct another chosen transaction]."

REMARKS: Give pointers on how to ask and receive directions, as above.

This lesson provides good practice in using the cane in an unfamiliar location. The student must be alert for unexpected obstacles, step-downs, etc.

EXAMPLE 4: *DROP-OFF ROUTES*
(*Advanced students*)

Challenge advanced students by taking them out in a car, driving around so as to mix them up, and dropping them off. Perhaps give a clue as to the direction in which a student is facing. The student must use his wits to get back. He may ask directions of others, but may not accept a ride, even from friends – a general principle in training. Students may be dropped anywhere from across the street to three miles from the school or home. The first drop-off may be done in a somewhat familiar area if desired. Some students may be up to more challenge.

Obviously, this should be done after a student has acquired basic technical competence, crosses at lights well, understands how to get and follow directions, and has overcome most shyness regarding asking others for directions. The purpose of drop-off routes is to convince a student that he can work his way out of anything. Most blind people will be left at the wrong address or street at a most unexpected moment. Prior experience of what to do in such a case is extremely valuable.

In the Module, "Malls," there is a detailed Example which emphasizes these same kinds of skills. It is called "Dealing With Confusion."

MODULE 68
UNCONTROLLED INTERSECTIONS

OBJECTIVE: (*Preschool and up*) The student will cross an uncontrolled intersection which has very little traffic.

OBJECTIVE: (*Upper elementary grades and above, in selected situations*) The student will cross an uncontrolled intersection which has a moderate amount of traffic at moderate speed.

OBJECTIVE: (*Very mature, advanced students only*) In selected situations, the student will cross an uncontrolled intersection which has heavy traffic moving at moderate speed.

AGE OF STUDENT:
Very little traffic: Preschool.
Moderate traffic: Intermediate grades and up.
Heavy traffic: Advanced, very mature students only.

PRIMARY SKILL EMPHASIS:
Street crossing
Traffic movement
Sound direction and meaning
Parallel and perpendicular

ADDITIONAL SKILL EMPHASIS:
Street patterns
Right and left
Compass directions
Moving straight ahead
Correcting a path
Flexibility and confidence

SEE ALSO (Other Modules):
Stop Signs
Street Crossing With Little Traffic
Driveways, Alleys, and Streets
Street Crossing With Lights – Basic Skills
Street Crossing – Developing Flexibility and Competence
Complicated Street Crossings

CAUTION: Unless there is very little traffic, the techniques described in this Module require mature judgment and experience. A knowledgeable adult must observe traffic patterns on a particular street carefully, at the time of day in question, before advising a student to cross significant continual traffic which is not controlled.

ACTIVITIES:

EXAMPLE 1: *VERY LITTLE TRAFFIC*
(*All ages*)
The Module, "Street Crossing With Little Traffic," contains detail on teaching this skill to a young child. Such a crossing is appropriate for a preschool child, with close supervision as for any child of this age. It should be learned easily and quickly by older beginners. The traveler simply waits until no traffic is heard in the vicinity.

See other Modules, as listed above, for suggestions about crossing smoothly and directly.

EXAMPLE 2: *HEAVY TRAFFIC*
(*Very mature, advanced students only*)
When an uncontrolled intersection has traffic which is heavy and continual, but which moves at only moderate speed, a special technique can be employed. Not all students will learn this technique, and it should be taught very near the end of training. Confidence and skill in judging traffic are essential.

The student waits until there is no imminent traffic in the lanes closest to her. She extends the cane *parallel to the ground, at about chest height,* as a signal for all to see; then she lowers the cane to normal position and proceeds to the center of the street, using the usual touch technique. In the center, she lifts and extends the cane again to alert traffic which might be coming from the opposite direction. She waits until traffic stops, then continues across the street.

This can be effective for a competent, confident traveler on a regular city street. However, the student must accurately judge when there is no traffic (in a particular lane), or how far away it is. She must remember that a receding car can mask the sound of an oncoming car from that direction. Also, it is especially important to do everything quite deliberately – no running back across the street or speeding up unexpectedly. Since drivers will anticipate what a traveler will do, the pedestrian must make her intentions clear with body language.

Other options should always be considered carefully – notably, walking to the nearest controlled intersection.

This technique is *not* appropriate for high-speed traffic. *No* pedestrian should be walking across a high-speed freeway at all.

EXAMPLE 3: *MODERATE TRAFFIC*
(*Intermediate grades and above*)

Sometimes an uncontrolled intersection will have a moderate amount of traffic moving at a moderate or slow speed. Such a street can readily be crossed by a blind traveler with some experience.

A simpler version of the technique for heavy traffic, above, is called for. If the student waits until there is relatively little traffic, and extends the cane (either in normal position or raised), she will easily cause traffic to stop in the lanes nearest to her. She proceeds to the middle of the street, where she pauses to listen and extends the cane again. Then she completes the crossing.

A knowledgeable adult should observe traffic patterns on a particular street carefully, at the time of day in question, before advising a student to take this approach. But in selected situations, this can be safe and effective even for a youngster in the middle grades. It can enable independence when otherwise the student would either have to receive help or walk many blocks to a light.

MODULE 69
MORE IDEAS
For Lessons
In the Community
Outdoors

AGE OF STUDENT: Elementary school and up

ABOUT THIS LIST:

Following is a representative list of outdoor objects, aspects, places, etc., typically found in the community. Examining different things at various times helps assure variety, interest, and a depth of experience. Many other suggestions appear in the Modules in this section and are not necessarily duplicated on this list.

Be alert to interesting things that are seasonal or temporary. If something would be especially valuable for your particular student, plan ahead.

CAUTION: Always be alert for possible hazards. These may be physical – contaminated trash, hot pipes, sharp edges, etc. Or they may be in the form of persons, such as loiterers in a vacant lot. If the student should not explore the area without an adult present, make this clear.

Be careful to respect private property. If you wish to explore an area where the public would not ordinarily go, ask permission.

IDEAS:

- Vendor carts (note that they are not permanent)
- Various signs, including those which hang in such a way that they may strike a person on the head
- Parking meters
- A mailbox
- Fire hydrants
- Parked cars (parallel parking vs. angle parking; on the street vs. in a parking lot)
- A "short cut" through a vacant lot, etc. (See Caution, above).
- An open manhole or construction hole (see Caution)
- A curb cut which is not at the corner as expected (e.g., for a bus stop)
- Live plants, especially if blooming
- A tree growing in an unusual place (as, with sidewalk surrounding it)
- Vending machines
- Ramps
- Benches
- Bicycle racks
- Places of special local significance, such as the bell tower and windmills in Pella, Iowa
- A window well without a cover
- Steps leading *down* to a door
- Various kinds of steps – wood, concrete, marble; with or without a railing; with or without risers; carpeted or not; straight or at an angle
- Piles or windrows of snow
- Unusual approaches to a doorway, as with a "maze" of sculptures or plantings
- A door that has been boarded over or converted to a window
- An abandoned building (See Caution. A person would *not* enter, but only observe that the building is abandoned.)
- A drop-off beside a ramp or stairway
- Arrangements for an outdoor concert or parade
- A curb that is higher than usual
- Construction or repair (See Caution)
- Doorknobs, door handles (Are they all the same?)
- Textures of various walls
- A long, straight, easy walk (important in maintaining the habit of brisk speed)

PUBLIC BUILDINGS GENERAL

MODULE 70
GENERAL OVERVIEW – BUILDINGS

NOTE: Stairs, Elevators, and Escalators are discussed in detail by the Modules of the same respective names.

OBJECTIVE: The student will visit and discuss three homes and three public buildings with varying characteristics.

OBJECTIVE: The student will describe a typical system for numbering floors and rooms in a public building. He/she will ask directions to find an office and a rest room in an unfamiliar building, and proceed successfully to each.

AGE OF STUDENT:
Beginning level: preschool and early elementary grades.
Overall understanding: upper elementary grades and above.

PRIMARY SKILL EMPHASIS:
Floor plans
Orientation overall
Doors and doorways
Elevators
Communication and instructions
Corners, turns, and angles

ADDITIONAL SKILL EMPHASIS:
Daily living skills
Stairs
Escalators
In a crowd or a line
Meeting the public
Structure of buildings
Careers

SEE ALSO (Other Modules):
    Routes for New Buildings and New Classrooms – Upper Grades Through High School
    An Office Building
    What Is a "Room"?
    Alternate Routes Within a Building
    PUBLIC BUILDINGS (GENERAL) Modules
    PUBLIC BUILDINGS (SPECIFIC EXAMPLES) Modules

STUDENT BACKGROUND: This Module is a good example of a continuing "strand" of learning. It is a topic which should be revisited continually, with ever-increasing sophistication and generalization.

ACTIVITIES: HOMES

EXAMPLE 1: *BASIC EXPERIENCE*
See other Modules in this book for detailed suggestions in learning about individual homes:

What is a "Room"?
Apartment House or Condominium
Unfinished Basement, "Crawl Space," or Attic
Home – Contents of Room
Outside and Inside the House
Porch or Deck

EXAMPLE 2: *GENERALIZATIONS*
(*Preschool and primary grades*)
Even a preschooler can answer questions such as:

(1) "Tell me four rooms that we would find in just about any home." (Kitchen, bathroom, bedroom, family/living room)

(2) "Tell me some other kinds of rooms you might find in a home." (Dining room, sewing room, laundry room, basement, attic, etc. Also, often there is more than one bedroom or bath.)

(3) "I can think of two things that are sort of rooms, but not quite part of the regular house. Sometimes they have a roof and a floor, but no regular walls." (Garage or carport; porch or deck)

(4) "Some big buildings have a lot of floors (stories), with a basement. But how many floors do most houses have?" (This will vary with locality. It will also tie in with a

discussion of apartments.)

(5) Discuss any features that are especially common locally. (Example: Porches with storage underneath)

An older student can review the above concepts, and discuss these and other generalizations on a mature level. He should also learn about important regional differences. For example, if homes in your area have no basements, he should learn that in other climates they may be nearly universal.

EXAMPLE 3: *VARIOUS KINDS OF HOMES*

See that your student visits each type of structure that is common in your area. Usually this will be apartments or condominiums, mobile homes, and single-family houses. Ordinarily this occurs naturally with the family, but the teacher should make suggestions or help when necessary. Note that a child who lives in a mobile home needs to visit houses.

Examples of homes that may be less common, depending on locality, include:

    Duplexes, town houses, row houses
    A houseboat
    A mobile home
    An apartment above a store
    A large, older house that has been divided into several apartments

ACTIVITIES: OTHER BUILDINGS

EXAMPLE 4: *COMMON MAJOR FEATURES*

The following features of buildings are discussed in detail in other Modules:

    Stairs in Unfamiliar Buildings
    Emergency Exits in Various Buildings
    Doors and Doorways
    Elevators
    Escalators

The student should have practice with each of these features in more than one building.

EXAMPLE 5: *SPECIALIZED DOORS*

Revolving Door: A revolving door may be a new experience. In a small town they may be uncommon. Or, the student may always have walked through an alternative regular door.

With a young or immature student, it may be necessary to give considerable assistance at first—possibly even having the student go through with you in the same compartment.

Explain the following recommended procedure:

Doors ordinarily rotate to the right (counterclockwise). Approaching from the left may be helpful. Listen for a moment, noting the movements of people and/or of the door itself. When the door is moving relatively slowly, reach out with the cane to check its motion. (This is safer than reaching out with one's hand, which could be caught and injured.)

Extend the cane on into the compartment, touching the wall ahead, and proceed into the compartment. (Push if necessary.) Note the change of air pressure which means you are inside, and feel the pressure change again when you reach the opening on the other side. Turn slightly to your right as you exit the door.

Discuss turnstiles, which are somewhat similar in concept but much simpler in structure.

An experienced traveler may prefer variations of this procedure.

CAUTION: A revolving door is safe for a person who uses good techniques. A person can be injured, however, by letting a hand or fingers get caught, or by being slammed by a rapidly-moving door. Give close physical guidance to young or immature students. Give appropriate directions to more mature students. If the student has special physical problems, consult other experts about the advisability of using revolving doors. A regular door should be available for those who need it (though blindness in itself should not preclude use of revolving doors).

An automatic (sliding) door, described below, ordinarily seems to have no hazard. However, I know an elderly, frail woman (not blind), who was knocked down by such a door when she moved slowly. She broke her hip. If your student has orthopedic problems, consult a physical therapist about any special considerations.

Automatic doors: Automatic (sliding) doors are very common in supermarkets and elsewhere. It is easy to tell whether the door is open by using the cane and listening.

Security doors: Many apartment buildings have a loudspeaker and buzzer system for entry. A visitor pushes the button for the desired apartment, communicates through a loudspeaker, then opens the door which has been "buzzed" unlocked. With experience, your student will not find this baffling. For example, if inquiring ahead of time, he will ask where the button in question is located (e.g., fourth from the left in the second row) since he cannot read the names. He will know he must open the door quickly before it locks again.

Discuss other common security systems if they are not actually encountered:

- Pushbutton combination locks
- Locks opened by a plastic "key" or card
- Metal detectors
- Showing identification to a guard

EXAMPLE 6: *REST ROOMS*
Locating the Rest Room: It is increasingly common to find a Braille or raised-print sign at a rest room door. This can be helpful. However, impress upon your student that this alone is not sufficient for finding a rest room in an unfamiliar building.

First of all, signs are not universal or consistent in nature or location. Even more important, the best sign is of no help until it is found. It would be most inefficient (even ludicrous) to feel all along a hallway, laboriously searching for a sign that may not even be in this particular hallway at all.

Usually, the most efficient approach is to ask someone. (See the Module, "Asking Directions and Figuring It Out," for detailed suggestions.) Also, sometimes architecture suggests where rest rooms are likely to be—e.g., near the stairwell on each floor.

The Cane Prevents Problems:
The matter of rest rooms is one of the most obvious reasons for using a cane *all the time.* Even if a person is with a friend, the friend may not want to go there at the same time, and may not use the same rest room. And if (as occasionally happens) the blind traveler inadvertently enters the *wrong* rest room, a visible white cane can make the difference between a somewhat embarrassing episode vs. a major incident which could even involve the police.

Security:
Especially with a younger student, consider beforehand what rest room would be used if needed. The Module, "Rest Rooms at School," offers suggestions for younger children.

Encourage the student to use the rest room before leaving the school building.

A student beyond preschool should not need actual help with toileting. But any child under 8 may occasionally have trouble fastening clothing.

Also, a beginner could possibly become disoriented in a large public rest room. If you and the student are the same sex, you can easily enter if you so choose, and discreetly check. But for an older student of the opposite sex, confusion in a large rest room is a touchy matter which the student may hesitate to mention. Try to prevent embarrassment. A temporary solution is to seek out a small, one-person rest room. Also, as necessary, arrange help from a tactful staff member of the appropriate sex. For example, the counselor might go along occasionally and help the student examine a large public rest room.

With experience, orientation inside the rest room should not be a problem.

Consider also where the student will wait if *you* need to use the rest room in a public building.

CAUTION: Vicious crimes have been committed in public rest rooms, in a very few minutes, while family or friends waited just outside. Note your surroundings and use security precautions appropriate for your area.

EXAMPLE 7: *THE "BIG PICTURE"*

Even a young child can begin to grasp generalizations and comparisons:

- "Tall buildings have elevators."
- "In a mall, we don't have to go outside to get to the next store."
- "The Post Office has automatic doors like the bank."
- "The County Building is a lot like City Hall, but bigger."

Refine and expand helpful generalizations. Also, watch for generalizations that are *not* correct, and for other kinds of misconceptions. Perry, for example, had always lived in a college town. He had been to the Drama Workshop at the college. But at age eleven, he was startled to discover that the campus had many different buildings. He had assumed that the college, being a school, was all in one building – just like the grade school and the middle school.

Mental mapping: Help your student form the important habit of "mental mapping." An overall description of an unfamiliar building might be: "This building is rectangular, and it faces south. The entrance is in the middle of the south wall. To the left of the main entrance is a reception area with seating. To the right is an escalator leading to meeting rooms on the second floor.

"On the second floor are meeting rooms with names such as 'Sierra Ballroom.' Above the second floor, there are offices; suite numbers begin with 3 for the third floor, and so on. Odd numbers are on the north side of the hall, with a few exceptions.

"At each end (that is, at the east end and at the west end) there is a stairway and an elevator.

"Floor 23 is the highest; it has an expensive restaurant."

Help your student build mental mapping skills. Give clear verbal descriptions which focus on overall patterns. Use simple tactual maps from time to time.

Practice, practice: Analyze typical patterns and features that can help in unfamiliar buildings. Discuss various systems of numbering and designation. For example, some buildings have rooms with N, S, E, or W added to denote compass directions.

Check understanding: ("If your dentist's office is in Suite 653, you would take the elevator to what floor?")

Note that there is often a guard or information desk near the main entrance. Also, there is usually a board or sign which lists the occupants and their room numbers. The blind traveler should know that the main entrance is a good place to ask for information. Even if there is no guard, someone could read the directory board.

Include experience in shopping malls (see "Malls" Module.) Discuss: Is a mall "all one building" or many?

EXAMPLE 8: *OTHER EXAMPLES*

This book includes a specific Module for each of several representative examples of public buildings:

    An Office Building
    A Doctor's Office
    Hotels and Motels
    A Restaurant
    A Grocery Store
    The Airport
    An Auditorium or Theater
    The Bank
    A Service Station
    Malls

Additional examples of typical buildings include:

    Post Office
    Library
    Large department store
    Large "discount" store
    Specialized stores
    Church or temple
    Bus terminal
    Health club or gym
    Bowling alley

Following are a few miscellaneous features that are helpful and/or interesting to examine:

- Pay lockers (A blind traveler who does not have a car for storing packages can find these very helpful in a mall or

elsewhere.)
- Mail chutes in tall buildings
- Different kinds of water fountains
- Unusual doors (Example: a Dutch door, in which the top opens separately from the bottom)
- Stairways with varying characteristics
- Various kinds of chairs, seats, benches, tables, etc. (Note: This can be very interesting to young children. Examining and sitting on a particular kind of seat can provide a helpful break and diversion.)
- Neon signs that hum noticeably
- Distinctive characteristics in regard to sounds, echoes, scents, etc.
- Local features related to climate or culture

MODULE 71
STAIRS IN UNFAMILIAR BUILDINGS

NOTE: The Modules, "Description of Basic Techniques" and "Introducing the Cane," describe the introduction of basic stairway techniques.

OBJECTIVE: The student will detect and recognize stairs in familiar and unfamiliar areas. He/she will walk up and down steps which have varying characteristics.

AGE OF STUDENT: Preschool and up (See individual Examples below)

PRIMARY SKILL EMPHASIS:
Stairs
Detecting step-downs or drop-offs
Posture, grip, gait, and arc

ADDITIONAL SKILL EMPHASIS:
Orientation overall
Carrying things
Corners, turns, and angles
Floor plans
Structure of buildings
Finding a seat
General travel (indoors)
Escalators

SEE ALSO (Other Modules):
>Introducing the Cane (Including Stairway Technique)
>Description of Basic Techniques (Including Stairway Technique)
>Escalators
>Elevators
>PUBLIC BUILDINGS Modules
>Unexpected Dropoff or Step-Down
>Exterior Fire Escape
>Obstacles (Noting Them and Proceeding)

TEACHER PREPARATION: When going to another school building, it is wise to arrange it ahead of time. It is a courtesy to the principal (who desires to know who is in the building) and helps to prevent arriving at unsuitable times. For a building which is not open to the general public (e.g., an apartment house with security), permission must be arranged.

However, if you are going to a place which is open to the general public, it is usually best *not* to make inquiries beforehand. The management might try to object to your coming, despite the fact that you and your student are part of the "public." Use your judgment, however; sometimes a prior explanation will encourage a pleasant and welcoming contact.

STUDENT BACKGROUND: These examples assume that the student already has a good start in the basic technique for stairs and has had practice in an easy location. Sometimes, of course, an unfamiliar building is the only logical place for beginning work on stairs. This is appropriate if the setting is carefully chosen.

ACTIVITIES:

EXAMPLE 1: *UNFAMILIAR SCHOOL BUILDING*

Often the best place to begin practice outside the student's own school is at another school. Varied practice is gained while in a particularly friendly and "sheltered" setting. If there are special health concerns or other problems, support is available from the nurse and other staff.

A preschool student can particularly benefit from practice in the school which she will attend later (with much more help and repetition than is suggested below for an eight-year-old).

Eight-Year-Old Student With Little Experience
Remain close to the student throughout the lesson. Rather than giving directions all at once, give directions for a short task and then discuss it. Sometimes guide the student through a task that is not being emphasized (e.g., walking down a series of hallways) to arrive speedily at the emphasized location (i.e., stairway).

Ask the student to follow you from the car to the door of Parker School, following your voice.

Explain that just inside the door are steps leading up to first floor and down to the ground floor. Direct the student to open the door, find the steps that go up, and proceed to first floor. Go with her to the office and greet the secretary.

Walk with the student, guiding her to cross the hall and walk toward the interior stairwell. Help her to cane the wall with each arc, looking for the stairwell door while continuing to make a complete arc each time.

Ask her to open the stairwell door, find the steps going up (being alert to the possibility of finding steps going down), and proceed to second floor. Note that halfway up, there is a landing, and the stairway turns to continue. The landing is small and not another "floor."

At the second floor, ask the student to walk ahead across the hall until the wall is reached. Then she should turn around, start down the stairs, and keep going to the ground floor, where the stairs end. Narrate while proceeding:

"This is the landing between second and first floor...Here's first floor...the landing between first floor and ground floor... the ground floor."

At the ground floor, walk together down the hall to the cafeteria. Say hello to the cooks and explain that you are visiting. What is the menu today? Is it the same as for the other school? Sit down at a table for a few minutes. Relax and discuss the trip.

Ask the student to follow you back to the stairs. Proceed all the way to second floor. Ask the student to narrate progress in the same manner that you did on the way down.

At second floor, direct her to walk straight ahead to the wall, then turn around and go back down.

Continue practice on stairs (interspersed with going elsewhere briefly) as much as time and energy permit.

Go back to the office. Thank the secretary and tell her you are leaving. Have the student follow you outside to the car.

Eleven-Year-Old Student With Experience
The advanced student practices tasks similar to those above, but with greater independence. In this instance, the teacher gives directions for a substantial route, follows at a distance, and meets the student later for further directions.

When ready to get out of the car, direct the student: "I will tell you how to go in and find the office. I'll follow you quietly and help you if you need help.

"When you get out of the car, walk straight ahead until you find grass. Turn left on the cement, just before the grass, and soon you will come to the door. There are steps just inside, leading both up and down.

"Go up–about half a flight–and you'll be on first floor. Turn left, then left again at the first hallway. In that hall, the third door on the left is the office. When you get to the office and start to introduce yourself, I'll come along in and join you.

"Now, would you repeat those directions? We'll talk them over until you're sure you have them."

After greetings in the office, give the student considerable blocks of directions in a similar manner as she continues:

"Cross this hallway and turn left. On your right, you will find a stairwell door. Go up the stairs to second floor. Turn right after you exit the stairwell, and you will find the media center at the end of the hall. Go on into the media center and take a seat. I will meet you there."

"Now, go back to the stairs and go all the way down to the ground floor. That's the same thing as the basement, but they call it the ground floor. When you get to the bottom, go on out of the stairwell, turn right, and go to the cafeteria. It's at the end of the hall, just like this media center–more or less right under us. I will meet you there."

"Practice going all the way up and all the way down, once more. Go up to second floor, to the media center again. But when you get there, just turn around and come back here. Sit down at a table here in the lunchroom, and I'll treat you to a Pepsi from these machines."

"OK, it's almost time to go back to your school. Let's review where the office is.... That's right, go back up to first floor and cross the hall to the office. Tell them we're leaving; this time I probably won't come into the office. I'll meet you outside the door to the parking lot... Review, please, how to go from the office to the door we came in...."

Meet the student at the outside door and proceed to the car.

REMARKS: The examples below are explained more briefly than those above. It should be assumed that a beginning student would have more help, and an advanced student less help, in a manner similar to the above.

EXAMPLE 2: *UNFAMILIAR HOUSE*
Arrange to go to a house other than the student's own home.

Walk up the steps to the front stoop. Are there railings on both sides of the steps? Note that a person need not always hold onto a railing. Practice sweeping the cane to the sides of the step, at least on the first step, to avoid stumbling off if there is nothing at the side.

Go inside and practice walking up and down the stairway(s). Note characteristics such as those below, and compare with other homes.

- A straight wooden staircase with a banister rail
- Complete front and back stairways in some larger homes
- More stories than the student has previously seen in a home
- A steep, narrow stairway to a basement or attic. (Sweep the steps with the cane to avoid stepping off the side. Are the steps "open," without riser panels?)
- Steps going up and/or down immediately inside a door
- A split-level home where a single step or two may appear between rooms

While practicing, the student should walk some distance on the level whenever she reaches the top or bottom, rather than simply turning around immediately. This provides experience in finding the stairs and verifying the step-up or step-down.

EXAMPLE 3: *WHAT CONSTITUTES A "FLIGHT" OF STAIRS?*
Review what the student knows about standard groupings of steps. People speak of a "flight" of stairs, or "going up one floor (story)."

Go up and down a fairly standard flight of steps. Although counting steps is not desirable as a technique for travel, it may be instructive to note how many steps are in a typical "flight" (about 13).

(NOTE: Although the sighted public tends to assume it is the normal method, *reliance* on counting steps should be strongly discouraged. It is inefficient and unreliable, and cane usage makes it unnecessary. Counting steps is tedious and inefficient; a person can easily be distracted and lose count.

Counting contributes to the idea that blind persons cannot negotiate all kinds of stairs without difficulty. Cane usage, in contrast, is reliable and efficient on both familiar and unfamiliar stairs.)

Discuss the typical height of a ceiling in buildings of recent construction (about 10 feet). Usually, one flight of stairs covers this distance.

Go up and down:

- A straight flight with no turn-back
- A divided flight with a landing and turn-back. (How do we recognize the landing as not being the next floor?)
- An extra-long flight, as in a public building with high ceilings.
- A set of steps that is less than one flight (see Example below)

EXAMPLE 4: *MISCELLANEOUS STEPS – NOT A FULL FLIGHT*
Look for opportunities for practice on steps that are not a full "regular" flight – e.g.:

- To the stage in an auditorium
- Steps to various levels in the audience portion of an auditorium. (Steps to the balcony may approximate a full flight.)
- To the front or back door of a residence
- Large, wide steps leading to doors of a public building

EXAMPLE 5: *UNUSUAL KINDS OF STEPS*

Practice on steps which have an unusual shape, height, pattern, etc. Discuss where such steps might typically be found, and how to recognize them. If the traveler suspects that the stairway may not be of typical size and/or may have nothing at the side, she should sweep across each step with the cane as necessary.

Examples include:

- Spiral staircase
- Extremely wide steps (often found at large, older public buildings)
- Steps with unusually high or low risers; "open" steps with no risers
- A flight which, in turning, has no landing but instead has some wedge-shaped or triangular steps
- Various surfaces, including wrought iron

EXAMPLE 6: *UNEXPECTED STEPS*

To a young child, almost any steps in an unfamiliar area may be "unexpected"; hence, valuable practice is possible almost anywhere.

A more mature student anticipates steps according to surroundings, sound clues, etc. This is desirable. But it is also important to remain alert for the unexpected (especially step-downs).

Many examples in this Module, as well as elsewhere in this book, provide a good demonstration of unexpected steps.

- Auditorium or theater (See the Module, "Auditorium or Theater.")
- "Miscellaneous" steps, as described above in this Module
- A basement entrance, especially one where steps lead down unexpectedly from the sidewalk
- Wide, decorative steps at a mall or large public building
- A "drop-off" greater than a standard step – e.g., a loading dock.

EXAMPLE 7: *ENCLOSED STAIRWELL WITH SEVERAL FLIGHTS*

The experience at the school, above, provided one example of a stairwell.

Go to a large building that has an enclosed stairwell with fire doors and at least three flights of fairly uniform stairs.

Walk up and down at least three flights. Name each floor (and each landing, if any) when you pass it.

At the top and bottom of the chosen distance, walk away rather than turning around immediately; this provides practice in locating the stairs. Preferably, ask the student to find a specific place at the top or bottom. For example, "Turn left and go to the end of the hall, then come back," or "The first door on the right is a meeting room. Go in and take a seat, and I'll join you."

How can a blind traveler know the floor number if she cannot read the number? She should know where she is upon arrival, and count flights (remembering to think about landings vs. floors and to be alert to overall distance). She can ask directions occasionally. A few modern buildings may have Braille labels.

Discuss why a person might use the stairs even when there is an elevator. Sometimes the stairs are faster or more convenient. Exercise improves health. Emphasize that elevators should never be used in case of fire, and that a blind person can use stairs as readily as anyone else.

Examine another stairwell (or another portion of the same one) where there is a different arrangement. For example, the basement stairs might be straight with no landings, and somewhat steeper and narrower. In a hotel, often the guest-room floors have a uniform stairwell, but the lower floors (where meeting rooms are) have a completely different layout. One should not make rigid assumptions.

MODULE 72
ELEVATORS

OBJECTIVE: The student will travel independently on two different elevators.

AGE OF STUDENT: Elementary grades and up (These Examples are described as for students in the intermediate grades unless otherwise noted.)

PRIMARY SKILL EMPHASIS:
Elevators
Doors and doorways

ADDITIONAL SKILL EMPHASIS:
Posture, grip, gait, and arc
Sound direction and meaning
Communication and instructions
Structure of buildings
Corners, turns, and angles
Daily living skills
Emergency procedures
Stairs
Examining things tactually
Floor plans
In a crowd or a line
Meeting the public

SEE ALSO (Other Modules):
>In a Crowd
>Doors and Doorways
>Escalators
>General Overview – Buildings
>Emergency Exits (In Various Buildings)
>Hotels and Motels
>Urban Rapid Transit

REMARKS: In a rural setting, especially in the Midwest, be sure the student understands that this kind of elevator is not the same thing as a grain elevator (a tall structure used for storage of corn, beans, etc.)

CAUTION: If the student has not ridden on elevators before, or is known to be susceptible to motion sickness, make riding very brief. With any student, avoid extremely lengthy elevator practice uninterrupted by other activities. If possible, integrate elevator practice with other kinds of practice over time.

Elevator doors can close suddenly. If the child has special medical problems such that being bumped by a door would harm him, take precautions.

Note that a door could close unexpectedly *between* you and the student, leaving one of you on the elevator and one not. With a very young child, make sure this does not happen: hold onto the student firmly and enter together. With a more experienced student, discuss this possibility and explain how you would get together if separated. (Example: Plan to meet at the floor which was your destination. If the other person does not arrive after quite some time, assume there was a mix-up and go back to first floor.)

Be extra-rigorous about always caning the floor of the elevator before entering. A malfunction could result in the door opening to reveal the floor of the car higher or lower than normal – or even no car at all.

Take care that discussions are age-appropriate and do not *cause* unnecessary fear of obscure dangers. Discuss safety in a matter-of-fact way, with assurance that modern elevators are well-designed and safe.

TEACHER PREPARATION: For a beginner, try to select a time when elevators are not crowded. An experienced student, however, benefits from experiencing crowded situations.

If the student cannot grasp the pattern of the buttons from a quick examination and discussion, make tactual diagrams which can be used anywhere. (Simple marks arranged in a pattern are sufficient; it is not necessary to make realistic "buttons.") Lengthy examination while on the elevator is difficult. Other people may interrupt. Also, the elevator will not stay in one place; and lengthy examination while the car moves up and down invites motion sickness.

Consider Cautions, above.

ACTIVITIES: Discuss experience and knowledge which the student already has about elevators.

Help the student as much as necessary at first, and then build independence.

EXAMPLE 1: *INTRODUCTION*

The student enters an office building, turns left, and approaches the elevator area. The sound of elevator bells may confirm direction.

Push the "up" button. (If other people are present, it is acceptable to ask, "Is the *up* button lighted?" But the student should have experience finding and pushing the button himself.)

When sound (bell, door opening, etc.) indicates an elevator car has arrived, briskly step toward it and enter.

If other people are present, the cane gently detects others' feet. The student must move quickly, yet not be rough with other passengers.

Examine the control buttons on the elevator. Are there any Braille labels? Raised print labels? If not, the pattern of the buttons on a familiar elevator can easily be memorized, and this is important for independence. With experience, one can also make an intelligent guess in an unfamiliar elevator. (Often another passenger will push the buttons; however, one should not have to depend on having other people around.) Note special buttons such as "alarm," and the emergency telephone panel.

Push the button for the desired floor.

Many late-model elevators "beep" when passing each floor—often in a pattern to indicate the floor number. Others have an actual spoken announcement (in synthesized speech) for each floor. As the elevator proceeds, notice whether there are any indicators of this kind.

When getting off, observe whether there is a tactual label on the doorway confirming the floor number.

If one is alone in an elevator, and no one else summons it, presumably the elevator will go directly to the floor desired. However, the traveler should realize that many factors could cause the elevator to go elsewhere first.

If there are no "beeps" when passing floors, and no confirming tactual label upon arrival, other methods can be used for checking the floor number. For example:

- If you are going up only one floor, the next stop should indeed be yours.
- If another passenger gets on at fifth, and you had pushed the button for sixth, your floor should be next.
- If you are going from first to fifteenth, and the car stops almost immediately, you are not there yet.
- You may know of identifying characteristics for various floors in a particular building—e.g., no carpeting in hallways above third.
- It is acceptable to ask other passengers for floor numbers, unless the teacher directs otherwise for practice.
- None of these (including information from other passengers, and including labels) is absolutely foolproof. The student, another person, or the equipment may make an error. Remain alert to the possibility that one might get off on the wrong floor.

Exit at the desired floor and proceed with the errand. (If no specific errand is planned, the student might walk to the end of the hall and back.)

Find the elevator and go back down to the ground floor. Exit the building, come back in, and repeat.

EXAMPLE 2: *ELEVATORS IN VARIOUS BUILDINGS*

Ultimately, the student should have practice with elevators in various buildings, going to various floors. Discuss situations and variations such as the following, if they are not available for actual experience:

- There are two or more elevators together. The traveler must listen carefully and hurry to the correct door before it closes.

– There are several elevators together. At the ground floor there is always one car waiting silently with its door open. In this case, the student should walk along and check each door with the cane. (Also, pushing the call button is likely to produce a sound at the open door.)
– Certain elevators go only to certain floors.
– Freight elevators are not for general use. Sometimes there are other elevators restricted to staff only.
– Occasionally one still finds a non-automatic elevator which is operated by an employee.

SAFETY NOTES: Emphasize that an elevator should never be used in case of fire. Observe where the stairs and other emergency exits are located.

Many persons believe, incorrectly, that blind persons typically have difficulty with stairs. Point out that, on the contrary, sometimes the stairs are more convenient and provide needed exercise, as well as being essential in case of fire.

EXAMPLE 3: *STRUCTURE AND MECHANISM*

Discuss, at least briefly, the structure of the car itself, the overall mechanism, and the elevator shaft. If practical, get as close as possible to the equipment at the top and at the bottom, and listen.

Discuss safety mechanisms and procedures. What is done if an elevator gets stuck? (See Caution, above, and be careful not to frighten a young child by unwise discussion of dangers. An older child will realize that such dangers could exist, and should find a matter-of-fact explanation reassuring.)

RELATED PRACTICE: Emphasize that blind persons have no more need for elevators, as such, than other people do. However, because of public attitudes, people may urge (or even try to require) that the elevator be used. For example, in an airport a blind person may be directed to the elevator instead of a nearby stairway or escalator. As the student matures, he should anticipate this possibility and head it off when possible.

An elevator in a tall building will be used by all. However, in a two-story building, it will probably be mainly for the handicapped.

MODULE 73
ESCALATORS

OBJECTIVE: The student will recognize an escalator, and travel up or down independently.

AGE OF STUDENT: Preschool (closely accompanied)
Elementary grades and up (experienced students need not be closely accompanied)

PRIMARY SKILL EMPHASIS:
Escalators
Stairs
Posture, grip, gait, and arc

ADDITIONAL SKILL EMPHASIS:
Detecting step-downs or drop-offs
Purchase or transaction
In a crowd or a line
Carrying things
Right and left
Sound direction and meaning
Floor plans
Corners, turns, and angles
Landmarks

SEE ALSO (Other Modules):
  Description of Basic Techniques (Including Stairway Technique)
  Introducing the Cane (Including Stairway Technique)
  Elevators
  PUBLIC BUILDINGS Modules
  In a Crowd
  Walking in a Line of People
  Walking Independently While Following Someone
  Urban Rapid Transit
  The Airport

TEACHER PREPARATION: For a beginning lesson, try to find a time when the area is not extremely crowded. However, an experienced student will benefit from practicing in crowds.

CAUTION: See that the student observes basic safety procedures—notably (a) not reaching or leaning over the rail, (b) not pushing toes against the risers, and (c) not touching the step with her hands.

ACTIVITIES: If the student is unfamiliar with escalators, describe them beforehand. Possibly have the student examine a regular staircase with her hands while discussing how an escalator moves. Explain that the steps fold flat at the top and bottom and return underneath—comparable to a conveyor belt. Explain that the handrail has a moving belt also. Discuss the concept of a pair of escalators—one going up, the other down.

EXAMPLE 1: *BEGINNING*
Finding the Correct Escalator
The student arcs her cane, and listens, to locate the escalator.

Touching the moving handrail indicates the direction of motion (i.e., up or down) instantly. At the same time or very shortly after, the cane touches the moving steps.

It is helpful to practice approaching an escalator going the wrong way. The student notes the wrong direction of the handrail, and that the cane moves back toward her when placed on a step. (Obviously, this should be done on an empty escalator.) This helps prevent later problems: the student would readily realize she is going the wrong way, and would not have an accident by attempting to get on, or by hesitating so long as to cause a collision with someone coming toward her.

Proceeding Up or Down
If the student is inexperienced, hold onto her at first as needed. Place her hand on the moving handrail while you stand behind or beside her and help. See that she keeps her cane touching the steps at all times.

Students often worry that they will step on between steps while they are flat at the beginning. Recommend that the student simply walk on, holding onto the handrail, and move her feet if necessary as she goes on up. It is hard for the traveler to tell immediately whether she is stepping squarely onto a step or not, but it is unwise to delay while trying to find out.

Once on the "up" escalator, the cane should be held vertically a step or two ahead of the student. She can then easily tell when the steps flatten out, and she is not likely to trip others.

Similarly, when going down, the cane should be touching a step or two ahead.

Stepping Off
The student is alert to notice when the steps flatten out and the cane touches the solid floor, indicating the time to step off.

EXAMPLE 2: *INDEPENDENCE*

Once the student understands how to proceed, do not accompany her closely. Instead, have her approach independently from some distance, practicing from various directions. Do not meet her immediately when she steps off. Instead, direct her to proceed to a designated location. ("When you get to the bottom, walk straight ahead until I meet you" may be a helpful plan in some situations.)

Include practice when others are present. Avoid crowding too close to the person ahead. (It may be helpful to practice with the teacher ahead.)

Discuss considerations for safety and courtesy:

- Do not run, lean over the side, or engage in other silly behavior.
- Walking at a moderate speed in the correct direction is usually acceptable on a moving escalator if it does not crowd other people. However, most people simply stand and let the escalator carry them.
- Do not push toes against the riser. When the steps fold, they could pinch or catch toes. Untied shoestrings can also get caught.
- Do not touch the step with your hands; a hand could be pinched or injured.
- Be alert to get on and off at the correct time. Hold the handrail. Losing one's balance is dangerous.
- There are some situations in which a person should use the stairs or an elevator instead of the escalator. These include carrying large objects, carrying a child, pushing a stroller, using crutches, etc. It may include using an *orthopedic* cane and walking with considerable difficulty. Occasionally someone becomes confused about this and asserts that a person must use the elevator because of blindness. The blind traveler should be prepared to explain (and insist, if necessary) upon the right to use the escalator.
- Usually there is an emergency "stop" button for emergencies.

EXAMPLE 3: *CHANGES AND VARIATIONS*

Go up and down two or more floors on a series of escalators. What is the pattern for continuing up or down? (e.g., keep turning right)

Recognize that escalators are not *always* in matched pairs of "up" and "down."

A given escalator may not always perform the same way. It may be shut off because of maintenance problems, in which case people walk on it like a stairway. Also, in a large meeting hall, an escalator may be "reversed" to accommodate crowd movements.

Usually, an individual escalator covers the range of one flight of stairs. But occasionally an escalator "skips over" a floor or mezzanine.

"Moving sidewalks" are used at some airports. These are somewhat comparable to escalators, but are flat – "a conveyor belt for people."

MODULE 74
MALLS

OBJECTIVE: (*Lower elementary grades*) In an enclosed shopping mall, the student will walk from one familiar location to another familiar location and back.

OBJECTIVE: (*Upper elementary grades and above*) In an enclosed shopping mall, the student will follow directions to two unfamiliar and non-adjacent locations. He/she will discuss the overall floor plan of the mall, naming at least two well-known businesses which are in landmark locations.

AGE OF STUDENT:
Early elementary grades: Readiness and partial independence.
Age 12 and up: Increasing independence, as age-appropriate.

PRIMARY SKILL EMPHASIS:
Orientation overall
Landmarks
Communication and instructions
Purchase or transaction
Escalators
In a crowd or a line
Sound direction and meaning
Interpreting odors
Right and left
Compass directions
General travel (indoors)

ADDITIONAL SKILL EMPHASIS:
Doors and doorways
Carrying things
Corners, turns, and angles
Floor plans
Flexibility and confidence
Responsibility and citizenship
Open space
Daily living skills
Careers

SEE ALSO (Other Modules):
In a Crowd
Alternate Routes Within a Building
Visually Confusing Appearance
Asking Directions and Figuring It Out
PUBLIC BUILDINGS, GENERAL Modules
PUBLIC BUILDINGS, SPECIFIC EXAMPLES Modules
Description of Basic Techniques (Including Stairway Technique)

TEACHER PREPARATION: Especially with an older beginner, it is important that the teacher examine the area beforehand – at least by looking over a floor plan, and preferably in person. If the teacher enters the mall for the first time while accompanying the student, the teacher cannot grasp the overall layout immediately, and therefore loses the chance to plan what the student will practice or discover at the beginning.

FIGURE(S):
FIGURE 74-1: Typical Enclosed Mall

ACTIVITIES:

EXAMPLE 1: *OVERVIEW OF A MALL*
(*Beginner*)
Beforehand, discuss the nature of a "mall." This example assumes that all businesses are enclosed together, with one continuous roof. The businesses open onto a large central "mall" (a large hallway or walkway which is also under the roof). There are several "main entrances" which go into the mall walkway. Some businesses may also have individual entrances directly from outdoors.

Especially with a younger student, discuss the overall layout of the particular mall beforehand. Consider using a simple map or tactual diagram. (This need not be detailed. If the mall is roughly in the shape of an "L," for example, a raised outline of the overall shape can be quite sufficient. Braille letters might indicate the approximate locations of a few major stores.)

When entering the mall, note a prominent business near that entrance. The easiest way to ask directions for getting back is to name a well-known business.

Help your student form a mental map of the overall layout, with well-known "anchor" businesses as landmarks.

In Figure 74-1, for example, the general shape is an "L," with the long "leg" extending north-south. At the north end is Sears, with the bus stop near its east door. If we walk south from Sears inside the mall, toward the corner of the L, we pass (among others) a shoe store and Ace music on the west side, and a bakery and another shoe store on the east side. If we turn the corner and walk west toward Wards, we pass the rest rooms on our right and a bookstore on our left. In this western portion only, there is also an upper level inside the mall; it is reached by ramps or stairs, and includes a dentist's office on the south side.

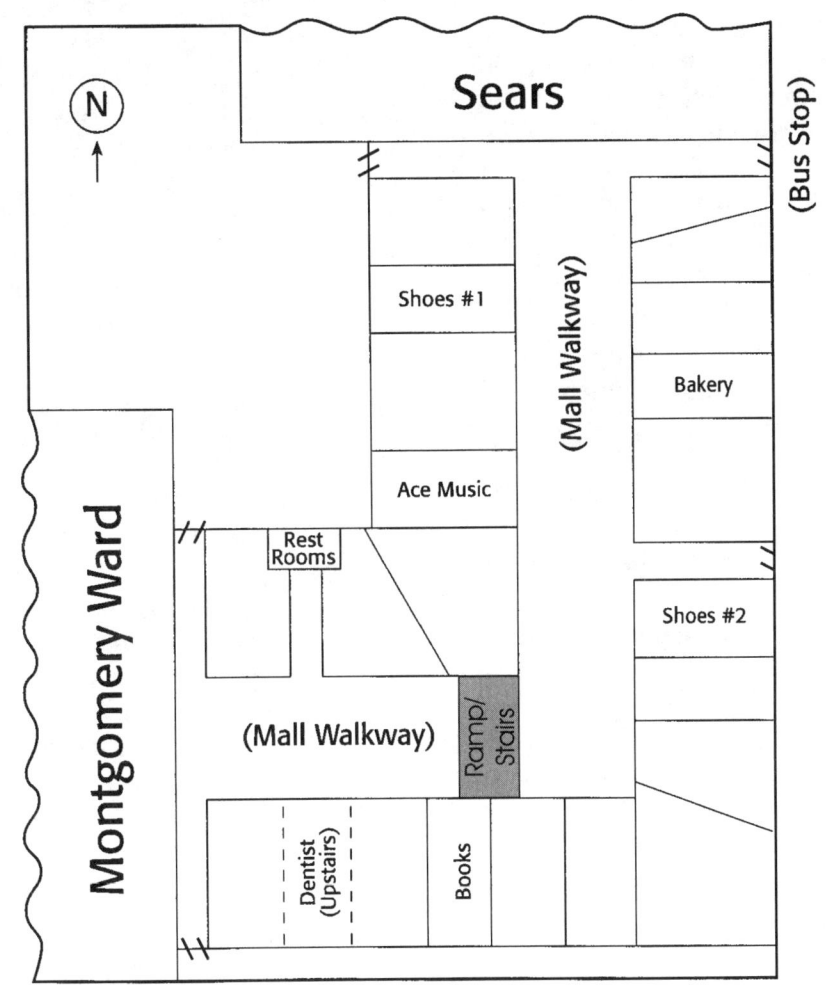

**Figure 74-1
Typical Enclosed Mall**

When introducing a student to this mall, emphasize that the general shape is an "L." (We call this an "L" shape even though the L is backwards.) The long "leg" extends north-south, with Sears at the north end. The shorter "leg" extends west, with Montgomery Ward at the west end.

Even if you and your student arrive by car, consider parking near the bus stop and simulating arrival by bus. Begin at Sears. Walk south and proceed along the west side of the walkway; turn toward Montgomery Ward and proceed along the north side of the walkway. Describe (or help your student recognize) some of the businesses or other features along the way: Ace Music, with its loud rock recordings; the stairs and ramps just west of the corner; the side hall with public rest rooms. Note the west end with the entrance to Wards.

Return in a similar manner, examining the south and east portion of the perimeter. Again note the ramps and stairs near the corner; make it clear that the west portion has a two-storied mall walkway, while the remainder has a mall walkway on one level only. (Individual stores, however, may have more than one level within the store regardless). Note scents from various shoe stores, the bookstore, and the bakery. Enjoy a small treat at the bakery.

Leave from the same entrance, near Sears. Afterward, discuss the trip in reference to the raised diagram.

EXAMPLE 2: *CLUES, LANDMARKS, FEATURES*

The first Example, above, describes walking around the perimeter of the mall as an introductory or general-information lesson. During such a lesson (and succeeding lessons), emphasize the types of clues or landmarks typically found at any mall. Also emphasize the features of the particular mall in question. The following list is helpful, but by no means exhaustive:

- Prominent odors: restaurants; candles; coffee; dentist's office; beauty salon; popcorn (may be with a theater); shoe stores; bookstores
- Prominent distinctive sounds: music (various kinds); pet shop; toy store; bowling alley; theater; fountain; loudspeakers
- Changes in texture underfoot – tile, carpet, etc.
- Ramps, steps, escalators
- Size and shape of mall walkway (e.g., echoes and air currents in a narrow hallway vs. a wide area with high ceiling)
- Small booths or kiosks in the middle of a wide mall
- Outside entrances (especially noticeable in inclement weather)

Also discuss effective strategies for gaining and using information:

- When first entering the mall, always learn the name of a prominent business near that entrance, to identify the entrance and find it again.
- Example 1 describes strategies for understanding the overall floor plan.
- Although prominent scents or sounds are good landmarks, one must recognize that there may be more than one beauty shop, restaurant, shoe store, etc.
- Keep track of what floor level you are on. The floor level within a store may differ from that in the mall itself. Also, outside entrances may vary: if there is a hill, the "second floor" may turn out to be at ground level.
- Walking around the perimeter, as described in Example 1, is often desirable. It is a good way to grasp the overall floor plan. Also, it is easier to keep one's bearings in this manner than by continually crisscrossing a hallway. Of course, it is not necessary to traverse the *entire* perimeter if the desired stores are within one area.
  For example, in Figure 74-1, suppose it is desired to visit Sears, Ace Music, some shoe stores, and the bakery. Proceed in this sequence: enter at bus stop; shop at Sears; proceed along the west side of the mall to the corner (stopping at the shoe store and Ace Music); cross over at the corner and proceed back up the east side, stopping at the other shoe store and the bakery; return to bus stop.
- Enter and leave a given business through

the *same door*. A major source of confusion is to go out a different door and find oneself in an entirely different place – even on a different level or facing a different direction.

- It is not essential to know exactly where you are at all times. Within certain limits (e.g., not going out into the parking lot), it is all right simply to keep moving along and looking around. Then after awhile, if information is needed and not apparent, ask directions.
- A good strategy for orientation is simply to walk into any business that is handy. In a familiar mall, one may immediately be re-oriented simply by learning which shop it is by brief examination. If necessary, one can easily ask directions. (Employees are more knowledgeable than the general public.)
- Fountains are landmarks, but often are more an annoyance than a help. They are a major interruption to a direct path, and they tend to be noisy.
- Do not over-rely on asking directions of other people.

Conveniences
A sighted person, burdened with shopping bags, may put them in the car and continue unhampered. Any shopper may use a backpack or other carrier. However, many persons are unaware of an excellent option which is especially convenient for the blind shopper: public lockers. As in airports, in many malls a person can insert a coin and rent a locker. It is handy for storing a heavy coat or a school bag, as well as purchases. Show your student these lockers and examine how they work. They are often near a bowling alley or a fitness gym.

Note other amenities and features that can add to a shopper's comfort and efficiency. Stop at a refreshment stand halfway through a long stint. When waiting for a companion, try to wait where there is a bench. Where are the rest rooms? Telephones? Floor plan diagrams?

EXAMPLE 3: *TO AND FROM THE BUS*
Even though you and your student may arrive by car, if possible park near the public bus stop and simulate coming and going from there.

Where is the bus stop? Is it in the parking lot, just a few feet from Sears? Or is it out at the street, a considerable distance from the store?

What routes serve the mall? Do all buses arrive there, or is the mall on a "route extension" which only operates at certain hours?

EXAMPLE 4: *GENUINE, INTERESTING ERRANDS*
It is highly appropriate and convenient to involve whatever daily living skills the student is now learning, and to provide practice and variety for skills already learned.

If it is not convenient for the student to buy something she herself needs, I provide a small amount of cash and ask her to buy an item for me – something which is easy to select. Examples include soap, pencils, packaged snacks, etc. I can always use items of this nature, and they can be assigned on the spur of the moment.

Also, most malls have other businesses besides shops. Often there are services such as dentists, beauticians, and banks. A logical errand is to ask about prices and hours. Often one can get a brochure or business card.

Except for introductory lessons, it is important for the student to have a concrete purpose for practice. Getting an object (even a brochure) provides a sense of accomplishment and practicality. In many locations this is difficult or impossible, but in a mall it is strikingly obvious.

EXAMPLE 5: *ASKING DIRECTIONS*
The best reference points are the "anchor" businesses – usually large department stores. Most people will know where they are and will mention them when describing less-familiar locations.

Compass directions, while useful, may not be very reliable when asking for information in a mall. Many sighted people will not be thinking in these terms – instead they will speak of "around the corner near Target" or "toward

McDonald's." Urge your student, nevertheless, always to maintain a mental map with compass directions at least assumed. If the true compass directions cannot readily be determined, one can mentally "assign" directions to form a working model (and alter it if more information is learned later). For example, if a traveler in Figure 74-1 assumed that Sears was to the east and Montgomery Wards was to the north, she could still follow directions such as "The rest rooms are around the corner toward Wards, off to the right."

A good strategy is to go to a posted diagram of the mall and ask directions from someone who is looking at it. Such maps are usually found at major entrances to the mall, and at mall intersections or corners. Another approach is to enter any business and ask. Also, of course, one may talk with anyone handy.

Most large malls have an Information Center. If this is easily found, it can be very helpful. Otherwise, however, it is usually not wise to spend time looking for it.

Asking "Where is the bus stop?" is also a poor strategy. Most people will not know. It is far better to inquire about a specific business. Even a small shop can easily be found on a diagram or index. This points up, again, the importance of learning the name of a significant business near the bus stop or entrance. "And," I tell my students, "just 'a restaurant' is not sufficient identification! There may be dozens of restaurants scattered around!"

Levels of maturity: I observe three levels of difficulty (or maturity) in regard to asking directions:

   a. For a very young student or a nervous beginner, I give complete directions and do not make the assignment complicated. The student may not need to ask directions at all. If she does have difficulty, she can enter any business and ask.
   b. For an experienced student, I often give partial information and expect her to ask, or figure out, the rest. For example, I might say, "There is a dentist's office in the west wing on the second level. Go there and get a brochure or business card. Find out whether the dentist accepts new patients."
   c. The Example, "Dealing with Confusion," below, describes an exercise for an advanced student in entering an unfamiliar mall with little or no information.

How much to ask: Structure the kind and amount of information for which a student may ask. The Module, "Asking Directions and Figuring It Out," discusses overall guidelines about asking for help during an assignment.

Even when "asking directions" is the skill being practiced, the student should expect to learn a great deal on her own. You might advise, "For at least [ten] minutes, try to figure it out on your own. Pretend you can't find anyone to ask. *Then* you may decide what information would be most helpful, and try to get it from another person."

EXAMPLE 6: *SECURITY CONSIDERATIONS*

Asking directions is often more necessary in a mall than elsewhere, because of the great variation in floor plans and the lack of standard city blocks.

If the student is so young that she would not be entirely independent (a parent would always be nearby), she may be told to talk only with employees inside a store. A student beyond elementary school, however, needs to approach the matter of "talking to strangers" more as an adult does. An older student should be able to (a) consider the circumstances – as, she is inside a mall and could not easily be kidnapped; (b) watch for possible clues that a person is acting inappropriately, and end the conversation in that event.

Also note that you, as a teacher working with a student who is not an adult, would intervene in case of real danger.

The Example, "Asking Directions," above, examines the question of "talking to strangers" in an age-appropriate manner. Discuss this, as well as other security considerations, with your student and her parents. More than one person has sat down to rest her feet, set her purse beside her, yawned – and found that the purse has disappeared. Talk about holding onto purse and bags, carrying expensive purchases in a modest and non-transparent bag, not counting money prominently, etc. Teach cautions appropriate for your locality.

If school rules require that you remain with your student, plan ahead to be sure that you do. For example, if the student is on an escalator headed for a crowded hallway, you should be close behind.

EXAMPLE 7: *EXPLORING INDEPENDENTLY*
(*High school and above*)

Many Examples in this Module deal with various degrees of independent exploration. A student of high school age should be able to enter a mall with virtually no knowledge (other than very general information, such as avoidance of high-crime areas of a large city) and explore independently.

One blind traveler explains, "If I go into a strange mall and have no easy way of getting an overall picture of it, or simply want to explore for myself – I find an unusual business as a reference point near the entrance where I went in, and then I proceed. I walk in a consistent direction by keeping stores on either left or right, and walk around the perimeter in that way. I keep track of stairs or escalators so as not to have trouble finding the entrance again. Once at the Brickyard in Chicago I did forget which level I was on and had a hard time figuring out how to get out again. But usually this approach works well.

"A student should become familiar with common patterns for mall layouts, and realize that there may be unusual patterns. In the Mall of America in Bloomington, Minnesota, each corner has a major store. They are: Sears, Nordstrom's, Bloomingdale's, and Macy's. In the center is Camp Snoopy, an amusement park. The transit center is in the middle of the east side.

"This square mall is actually quite easy to get around in, as long as you know these things. Sears is in the northeast corner, Nordstrom's is in the northwest corner, Bloomingdale's is in the southwest corner, and Macy's is in the southeast corner. You can walk through Camp Snoopy to take shortcuts, but you can do that only on the first floor.

"The mall has four stories. On the other three floors, you simply can walk all the way around the mall by keeping Camp Snoopy on your left or right. You can keep track of what direction you are going by noting which major stores you are between."

EXAMPLE 8: *DEALING WITH CONFUSION*
(*Upper elementary grades and above*)
In a familiar mall

Even in a familiar mall, it is easy to get "turned around" and be temporarily unsure of one's location. It is excellent practice to take a student to a partially familiar location, and ask her to figure out where she is and proceed with an errand.

This exercise provides excellent and realistic practice which adds to experience and self-confidence. If properly done, with a student who is sufficiently prepared, it does not cause fear or distrust.

It is important to discuss such an exercise beforehand – certainly with the student, and perhaps with others also to prevent misunderstanding. I explain as follows:

- This is realistic and valuable practice. A person may easily become confused and be unsure of where she is. Also, a driver may be misinformed or absent-minded and give a passenger wrong information. This exercise gives practice in recognizing such a situation and recovering one's bearings.
- I would never knowingly give a student wrong information (without indicating it might be wrong). However, I could be misinformed or absent-minded and

make a mistake. Furthermore, for instructional purposes I will sometimes "label" information as possibly incorrect or incomplete. I will do it by saying, "I am the taxi driver, and I'm telling you... [this door faces northeast.]" The student should take this expression as the introduction of questionable information.

- I review various techniques for orienting oneself.
- I tell the student to wait a certain length of time (using a Braille watch or talking clock, or estimating) before asking directions of anyone else. (This might be five minutes for a relatively young student, or fifteen or more for an advanced and mature student.) During this time the student must be walking around and trying to find clues herself. Any time spent standing or sitting in one place does not count.
- I will follow and watch, as usual. I will expect to help if it is really needed, to the same degree as for any other lesson.
- I point out that everyone, including this student, can recall times when she was momentarily confused about where she was. This new assignment is different only in that it is a "planned confusion." It is not really so different, and is excellent practice for dealing with confusion which occurs naturally.
- Although asking directions of other people is frequently appropriate, often no one can be found immediately. Or, people may not be helpful. This exercise provides excellent practice for when one *cannot* immediately get directions from someone else. And even when helpful people are available, over-reliance on such help is a trap which can reduce independence to zero.

The easiest way to arrange this experience is to drive around in the parking lot for a few minutes in an unpredictable path. Circle, back up, make various turns, etc. Then send the student through an entrance of your choosing.

CAUTION: If school rules require you to remain near the student at all times, be careful not to "lose" her at this point. If you drop her off at the door while you park the car (perhaps because walking through the parking lot would give her a clue you do not wish her to have), ask her to wait outside until you arrive and say "Go ahead."

In planning what door to use, I may look for the following "confusers":

- An entrance the student has rarely or never used
- A door directly into a business, rather than an entrance into the mall
- An entrance which has conspicuous similarities to another entrance
- Facing a different direction than expected (e.g., on the west side if we usually come in on the east)
- A familiar entrance where something has changed – construction, a special exhibit in the hallway, etc.

In an unfamiliar mall

For an advanced older student, if possible, assign a route in an entirely unfamiliar mall. (This may not be possible if all malls within commuting distance are somewhat familiar.) Give an assignment such as: Purchase toothpaste; get a menu from the Greek Deli; and find out what is showing at Theater #3. The student must determine how to get to the mall by bus, and start from "scratch" in finding the businesses.

It is assumed that the student will need to ask directions.

VARIATION(S): Visit or discuss various kinds of malls, such as:

- A mall much larger or smaller than the most familiar one(s)
- A "strip mall": Typically this is a long strip of businesses which are contiguous, but which all open directly outdoors rather than having a covered walkway. It is much like a traditional

downtown city block, but often is longer than a typical block. Also, it has a parking lot in front, instead of fronting onto the sidewalk and street.
- A street which is called a "mall" because no vehicles are permitted (except perhaps buses), but which does not have a roof over it.
- In Washington, D.C., "The Mall" is a large, grassy area – essentially a park – near the Washington Monument.

RELATED PRACTICE:
Map skills
Daily living skills

MODULE 75
EMERGENCY EXITS
In Various Buildings

OBJECTIVE: The student will exit independently from any part of the school building. He/she will examine and discuss emergency exits in two different public buildings.

AGE OF STUDENT: Elementary grades (with follow-up for older students)

PRIMARY SKILL EMPHASIS:
Emergency procedures
Doors and doorways
Floor plans
Flexibility and confidence

ADDITIONAL SKILL EMPHASIS:
Stairs
General travel (indoors)
Structure of buildings
Responsibility and citizenship

SEE ALSO (Other Modules):
  Fire Drills
  Exterior Fire Escape
  Alternate Routes Within a Building
  School Bus
  PUBLIC BUILDINGS Modules

TEACHER PREPARATION: Look for good representative examples of emergency exits. Include at least one which has an alarm, and at least one which can be used without causing an alarm or other problems.

STUDENT BACKGROUND: Understand the concept of emergency exits. Participate in fire drills at school.

ACTIVITIES:

EXAMPLE 1: *EXIT DOOR WITHOUT ALARM*
At the city office building, turn left at the first hallway inside the front door. Find the third door on the right.

"This is the Public Safety Office. Go on in and greet the receptionist. Tell her we're studying emergency exits. Ask if we may go out through the exit behind this office."

Observe that this office has an outside door which has no alarm but is locked from the outside. Go out this exit, imagining an emergency. Return to the regular front door and re-enter the building.

EXAMPLE 2: *EXIT DOOR WITH ALARM*
"Now turn *right* at the first hallway. Go to the very end of the hall and wait. Do not try to open the door at the end of the hall."

Describe the alarmed emergency exit. Help the student examine it very gently by touch without setting off the alarm. Discuss situations where you would open the door.

"If you worked here, or came here often, you should learn the location of emergency exits."

RELATED PRACTICE: Examine other safety equipment, such as fire hoses or extinguishers.

Note emergency exits in various buildings – theaters, stores, hospitals, etc.

Review emergency procedures at school.

Locate emergency exits on the school bus.

Plan home fire drills.

FOLLOW-UP: With older students on advanced routes, sometimes call attention to emergency exits.

PUBLIC BUILDINGS
SPECIFIC EXAMPLES

MODULE 76
AN AUDITORIUM OR THEATER

OBJECTIVE: (1) The student will detect step-downs and drop-offs with the cane, and proceed appropriately.
(2) The student will locate an appropriate seat, sit down, and stow the cane, in varied situations such as auditoriums, libraries, and restaurants.

AGE OF STUDENT: Preschool and up (see individual examples)

PRIMARY SKILL EMPHASIS:
Detecting step-downs or drop-offs
Floor plans
Finding a seat
Stowing cane
In a crowd or a line
Stairs
Sound direction and meaning

ADDITIONAL SKILL EMPHASIS:
Structure of buildings
Human guide
Walking in company with others
Meeting the public
Corners, turns, and angles
Orientation within a room
Obstacles in path
Purchase or transaction
Flexibility and confidence
Careers

SEE ALSO (Other Modules):
 In a Crowd
 Walking Independently While Following Someone
 Alternate Routes Within a Building
 Orientation Inside New Classroom
 Human Guide
 Unexpected Drop-off or Step-Down
 Visually Confusing Appearance

REMARKS: Show parents and school staff how reliably the cane finds the edge of the stage. Urge that the student be expected to use her cane when she is on stage – when she walks up to receive an award, give a real speech, sing with the chorus, etc.

A blind student may act in a play or take part in any other activity.

Many blind adults recall that their strongest feeling at their own graduation was fear of falling off the stage. How sad – how unnecessary.

TEACHER PREPARATION: Look around the auditorium and the stage. Note overall characteristics and interesting features. Determine whether the student is already somewhat familiar with the area; if so, build on any existing knowledge.

ACTIVITIES:

EXAMPLE 1: *GENERAL ORIENTATION*
(*Elementary grades*)
(This Example assumes a school auditorium with built-in seating.)

Ask the student to enter and find any seat, sit down, and place the cane where it is out of the aisle and won't roll away. (Each time the student takes a seat during this lesson, she should put the cane down and pretend she is going to stay.)

"Think about how it is when other people are here. When you're walking down the aisle past the rows of seats, how can you tell if a seat is already occupied? ... Yes, you might listen; gently touch the back of the seat; touch people's feet gently with your cane; ask if there is an empty seat nearby.... And, of course if it's a school assembly, you might have assigned seats.

"Practice that, please. I will walk on down the aisle and take a seat on the end of a row, on the left side of this aisle. You come along down, notice where I am, and take a seat farther forward.

"Now, please imagine that you need to climb over a couple of people to get to a seat inside the row. Your cane can help you find where to step, and at the same time it can tell you where there is an empty seat.

"I'm going to move three rows back on this same side of the aisle. I'll sit near the end, but perhaps not quite at the end. I'll tell you when I'm ready. Then you count three rows toward the back, walk on in past me, and take the next seat on the other side of me. This is good practice for crowds."

Continue with practice such as the following:
- "Walk all the way down this aisle toward the front, and find the stage area. But don't go up on the stage now. Use your cane well, and be alert for steps and other things."
- When the student arrives at the front, discuss the slope downward from the back of the auditorium. Were there steps, or was it just a gradual slope?
- Explore the area in front of the stage. Examine the orchestra pit if there is one; otherwise, describe what an orchestra pit is. (It does not always have a railing in front. Careless blind persons, often with useful sight, have fallen into such places when not using a cane.) Find the front of the stage, and the steps leading up.
- Walk around the perimeter of the room, getting as close to the side walls as the seating permits. Discuss how many people can be seated.
- Do the outermost sections reach all the way to the wall, without an aisle next to the wall? Take a seat next to the wall.
- Go to the front row and sit down.
- Go to the back of the auditorium and take a seat in the last row.
- "Have you noticed how many aisles there are that go from back to front? Check this by walking behind the back row and counting aisles."
- "Are there any aisles, or major breaks, where you can easily walk from side to side in the audience? Walk down the middle aisle, and keep touching the nearest seat on one side as you walk by. See if all the rows are evenly spaced."
- Find the center section, and take a seat.
- Discuss whether row numbers start at the front or the back. Then say, "Go to Row 4. Take the third seat to the right of the center aisle."
- The student acts as "usher" and shows the teacher to a seat.
- The student should easily be able to go to a seat which is far from the aisle, even if the rows are crowded together and if she must step over the feet of others already seated. Practice this, with the student actually climbing past at least one person (the teacher) some of the time. For example, "I will direct you to some more seats. This time, I will be sitting in a seat near the aisle. You will climb over me and sit in the third seat." (The teacher makes a point of sitting in various positions, some not very convenient for the person coming in.)
- Locate emergency exits.
- The teacher acts as an "usher" and shows the student to a seat. The cane should continue to be used at all times.
- Imagine that the aisles are very crowded. The student walks a considerable distance and finds a given row, while using her cane close to the body with a pencil grip. (See the Module, "In a Crowd.")

EXAMPLE 2: *A STAGE*
(*Elementary grades*)
Note: Even if there is no regular auditorium, there may be a stage. Many elementary schools have a stage in conjunction with the gym. Children sit on the floor, or chairs may be brought in. The blind student should understand where the stage is and its general layout.

CAUTION: Before going onto a stage, consider the maturity and behavior of the child. If she is very impetuous, heedless, or uncertain, hold onto her.

- In the seating area, face the stage. Examine the area between the seats and the stage, as in the above lesson.
- Find the steps and go up them. Sweep the cane across the steps, more than would ordinarily be done; often such steps do not have a wall or railing on each side.
- On the stage, find the front. Note how easily the cane detects the drop-off. Be sure the student understands where she is in relation to the seating area.
- On the stage, walk from side to side at the front, caning the edge of the stage with each step. Is it straight or curved?
- Find the steps again. Are there other ways on and off the stage? Practice going up and down.
- The student walks along at floor level, in front of the stage. She talks with the teacher, who is above her on the stage. The student reaches up to examine the height.
- On the stage, walk from back to front. Find the front edge confidently.
- The student walks diagonally across the stage. Note one reason for arcing the cane well: the drop-off may be encountered somewhat to one's side, rather than straight in front.
- Examine the stage curtain. Open and close it if possible. Practice coming from behind a closed curtain and walking through to the front of the stage. Discuss how the curtain is used in performances.
- Examine other interesting things that may be present: sports equipment, backdrops, sets or properties for drama, lighting controls, etc. Discuss stage lighting.
- Is there a movie screen? Where would the projector be placed?
- Explore backstage areas.
- If possible, go under the stage. What is there?
- Assisted as needed, the student takes a position on stage facing the "audience." The teacher goes to a seat. The student then "gives a speech" (tells a joke, recites a poem, or makes impromptu remarks). The cane is at her feet. (Keeping her foot on the cane may be a wise precaution against its rolling away). Alternatively, she holds her cane as she would when standing elsewhere.
- Reverse roles: The student walks down and takes a seat while the teacher goes up and gives a "speech."
- Both student and teacher take a seat. Without assistance, the student walks up the steps, faces the audience, and "gives a speech" as above.

EXAMPLE 3: *READINESS*
(*Preschool age*)

Students below kindergarten age, whether blind or sighted, will be closely supervised while in an auditorium. They will be permitted very little independence.

Nevertheless, selected portions of the above activities are very appropriate for a preschool-aged child:

- Walking around various areas, gaining valuable experience in using the cane on unusual terrain
- Beginning to gain understanding of the overall layout of a theater, including the stage
- Determining whether or not a seat is occupied
- Coming in past other people's feet to enter a row
- Exploring the auditorium where the child will go regularly in kindergarten or first grade
- Enjoying an unusual environment; avoiding boredom

EXAMPLE 4: *SURPRISE!*
(*Elementary grades and up*)

Sometimes, especially for a theater-arts class, there is a stage entrance directly from a hallway. The door may look just like other doors.

If such an arrangement exists, and the student is not already familiar with it, consider asking her to enter the door without being told exactly what is within. Depending on the student's experience and ability, she may be given various degrees of warning. After the drop-off is found and discussed, you can say, "This is a good example of why the cane should be used even after entering a room. You could even say that this is a *dramatic* example – oooh, terrible pun."

EXAMPLE 5: *A PUBLIC THEATER*
(Elementary grades and up)

Often a tour can be arranged at a time when there is no show, especially at a "live" theater. Explore as much as is practical, in the manner suggested for the auditorium above. (A theater employee should be with you if you go to a non-public area, including the stage itself.) Look at the ticket window, the lobby area, the snack counter. Walk around on the balcony; examine the front of it, and be sure the student understands the balcony's relationship to the main floor. Find the emergency exits.

EXAMPLE 6: *CHECKING AND EXPANDING SKILLS*
(Fourth grade and above)

The competence of students above the primary grades in regard to this Module will vary considerably. At any given age, some students will have a good grasp of the skills and a good understanding of the general layout of a theater. Others – even those who are competent elsewhere – may have major misconceptions or lacks. For example, one student may have always gone only to the assigned seating with her class, and may have no idea how many aisles and rows there are. Another student may know how to get onstage from the front, but not realize that there are entrances from behind the stage.

Many students are fearful of falling off a stage. Many believe incorrectly that the cane is "in the way," too conspicuous, and not very helpful in any part of a theater.

It is wise to "spot-check" even an advanced student. Try a few selected exercises from the Examples above (presented in an age-appropriate manner). If many problems and needs emerge, the student should have detailed practice.

Moving about comfortably in theater-style seating is important for anyone. Furthermore, most people, at one time or another, find themselves on a stage – perhaps only briefly and as part of a group, but nevertheless on the stage.

Integrate and reinforce skills:

Recently, I complimented one of my students for an excellent talk about Braille at the citywide PTA meeting. But I was disappointed that her cane had been nowhere in sight.

"I could never have found my way around that auditorium at South High alone," she protested. "Someone had to guide me up to the podium. And I didn't know where I'd put my cane. In some theaters there's no way you can get it under the seats."

Looking around the student's own school, I located a theater-arts classroom with which she was not familiar. We found a time when it was vacant, and I (with exaggerated fanfare) simulated the PTA program: "May I show you to a seat, Ms. Ainsworth? ... And now it's time for the next item... Ms. KAREN AINSWORTH! Would you come on up to the podium, Ms. Ainsworth? Right up here...."

Thus she walked toward my voice, here and there in the large room which had unexpected step-downs. To her delight and surprise, she easily succeeded without ever taking my arm. (I explained that in a real situation, she might indeed choose to take someone's arm for a time, but this did not exclude the cane.) She practiced placing the cane under her seat and by the podium. During "informal moments after the program," she walked around the room alone. Later we repeated all this while her mother watched.

With a cane, one may choose to accept various degrees of help from time to time. Without a cane, there is no choice but dependency.

VARIATION(S): Introduce your student to various kinds of settings, formal and informal. Compare the seating in a church or temple. Examine an outdoor amphitheater or stadium. Discuss definitions and gradations – e.g., when does a "meeting room" or "classroom" become an "auditorium" or a "theater"?

MODULE 77
THE BANK

OBJECTIVE: The student will complete errands independently in [four] public buildings. (Note: Objectives relating to daily living skills may also apply.)

AGE OF STUDENT: Kindergarten and up (See Examples)

PRIMARY SKILL EMPHASIS:
Purchase or transaction
Carrying things
General travel
Communication and instructions
Finding a person

ADDITIONAL SKILL EMPHASIS:
In a crowd or a line
Doors and doorways
Meeting the public
Daily living skills
Responsibility and citizenship
Sound direction and meaning
Careers

SEE ALSO (Other Modules):
>PUBLIC BUILDINGS Modules
>Carrying Things
>Errands
>In a Crowd

TEACHER PREPARATION:
Plan an appropriate transaction, such as asking for change.

If extra attention is to be requested, such as a tour of the deposit boxes, plan for a time when staff are not too busy.

STUDENT BACKGROUND: Discuss banking services in general.

ACTIVITIES:

EXAMPLE 1: *GENERAL OVERVIEW*
(*Kindergarten and elementary grades*)

In this example, it is assumed that the student is walking with the teacher to tour the bank and become familiar with it. An independent errand is described in Example 2, below.

Exit the vehicle and listen for cars moving. Walk to the building and find the door. (Is it a revolving door, an automatic door, or a regular door?)

Proceed to a teller's window. (The location may be explained beforehand, or the student may ask directions. In a small bank it may be easy to figure out.) Listen and use the cane gently to determine whether other customers are waiting.

Ask the teller to show you a sample of wrapped coins (i.e., coins wrapped in predetermined quantities to prevent laborious counting). Ask for a sample wrapper to study.

Walk to the Customer Representative desk and explain that you are studying bank procedures. Ask the Customer Representative to explain what services he/she performs—e.g., what a teller cannot do.

Go to the safe deposit area. Ask the attendant to show you a sample deposit box. Examine the vault and its heavy door.

Walk around the outside of the building. Examine and discuss the night depository, the Automatic Teller Machine (ATM), etc.

Observe the drive-up window. Would it be safe and practical to walk to it, if the bank as a whole were closed but the window still open? Often it is possible for a pedestrian to use such a window. (If it is not practical to walk to the drive-up window at this time, the teacher should describe it. Also, perhaps the drive-in teller can be heard talking to drivers.)

As time permits, examine other features of interest, such as tables with pens attached.

When exiting, again listen for traffic.

EXAMPLE 2: *AN ERRAND AT THE BANK*
(*Intermediate grades and up*)

Plan a transaction to be accomplished. Examples include:

- Get change (e.g., ten dimes for a dollar)
- Get coin wrappers (these may be free in small quantities)
- If an older student has an account, she can make an actual deposit or withdrawal.
- Get brochures and information about how to open an account.

Plan the errand in as much detail as required by the student's experience. For example, plan how the money will be carried; discuss why one should not carry it loosely in one's hand. (Money is easily dropped, and it is unwise to show one's cash in public. Also, if this is not the student's own money, it should be in an envelope instead of being mixed in with other cash or loose in a pocket.)

The student should travel to and from the bank independently. If it is not practical to take public transportation or walk the entire distance, the student should leave the teacher a block or more away. (As always, "leaving the teacher" means that the teacher may follow and observe, but will not plan to assist.)

RELATED PRACTICE: Practice or review the legal signature and discuss its importance. Learn to print the word VOID.

Study how to fill out checks and keep records.

Review ways to fold and organize money in one's billfold.

Discuss Braille labels and other methods for organizing materials in a deposit box. Note that some banks have tried to discriminate against blind customers. Some have tried to say, for example, that a sighted person must participate whenever a deposit box is rented or accessed. This is illegal discrimination.

MODULE 78
A DOCTOR'S OFFICE

OBJECTIVE: (1) The student will use his/her cane appropriately while walking with another person, whether following someone's voice or holding someone's hand or arm.
(2) In varied locations, the student will locate a seat, sit down, and stow the cane appropriately.

AGE OF STUDENT: Preschool through second grade

Note: This activity is presented as for a younger child. Preschool and kindergarten groups commonly visit a doctor's office; this Module will be helpful whether or not the blind child visits with a group.

Older students may already have sufficient experience. However, they may benefit from reinforcement of independence at the doctor's office – e.g., finding a seat in the waiting room.

PRIMARY SKILL EMPHASIS:
Walking in company with others
Human guide
Finding a seat
Stowing cane
Finding a person

ADDITIONAL SKILL EMPHASIS:
Doors and doorways
Meeting the public
Examining things tactually
Interpreting odors
Sound direction and meaning
Daily living skills
Careers
Floor plans

SEE ALSO (Other Modules):
    PUBLIC BUILDINGS Modules
    Human Guide
    Distinctive Odors
    Distinctive Sounds
    Walking Independently While Following
        Someone

REMARKS: Often this Module is not necessary or appropriate for the cane travel teacher specifically, unless he/she is also a classroom teacher of young children. However, this Module can serve as a helpful guide to parents or other teachers.

Encourage parents to provide opportunities such as these during visits for medical checkups or care, and to consider an extra visit for educational purposes. Blind children are often lacking information which others gain through sight. Children tend to fear things they do not understand.

In preschool and the early grades, it is common for groups to tour the office of a dentist or doctor. Again, this Module can serve as a guide for including a blind child meaningfully.

If the cane travel teacher (or any other teacher) is arranging the tour, stress to all that no medical procedures will be involved. Consult the school nurse and parents to assure that no aspect might be considered an unauthorized "examination" (e.g., measuring blood pressure; looking into the mouth).

TEACHER PREPARATION: See Remarks, above.

Inquire about gaps in experience.

If at all possible, arrange for the child to visit at a time when no treatment will occur. This helps the child concentrate on learning about the environment; and this in turn lessens fear and misunderstanding later when treatment does occur. If the child is extremely fearful, consider visiting a *different* doctor (i.e., not the child's own doctor) for purposes of this Module.

Arrange to visit at a convenient time so that someone can help you tour the examination room.

ACTIVITIES:

Explain that you will visit the doctor to look at the interesting things in his or her office.

The child walks up the sidewalk or hallway. Using his cane, he finds and opens the door. He walks toward the receptionist (listening for her voice), introduces himself, and asks for a tour.

When going with the staff member into examination rooms, the child continues to use his cane. Sometimes he independently follows (or walks beside the person), while listening to voices and footsteps. Sometimes he holds someone's hand or arm. However, he continues to use the cane to note obstacles, steps, terrain, etc.

EXAMPLE 1: *PEDIATRICIAN*

Guide the child through experiences such as the following:

- Play with toy animals that the doctor uses to help young patients feel comfortable.
- Go into a treatment room, and get onto the examination table. Stow the cane on the floor or otherwise close by.
- Examine the stethoscope. Put it on and listen to your own heart and/or someone else's. Look at the blood pressure cuff and see how it is inflated. Examine other instruments as time permits.
- Analyze distinctive odors and sounds.
- Go behind the counter at the receptionist's desk. See the shelves of patient records.
- Walk around the waiting room (using the cane), find an empty chair, and sit down.
- If there is a toy corner, go there and play for a few minutes.

If a wait is necessary before touring the examination area, the waiting room would be visited first. However, if there is a choice, the waiting room is a good place to look at last. Less self-discipline and concentration is needed.

EXAMPLE 2: *DENTIST*

Guide the child to proceed in a manner similar to the above example, including:

- Walk around the treatment chair and examine it thoroughly. Sit in the chair and enjoy riding up and down. (The cane is placed on the floor or otherwise close by.) Recline in the chair, then sit up straight.
- Examine models of the teeth. Examine various tools and brushes. If possible, pretend to use the tools on the model.
- Analyze distinctive odors and sounds.
- The dentist or technician looks into the child's mouth briefly and gently.
- Get out of the chair. If possible, *the child* takes a turn at making the chair go up and down. Examine where the drill or brush is attached by an arm to a machine.
- Look at the X-ray machine and a display of finished X-rays. (The student may touch an X-ray print while it is described aloud.)
- Continue the tour in the office area and the waiting room, as in the above example.

FOLLOW-UP:

Write a thank-you note.

Report to the class about the trip. Relate it to social studies, vocations, and other topics.

MODULE 79
A GROCERY STORE

OBJECTIVE: (1) The student will tour a grocery store and describe the general layout.
(2) [If appropriate for age] The student will independently enter a grocery store and make a purchase.
(NOTE: Objectives for Daily Living Skills may also apply.)

AGE OF STUDENT: Preschool and up

PRIMARY SKILL EMPHASIS:
Purchase or transaction
Carrying things
Walking in company with others
Floor plans
In a crowd or a line
Human guide

ADDITIONAL SKILL EMPHASIS:
Sound direction and meaning
Interpreting odors
Examining things tactually
Weather and temperature
Meeting the public
Communication and instructions
Daily living skills
Careers

SEE ALSO (Other Modules):
   Carrying Things
   In a Crowd
   Walking in a Line of People
   Asking Directions And Figuring It Out
   Human Guide

TEACHER PREPARATION: Confer with parents about where the family shops. Discuss the student's previous experiences.

ACTIVITIES:

EXAMPLE 1: *FAMILY SHOPPING*
Encourage parents to include the child in grocery shopping as much as possible, from infancy. As circumstances permit, the child can examine various items tactually.

It is also desirable to arrange an occasional session with extra time, when the child can examine many things in a planned way. This may be done with the parent or the teacher.

The student may walk with the cart much of the time. She might hold onto it from behind while someone else pulls the cart and guides it. (She may carry her cane or stow it in the cart.)

Sometimes the student might push the cart without someone else's actually holding onto it.

If the student *pulls* the cart, she can use her cane normally. This valuable option is often neglected under assumptions that the cart should be pushed.

The child should understand the parent's method of shopping. Is there a written list? Is there a mental plan, adapted according to availability and prices? Sometimes provide a Braille list.

EXAMPLE 2: *A TOUR*
Discuss each area of the store as you pass through it. Groceries are grouped in categories, not placed at random.

Fresh Produce
Examine several kinds of produce by touch. Identify an apple, banana, peach, etc.

Note how the cane sounds when striking the bottom of the display as you pass. Compare to the sound made in passing refrigerators, shelves, freezers, etc.

Is the produce cooled? Is it sprayed with water?

Canned and Packaged Goods
Note the sound of the cane in striking shelves as you pass. Examine various packages, cans, etc. There are several brands of each product.

Refrigerated Products (Dairy, Meat, Etc.)
Note the sound of the cane in striking the bottom of the cooler. Hear the refrigeration motor.

Feel the cold. Touch the inside of the cooler, and some of the refrigerated products. Is the outside of the cooler cold also?

Handle packages of eggs with great care.

Is meat prepackaged, or is it prepared "to order" at the butcher's counter?

CAUTION: Watch for safety hazards in examining refrigeration. It is instructive to examine the structure of the cooler, but there may be electrical or heat hazards with some parts. In a freezer, frostbite can occur with lengthy contact, and wet skin can stick to cold metal.

Frozen Foods
How are *frozen* foods different from those that are merely cooled?

Touch some packages. Feel how cold and hard they are. Put them back immediately so nothing will melt.

Baked Goods
Handle bakery products carefully. Avoid squeezing.

Is there the delicious smell of fresh bread?

Non-Foods
Note the scents of various areas—soap, stationery, flowers, etc.

What non-foods are typically available in a "grocery" store?

Check-out Counter
The child walks ahead of the cart, approaching the check-out counter. Her cane gently touches the feet of the person ahead in line.

The child helps place the goods on the counter or conveyor. Help her safely examine the conveyor and other aspects of the check-out counter.

Is the "bar code" on each item passed over a specialized surface for automatic charging? Or are prices rung up manually? How does the cash register sound?

Let the child hand the money or credit card to the clerk. Examine the sales slip or register tape.

Walk with the cart to the car. Listen to traffic patterns in the parking lot.

EXAMPLE 3: *BEHIND THE SCENES*
Arrange a "backstage" tour at a time convenient for employees. Examine storage areas, meat packaging machines, ovens, etc. Walk out onto the loading dock. (See the Module, "Unexpected Drop-off or Step-Down.")

Is the dairy display replenished from behind the shelves? If so, go back there. (A bit of humor: Many a customer, not realizing what is behind, has been startled to see a hand reaching out mysteriously between milk cartons. If possible, have the student reach out from behind and touch the hand of the adult who has gone out in front; then trade places.)

Include things which sighted children see visually—the cash register, customer service counter, deli work area, etc. How much space does the clerk have behind the counter?

EXAMPLE 4: *TECHNIQUES FOR SHOPPING*
Discuss how a mature blind person shops.

In some situations, no assistance at all is needed (e.g., getting bread at a familiar store).

Often sighted assistance is used—a friend, relative, driver, store employee, etc. But the assistant is just that—an assistant. The blind shopper has a list (mental or written) and decides what will be bought.

See that the student builds skills to enable her to shop independently. By fourth grade, she should be able to enter a grocery store and make a purchase, if the store is familiar or other circumstances make the task easy. By eighth grade the student should be able to shop at any grocery store—even if it is large and impersonal—with proper planning. (She might decide to take a sighted assistant, or to choose a time when personnel are not too busy.)

Also, discuss how a blind customer identifies cans and packages at home.

Place Braille labels (or other simple tactual labels) on some products in the child's home. Note that some items already have distinguishing characteristics, such as a distinctive bottle.

The child can be responsible for storing certain items in the cupboard and getting them when needed.

FOLLOW-UP: If a tour was given by store personnel, write a thank-you note.

MODULE 80
HOTELS AND MOTELS

OBJECTIVE: The student will complete errands independently in [four] public buildings. He/she will explain a typical room- and floor-numbering system for a large public building.

AGE OF STUDENT: Junior high and up (younger if less independence is expected)

PRIMARY SKILL EMPHASIS:
Floor plans
Communication and instructions
Elevators
Escalators
Stairs
Doors and doorways
In a crowd or a line
General travel (indoors)

ADDITIONAL SKILL EMPHASIS:
Right and left
Compass directions
Meeting the public
Walking in company with others
Purchase or transaction
Finding a seat
Finding a person
Careers

SEE ALSO (Other Modules):
   Walking Independently While Following Someone
   In a Crowd
   PUBLIC BUILDINGS Modules

STUDENT BACKGROUND: Discuss personal experiences of staying overnight away from home. Discuss camps for groups, family camping, and staying with relatives, as well as hotels and motels.

TEACHER PREPARATION: Look over the hotel/motel beforehand to examine the layout and be sure it is a suitable example. If possible, make arrangements to enter a guest room. Consider taking several students together.

ACTIVITIES:

EXAMPLE 1: *JUNIOR HIGH AND UP*

The student enters the hotel and finds the front desk (by following directions from the teacher, by asking directions, or by listening.) Discuss the check-in procedure.

If possible (having arranged for this ahead of time), have an employee take you to a guest room. The student follows the employee, but uses the cane independently. The student examines the key (or electronic card), and practices unlocking the door. She walks around inside the guest room, examining and discussing what is there. The door locks as you leave.

Practice walking back to the lobby and then back to the guest room. Discuss the route, and how to find the right room. (Example: From the front desk, go to the left, then turn right at the hallway. Note when the hallway curves sharply. Beyond the curve, your room is the second one on the right after the stairwell.) Begin to analyze the room numbering system.

Meet a member of the housekeeping staff and discuss that job.

Locate an emergency exit.

Throughout this Module, emphasize the overall floor plan and room numbering system, together with cardinal directions. A hotel is a particularly good place to explain and demonstrate how important it is to know north, south, east, and west. For instance, where is the pool from a given room? In what corner of the building is the restaurant located? Where is the front desk from the elevators?

Go to another guest floor. Is the floor plan the same as for the floor previously visited?

Return to the lobby and find a seat. Usually there are soft, comfortable seats where guests may relax, chat, watch TV, etc.

Go to the "bell desk" and discuss the work of carrying bags and assisting guests. What percent of income comes from tips in this job?

Go to the restaurant and purchase refreshments.

Discuss security for a hotel guest – e.g., don't open the door to an unknown person; don't leave money in your room.

EXAMPLE 2: *ELEMENTARY GRADES*

For younger or less mature students, plan the sequence of activities as advantageously as possible. For example, refreshments may provide a needed break. The student may practice the way back and forth to the guest room more diligently if she may enter only *after* she has learned to find the way.

With younger students it is probably not practical to include all the activities in a single session. A general overview, emphasizing cane usage, is one approach. With very young children, it may be best to select just one area to be explored.

A different environment such as this can provide excellent variety and interest while the student is practicing basic skills.

MODULE 81
AN OFFICE BUILDING

OBJECTIVE: The student will complete errands independently in [four] public buildings. He/she will explain a typical room- and floor-numbering system for a large public building.

AGE OF STUDENT: Preschool and up (see Examples)

PRIMARY SKILL EMPHASIS:
General travel
Floor plans
Doors and doorways
Finding a person
Elevators
Purchase or transaction

ADDITIONAL SKILL EMPHASIS:
Stairs
In a crowd or a line
Responsibility and citizenship
Human guide
Addresses
Carrying things
Communication and instructions
Meeting the public
Careers

SEE ALSO (Other Modules):
   PUBLIC BUILDINGS Modules
   Asking Directions And Figuring It Out
   Elevators
   Errands

TEACHER PREPARATION: When possible, correlate with civic matters being studied in various classes. However, a valuable practice route to an office building—government or private—can always be given a purpose appropriate to the child's age and ability.

STUDENT BACKGROUND: Discuss the nature of the offices to be visited.

Practice shaking hands. If the cane is in the right hand, it needs to be moved to free that hand.

ACTIVITIES:

EXAMPLE 1: *PRESCHOOL THROUGH THE PRIMARY GRADES*

"We talked about who the mayor is. You might say he's the president of our town. We're going to his office now. And someone who works for him (or maybe the mayor himself) will show us around the office."

As the student walks along on the main sidewalk, she arcs her cane while using it to look for a sidewalk branching to the left. She follows that smaller sidewalk to the City Hall building. She walks up several steps, enters, and proceeds down the hallway (continuing to arc the cane) to the set of doors straight ahead. She enters, introduces herself and the teacher, shakes hands, and asks to see where the mayor works.

The student takes the arm of the secretary during the tour, but continues to use the cane while walking. (The teacher follows.) The mayor's desk is examined, with its pile of papers and fancy set of pens. The mayor is out greeting visitors from Mexico. The student receives a brochure listing city officials; she will show it to her classmates when telling about the visit.

The student thanks the secretary for the tour, and walks to the outer door of the mayor's office area. With as little help from the teacher as appropriate, she retraces her steps, exits the building, and returns to the area where the car is parked.

EXAMPLE 2: *JUNIOR HIGH AND UP*

The student determines which city bus line will take her to the Federal Building. (The teacher has already explained where the Federal Building is in relation to the bus stop, and where the Internal Revenue office is located in the building.) The student takes the bus, walks to the building, and enters. Following the teacher's directions, she locates the elevators and goes to the seventh floor. She turns left when exiting the elevator, and left at the first branch hall, then goes to the first door on the right.

She gets four copies of the new income tax forms. (Note: A sighted person would ordinarily go to the rack and get the forms without saying anything or asking for help. A blind person, however, would usually ask an employee to give them to her.)

The student then retraces her route to the elevator, back outside to the bus, and back to the school. She gives one copy of the form to the cane travel teacher, takes one to social studies class, and sets one aside to take home.

MODULE 82
A RESTAURANT

OBJECTIVE: The student will independently enter a restaurant, place an order, eat with appropriate table skills, and pay the bill.

(NOTE: Objectives for Daily Living Skills may also apply.)

AGE OF STUDENT: Third grade and up

PRIMARY SKILL EMPHASIS:
Purchase or transaction
Communication and instructions
Daily living skills
Finding a person
Finding a seat
In a crowd or a line

ADDITIONAL SKILL EMPHASIS:
Doors and doorways
Meeting the public
Attitudes toward blindness
Carrying things
Etiquette
Orientation within a room
Careers

SEE ALSO (Other Modules):
PUBLIC BUILDINGS Modules
Carrying Things
Walking in a Line of People
Lunchtime

TEACHER PREPARATION: Consider the best way to work this Module into the schedule. It may be correlated with a subject such as home economics. It can be a reward or treat.

ACTIVITIES:

EXAMPLE 1: *THE ICE CREAM STORE*
This Example assumes an experienced student who knows how to make purchases. A trip to the ice cream store will review and extend skills, and serve as a treat for the end of the semester. See that the student has money for her treat. This lets the two of you play the roles of independent individuals who choose to sit near each other after they enter.

Give directions to the store (if needed). This Example assumes the store is not familiar.

The student enters the store alone. She hears the cash register, walks toward it, and asks where to place an order. The cashier directs her to the counter at the left.

At the counter, the student asks about chocolate and banana flavors. She chooses a Cool Banana Crunch Sundae. Noting there are seats along the counter, she chooses one and sits down. (Otherwise she would have walked around or asked a clerk.) The cane is placed between the seats and the counter.

You order a soda and sit down on the student's left. You enjoy the refreshment and discuss the coming vacation.

The man sitting to the right of the student asks, "Do you go to school here?" The student replies and enjoys discussing sports teams. (Note: Later, talk with the student why it was all right to go ahead and converse, even though she did not know the man. The conversation was inside a business, and in this small town there is little danger of crime. In a large city it might have been wise to say much less.)

When finished, the student leaves a tip and returns to the cash register with her bill. The cashier says to you (standing behind), "Are you helping her?"

You pretend not to hear, and study your own bill. The student (prepared for this) says to the cashier, "I guess I'm next. Here's my check—would you tell me how much it is, please?" and proceeds to pay.

The student leaves independently. She meets you at the school and returns the change. You compliment her on handling the nervous cashier, and affirm that the conversation with the customer was all right also. The student thanks you for the treat and wishes you a good summer.

VARIATION(S):

(1) *To demonstrate independence more fully:* Sit entirely apart from the student, or do not enter the restaurant at all.

(2) *For a less independent student:* Stay together. The teacher takes some or all of the responsibility, while the student observes and/or assists.

(3) Go to restaurants and snack bars with varying degrees of formality/informality. Discuss customs and manners suitable for each. How does one decide whether or not to tip?

(4) Go to a cafeteria.

(5) Purchase carry-out food.

MODULE 83
A SERVICE STATION

OBJECTIVE: (1) The student will detect obstacles with the cane and proceed appropriately.
(2) The student will walk from a car or bus to a building, crossing a parking/loading area where vehicles may move in erratic patterns.
(Note: Objectives relating to daily living skills may apply also.)

AGE OF STUDENT: All ages (see Examples)

PRIMARY SKILL EMPHASIS:
Obstacles in path
Purchase or transaction
Daily living skills
Interpreting odors
Sound direction and meaning

ADDITIONAL SKILL EMPHASIS:
Examining things tactually
Finding a person
In a crowd or a line
Overhanging objects
Weather and temperature
Traffic movement
Careers

SEE ALSO (Other Modules):
  PUBLIC BUILDINGS Modules
  Utilities and Trash
  Distinctive Sounds
  Distinctive Odors
  Walking Across Open Space

TEACHER PREPARATION: Ask permission before taking a student behind the counter or into a work area. For a detailed tour, arrange a time convenient for employees.

CAUTION: In this environment, a young or immature child needs close supervision for safety reasons.

REMARKS: In many families, children typically remain in the car while an adult pumps the gas and pays the bill. A sighted child will see what is going on, but a blind child may have no understanding. Encourage families to provide a blind child with opportunities such as those below, at least now and then. A planned trip to a gas station with the teacher is valuable also.

ACTIVITIES:

EXAMPLE 1: *OBSERVING AND ASSISTING*
(*Preschool and early elementary grades*)
The following description assumes that the young child is closely accompanied by an adult at all times in this environment. However, this is a good example of valuable experience gained by using the cane while holding someone's hand. When moving cars are not close by, the child can walk alone with verbal direction.

The student steps out of the car and walks to the gas pump. His cane finds the step up to the concrete "island," and then finds the gas pump.

Help the child examine the pump overall, and specific parts: on/off switch, cradle, hose, and nozzle. He touches the window of the register dial while the adult describes it.

The child helps to take off the gas cap, lift the nozzle from the pump, place the nozzle into the opening, and turn on the gas. Listen to the gas pumping. Can we hear a separate sound from the dial as it clicks off the price? Note the smell of gasoline; discuss safety and fire prevention.

Hear the gas stop pumping. The child helps to replace the nozzle and the gas cap.

Listen for moving cars. When it is safe, walk toward the building. The child's cane finds the concrete "islands," pumps, waste receptacles, and other items.

A display of tires for sale is a fine opportunity to examine tires thoroughly without getting dirty.

The cane finds the building and the door.

Inside the building, listen for the clerk's voice and the sound of the cash register; walk toward the clerk. The child assists in paying with cash or credit card.

Walk back toward the door; the cane finds the door. Listen for cars moving before proceeding outside the door. In which direction is our car? Walk back to the car – again, the cane finds any obstacles, and finds the car itself.

EXAMPLE 2: *INSIDE TOUR*
(*Preschool and up*)

This activity is an extension of the above Example.

Walk around inside the station and note products for sale. Go behind the counter and examine the cash register, credit card processing equipment, etc.

Accompanied by an employee, tour the service area if possible. Look at service bays and hydraulic lifts. Examine tools and equipment.

EXAMPLE 3: *RESPONSIBILITY*
(*Fourth grade and up*)

Review or select from the above Examples as appropriate for the individual student.

An older youngster can learn to pump gas and pay for it independently, with some guidance from an adult.

A blind teenager or adult can take the entire responsibility for getting gas and paying for it; the driver can remain in the car. This is important both in regard to family roles and in using a paid or volunteer driver.

Build experience with different gas stations, different kinds of pumps, etc. Discuss various kinds of gasoline – how does one decide? Note price differences between self-service and full service.

Many service stations are also convenience stores selling snacks and other general merchandise. Is there such a station in the student's neighborhood, where he may wish to go for such purchases?

RELATED PRACTICE:

Encourage your student to learn basic skills in automobile maintenance. Check the oil and other fluids. Add air to a tire.

See page 301 in the *Handbook for Itinerant and Resource Teachers of Blind and Visually Impaired Students.*

REFERENCE(S):

Willoughby and Duffy. *Handbook for Itinerant and Resource Teachers of Blind and Visually Impaired Students,* pp. 297-306.

MODULE 84
VISITING A BLIND ADULT AT HIS/HER WORKPLACE

OBJECTIVE: (1) The student will describe methods used by three blind adults in their work (three different occupations).
(2) The student will tour an unfamiliar place, with independence appropriate for his/her age.
(Note: Vocational and Daily Living Skills objectives may also apply.)

AGE OF STUDENT: Elementary grades and up

PRIMARY SKILL EMPHASIS:
Careers
Attitudes toward blindness
Understanding vision and partial vision
General travel
Walking in company with others
Human guide
Daily living skills
Responsibility and citizenship
Finding a person
Stowing cane

ADDITIONAL SKILL EMPHASIS:
Elevators
Addresses
Finding a seat
Public transportation

SEE ALSO (Other Modules):
>Unfinished Basement, "Crawl Space," or Attic
>Lunchroom and Kitchen
>Utilities and Trash
>PUBLIC BUILDINGS Modules
>Rural Environment

TEACHER PREPARATION:
Become acquainted with the nearest chapter of the National Federation of the Blind, individual blind persons, and other contacts. Meet competent, personable blind adults who are working in various jobs, and who are willing to meet students.

If the visit will involve an unusual time schedule, arrange permission with the principal and/or parents.

STUDENT BACKGROUND: Discuss alternative methods used by blind adults in their employment. Begin to understand ways to achieve equality and overcome discrimination.

REMARKS: For the student who has considerable independence in travel skills, this Module provides excellent motivation and variety. However, it can be used at any point in the student's progress, since the human guide technique can be used as much as necessary. For a student who has never met competent blind adults, it may be important to include this at the beginning.

REMARKS: The student needs to have direct knowledge of blind adults in *all* major categories of work illustrated here: professional, non-college vocational, and homemaking. It is often assumed, perhaps unconsciously, that only certain categories of work are practical for blind persons.

The college-bound student should choose college because of genuine ability and interest, not emotional assumptions. Similarly, the student who is not planning on a college degree should be sure he/she is ruling it out for the right reasons. He or she should also consider post-secondary education which is not heavily academic.

Every person should learn skills of homemaking and child care.

ACTIVITIES:

EXAMPLE 1: *ELECTRICAL ENGINEER*

(Note: This Example assumes that the student is in sixth grade and learning to use the city bus system.)

Beforehand, the student telephones to make the appointment (assisted by the teacher if necessary), and gets directions to the workplace.

The student checks the city bus schedule and determines that it is possible to go there by bus.

Permission for the special trip is verified.

The student goes downtown independently via the bus, with occasional guidance from the teacher. As arranged, the student enters the telephone company building and asks the guard to call Mr. Willoughby. (The teacher follows behind, encouraging the student to be independent.)

Mr. Willoughby comes to the guard station, signs the guests in, and accompanies them to his office: up the elevator to fifth floor, down a hallway, and into a complex area with partial room dividers.

Mr. Willoughby shows the teacher and student his office. He lays his cane down while inside his individual office, but uses it at all other times, even when just going to the cubicle next door. He demonstrates his Braille watch, talking clock, and talking computer. He shows his Braille books, Braille telephone-number file, and other Braille notes. His briefcase, carried home each night, helps to leave one hand free for the cane.

He explains his job, trying to use words understandable to the layman. The teacher joins the conversation enough to be sure that all main points are brought out and understood.

Afterward, Mr. Willoughby leads the guests back down to the guard station and signs them out.

The student returns to school via the public bus, with minimal coaching from the teacher.

A thank-you note is sent.

RELATED PRACTICE: Discuss college and professional jobs.

EXAMPLE 2: *INDUSTRIAL LATHE OPERATOR*

NOTE: Since the overall preparation, activity, and follow-up would be similar to that with Example #1, much of that will not be repeated here.

Points specific to this Example include:

Ms. Secora turns on her machine and produces a sample object which the student may keep. She turns off the machine, both at the normal controls and at the extra safety switch. Then she guides the student to examine the machine by touch, as she describes its use. She explains how she operates the machine, using her sense of touch and her knowledge of machine operation, but not requiring extra safety attachments.

Braille measuring instruments, jigs and templates, and other interesting materials are examined.

She explains how she receives directions for specific assignments. In the office, there is a computer with speech capability, and sometimes she reads specifications there. At other times, she arranges for a co-worker or secretary to read things aloud. She takes Braille notes as needed.

The sounds and odors of a factory environment are very noticeable. Is ear protection ever required because of the machine noise?

RELATED PRACTICE: Go to an Industrial Arts classroom or home workshop, and examine various machines.

Discuss vocations which do not require a four-year college education. How does a person prepare for work as an industrial lathe operator?

EXAMPLE 3: *HOMEMAKER WITH YOUNG CHILDREN*

(Note: The homemaker may or may not hold a job outside the home also.)

Since the overall preparation, activity, and follow-up would be similar to that with Example #1, much of that will not be repeated here. Instead, points specific to this Example are summarized below.

Examine Braille labels and other devices which aid in food preparation, care of clothing, and other tasks. Note examples where no special materials are required, or a "regular" arrangement is advantageous—for example, a knob with clearly-defined "clicks." Are there ideas which could be applied to the student's own home?

Discuss child-care methods. Note alternative techniques such as bells on toddlers' shoes. Note techniques used also by sighted parents, such as gates at stairways.

Discuss the importance of homemaking and child care skills. If one works outside the home, how can responsibilities be balanced? If one works as a full-time homemaker, what are the advantages and disadvantages?

Homemaking—especially the care of young children—is work from which one never is truly "off duty." It is work which is very important to individuals and to society, but which sometimes seems to have low status, probably because one does not receive wages for managing one's own home.

RELATED PRACTICE: Discuss techniques for home management and child care.

If appropriate, discuss the question of heredity in relation to blindness.

OUTDOOR LOCATIONS

MODULE 85
SWIMMING POOL
OR BEACH

OBJECTIVE:
The student will detect step-downs and drop-offs with the cane, and proceed appropriately.

OBJECTIVE:
The student will walk on varied surfaces, including sand, pebbles, and grassy hills.

OBJECTIVE:
When planning to engage in a sport, the student will use the cane to a point as close as practical, and then stow it appropriately during the activity.

AGE OF STUDENT: Preschool and up (This Module is presented as for the intermediate grades.)

PRIMARY SKILL EMPHASIS:
Varied terrain
Detecting step-downs or drop-offs
Boundaries
Landmarks
Stowing cane
Purchase or transaction

ADDITIONAL SKILL EMPHASIS:
Emergency procedures
Barefoot walking
Sound direction and meaning
Interpreting odors
Air currents and echoes
Weather and temperature
Examining things tactually
In a crowd or a line
Hills and inclines
Open space
Meeting the public
Careers

SEE ALSO (Other Modules):
Other OUTDOOR LOCATIONS modules
Apartment House or Condominium
Back yard (Overall)
Walking Across Open Space
Unexpected Drop-Off or Step-Down

REMARKS: It may or may not be practical to get into the pool during a lesson. But it is easy to practice the associated skills around the pool, and to discuss actual swimming.

CAUTION: A teacher who is not a qualified swimming instructor should never take a student into the water (even shallow water) without a lifeguard present.

Also, a teacher should not go alone with a student where help could not be found quickly if the student fell in.

In all activities below, a young or inexperienced student should be accompanied closely at all times.

ACTIVITIES:

EXAMPLE 1: *PUBLIC SWIMMING POOL*
(This description assumes the pool is with a large apartment complex. The general approach is the same for a beach, river, or public pool.)

Practice approaching the pool from various directions and recognizing immediately when the cane finds the edge. Include practice in approaching from various angles (with the pool not always straight in front of the student). This is important because the student may reach the pool unexpectedly.

See Cautions, above.

"How does the pool smell? What sounds do you hear? Bend down and put your hand in the water. How does it feel?"

Practice going to and from the pool, from the student's own apartment and from other appropriate areas.

Find an unoccupied deck chair and sit down. Set the cane down as usual. Note that in a pool area, anything (floor, chairs, etc.) may be wet. That will not hurt the cane. If a person does not want to get clothing wet, he needs to check tactually before sitting.

At poolside, people often sit down without chairs. [Blind children may believe that this is never done.] Sit down on a towel or directly on the deck or ground. Again, consider whether clothing will get wet or dirty.

Examine lifesaving equipment – ropes, floats, etc. – that may be thrown to a swimmer in trouble. Note that a blind person can throw a float to someone in trouble, or (with proper training) perform a rescue by swimming.

Study the rules and procedures of the pool.

The student should become familiar with the changing room. He should walk around and examine the location of the showers, benches, baskets, foot bath, toilets, sinks, etc., with explanation being given as necessary. If the teacher is the opposite sex from the student, a friend or family member may be asked to help. Or, an experienced student can simply go in by himself and look around.

The cane should be taken into the dressing room. It should be used inside, unless the room is very small and familiar. The cane can be set down (or leaned against the wall) beside the shower, under a bench, etc. Is a shower required before swimming?

Where is clothing placed? Is there a key or token for retrieving one's own basket?

Walk with the cane while barefoot. Again practice approaching the pool itself from various directions and recognizing when the cane finds the edge.

Analyze landmarks for orientation while swimming. Examples include loudspeakers, dressing rooms, whirlpool, ropes, buoys, water input, diving board, etc. Usually some such landmarks are noticeable by sound, feel, or odor while the person is in the pool. Also, a person may get out of the pool and then walk around to determine location.

Particularly note the deep end of the pool vs. the shallow end. If there is a rope delineating the shallow area, reach down and touch it.

Discuss where to place the cane while actually swimming. Select an identifiable spot close to the pool – for example, at the edge of the grass, in the corner nearest one's own apartment. If it is necessary to walk a short distance without the cane, this should be done cautiously and not quickly.

Discuss where to leave wallet and keys. Mention wearing a key on a bracelet, or pinning it to the suit.

If possible and appropriate, bring bathing suits and actually go swimming or wading. Alternatively, the teacher may orient the student to the pool and offer suggestions to the family and the swimming teacher.

EXAMPLE 2: *SWIMMING CLASSES AT SCHOOL*

If there is a pool in the school building, the student should become familiar with it immediately as part of general orientation. He should know the pool's location in the building and be able to detect the drop-off reliably.

Until he is actually anticipating a swimming class, examining the locker rooms or other detail may not be important.

If classes go to a pool somewhere else, it is helpful to explore that area in advance.

Offer suggestions to the swimming instructor.

EXAMPLE 3: *THE BEACH*

Practice walking on varied terrain – grass, rocks, and sand. Find the water's edge, noting that it is not a clear-cut drop-off. At the ocean, discuss tides.

Walk barefoot in appropriate places.

The student must understand that the body of water is very large. Except in a very narrow river or lake, a person cannot "swim to the other side."

How is the safe-swimming area delineated? An experienced blind swimmer can find rope barriers, and can learn to estimate distance if intermittent buoys mark boundaries. In a crowded area, others' voices help in orientation.

REFERENCE(S):
David Walker. "Hook, Line, and Golf Balls."

MODULE 86
BRIDGES AND OVERPASSES

OBJECTIVE: The student will state the purpose of a bridge, discuss its structure, and name two bridges with which he/she has experience.

OBJECTIVE: The student will walk on varied surfaces – including sand, grass, and pebbles – at a speed appropriate for the situation.

AGE OF STUDENT: Preschool through primary grades

PRIMARY SKILL EMPHASIS:
Varied terrain
Orientation overall
Detecting step-downs or drop-offs
Street patterns
Hills and inclines

ADDITIONAL SKILL EMPHASIS:
Sound direction and meaning
Interpreting odors
Air currents and echoes
Overhanging objects
Examining things tactually
Boundaries
Climbing, clambering, crawling, etc.
Landmarks
Weather and temperature
Barefoot walking
Parallel and perpendicular

SEE ALSO (Other Modules):
   Rough Terrain
   Unfinished Basement, "Crawl Space," or Attic
   Porch or Deck
   OUTDOOR LOCATIONS Modules

ACTIVITIES:

EXAMPLE 1: *SMALL FOOTBRIDGE*
Go to a small footbridge, perhaps in a park or on an acreage.

NOTE: See Caution, below.

Walk down to examine the stream or gully below the bridge. Note how the cane indicates a steep slope.

Wade or step across to the other side if possible. The cane can be used in water, on rocks, or with any terrain. (Alternatively, a young child might lay the cane down while at the stream and be assisted by the teacher.)

Get under the bridge if possible. How can one tell when one is underneath? Note changes in sound, shade, wind currents, etc. Touch the bridge and its supports.

Walk across on the footbridge. If possible, extend the cane down over the side to examine the drop-off. Note that the cane does not touch bottom; discuss the distance in terms the student understands.

Does the tapping of the cane sound interesting on the bridge? (There may be a "hollow" sound because of empty space below.) The cane detects surface changes when entering or leaving the bridge.

Emphasize that you are above the stream that was previously examined. If possible, call down to someone who is below.

CAUTION: Extending the cane down over the side helps the child understand that he must not step off. However, on a footbridge without a solid fence on each side, other possible problems remain:
(1) The cane might be dropped.
(2) The child might find it great fun to reach down, and try it continually.
(3) The child might fall by leaning over too far.
(4) An inexperienced or immature child might step off accidentally despite instruction.

Therefore, accompany the child closely. Help him hold onto the cane, or remind him to hold tightly. He should never reach down without permission.

If behavior is particularly problematic, hold onto the child continuously, or delay the activity until later.

Also note: A teacher should never go alone with a child near water deep enough to be dangerous, unless help is available immediately in case of an accident.

EXAMPLE 2: *LARGE BRIDGE*

In a car or bus, ride over a bridge or viaduct. Leave the windows open. Are sounds and air currents different while on the bridge? Can you smell the river?

Discuss what is below. Note that some bridges (viaducts) go over railroad tracks or other features, rather than over water.

If possible, walk down below the bridge. Note how the cane indicates a steep downslope. From under the bridge, listen to the traffic above. Examine the structure of the bridge, and the terrain underneath.

NOTE: See Caution, above.

If possible, walk across the large bridge on foot. Note sounds and air currents. Discuss and examine as for the small footbridge, above.

Note expansion joints. (These are thin structural openings at right angles to the roadway. They allow a large bridge to expand and contract with temperature variations, without buckling or breaking.)

VARIATION(S):

- Sometimes play equipment features a jiggly suspension bridge. This is an enjoyable version of a bridge for the child to explore. (Note: If the child has had experience with one of these *before* he goes to a conventional footbridge, emphasize that a regular bridge does not jiggle.)
- Often a large pipe or culvert goes under a road, providing drainage continually or during heavy rains. This actually makes a very simple "bridge."
- On a navigable river, study a drawbridge.

MODULE 87
THE GREAT OUTDOORS

OBJECTIVE: The student will walk on varied surfaces, including sand, pebbles, and grassy hills.

OBJECTIVE: In an outdoor setting such as a park or campground, the student will follow directions to walk independently between two given points.

AGE OF STUDENT: Preschool and up
NOTE: Consider, and help parents consider, what is typically expected of a child of a given age. For example, any four-year-old is closely supervised and would not be completely alone in a public park. It does not follow, however, that a four-year-old always needs to hold someone's hand. At a picnic, for example, he may be allowed to roam nearby if his parents can see him. They will insist on holding his hand only when near an imminent danger such as a cliff. It should be the same for a blind child.

A ten-year-old, in contrast, is typically allowed to go alone to areas which his parents have deemed safe. For example, in a town of moderate size, he may be allowed to wander along the creek and play on swings at the park. But on a visit to a large city, he will be required to remain near the family. It should be the same for a blind child.

A young child should learn techniques which give him the independence appropriate for his age. If one particular park is nearby or often visited, he should begin to learn its characteristics. An older child should learn advanced techniques and how to apply them in varied situations.

FIGURE(S):

FIGURE 87-1: Loose Grip for Rough Terrain
FIGURE 87-2: The Great Outdoors

PRIMARY SKILL EMPHASIS:
Varied terrain
Boundaries
Orientation overall
Detecting step-downs or drop-offs
Hills and inclines
Open space
Posture, grip, gait, and arc
Landmarks

ADDITIONAL SKILL EMPHASIS:
Overhanging objects
Stowing cane
Air currents and echoes
Sound direction and meaning
Interpreting odors
Barefoot walking
Examining things tactually
Climbing, clambering, crawling, etc.
Compass directions
Maps
Walking in company with others
Obstacles in path
Weather and temperature

SEE ALSO (Other Modules):
    Walking Across Open Space
    Rough Terrain
    Walking Toward a Sound
    Distinctive Sounds
    Distinctive Odors
    Back Yard Boundaries
    Back Yard (Overall)
    Playground
    What's Out There? (On the School
      Grounds)
    OUTDOOR LOCATIONS Modules

ACTIVITIES:

EXAMPLE 1: *ROUGH TERRAIN*
Grip and Techniques
The long white cane is very effective on rough and varied terrain – even steep mountains with

boulders and gullies. But some variation of technique is required.

The Module, "Introducing the Cane," describes the regular technique for a level surface. It also describes the regular technique for going up or down standard steps. When the surface is otherwise – even ordinary grass – some degree of the following variations should be employed:

- Hold the cane with a somewhat different, looser grip. (Figure 87-1) This has been compared to the way young children hold their forks.
- With the looser grip, allow the cane to bounce somewhat higher than for cement.
- Walking in snow is similar to walking on grass. Again, hold the cane loosely and allow it to bounce gently. Do not slide it.
- *For very rough, steep terrain which may be hazardous:* Shorten up the cane and use a "pencil grip" as for a crowd. This enables the traveler to examine the terrain immediately ahead with greater detail. (At the same time, he should be walking rather slowly, as should anyone in this situation.) Sliding the cane may be desirable for precise examination of the terrain and for keeping track of the path if there is one. Watch carefully for drop-off edges. Consider tapping the cane double-time – i.e., *twice* for each step.

Have your student practice by following you across varied surfaces in a non-obvious pattern.

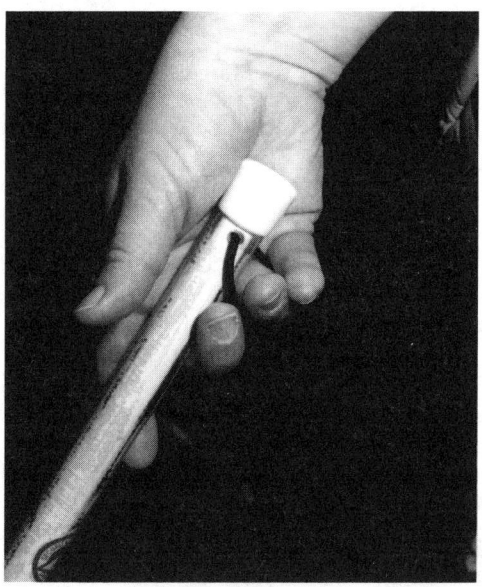

Figure 87-1
Loose Grip for Rough Terrain

EXAMPLE 2: *WALKING WITH OTHER PEOPLE*

Go to a park or an area resembling a park. A large, unfamiliar school playground is an especially secure and available possibility. (NOTE: When visiting another school or its grounds, always call ahead and discuss plans with an administrator. This is an important courtesy and also helps to prevent your arrival during a special event.)

Simulate a family outing. With a younger child, dramatize a bit and make it a game. (Pretend to eat a picnic lunch when a suitable location is reached, pretend to hear geese, etc.) With an older student, discuss places where he typically goes.

Ask the student to follow you. Deliberately walk across varied surfaces, in a non-obvious pattern. (Cross a corner of a pebbled area, walk down a path for awhile, then cut across the grass, go over a hill, etc.) Deliberately pass close to utility poles or other obstacles. Keep talking if your footsteps are not noisy. (See the Modules, "Rough Terrain" and "Walking Independently While Following Someone.")

Then ask the student to take your arm and walk with you. Review why this might be done, and why he should continue to use the cane. (See the Module, "Human Guide.") Walk briskly together across varied terrain, as above. Next, imagine that a large crowd is assembling to watch fireworks; walk slowly and practice the "pencil-grip" cane technique.

Practice walking in tight single file, as on a narrow mountain path.

Discuss various circumstances and their implications. Often a person chooses to be with others, but this need not mean dependence. In other situations, a person might indeed be alone or at a considerable distance from others.

EXAMPLE 3: *SOUNDS AND ODORS*
Often the most available sound for guidance is the voices of one's companions. Examples include following along in a structured line of Scouts, and walking casually with a family group. A child may be exploring an area while noting voices of adults nearby.

Help your student consider other sounds that also provide clues for orientation:

- Shouting, cheering, and other sounds associated with a given sport
- Large groups of people (e.g., at the entrance to an attraction)
- Footsteps on a paved path vs. on soft ground
- Loudspeakers
- Squeaking, etc., of swings and other play equipment
- Rides in an amusement park
- Vehicles on park roads
- Traffic on a nearby street or highway
- Bicycles on a path (the sound may be more easily noticed here than it is on a public street)
- Skaters
- Small sightseeing train
- Regular railroad train
- Splashing water, and the shouts of swimmers
- Water flowing in a river or brook
- Boats
- Geese or ducks
- Various animals at the zoo
- Leaves rustling in the breeze
- Echoes and air currents near a shelter, under an arcade, by a towering cliff, etc.
- Distinctive sounds from neighboring homes or farms (as, a yipping dog)

Odors can be helpful for orientation also:

- A lake or river
- Chlorine from a swimming pool
- Animals at a zoo
- Particular flowers or other vegetation
- Food concessions
- Campfires or grills

The Modules, "Walking Toward a Sound," "Distinctive Sounds," and "Distinctive Odors" offer additional detail.

EXAMPLE 4: *FOLLOWING A PATH*
Most parks have some clearly-discernible paths. The surface may be wood chips, fine wood mulch, pebbles of a given size, or packed dirt. It may have a row of stones along each side. It may even be paved. Usually there is a substantial difference from the surrounding terrain (grass, forest undergrowth, etc.)

Provide practice on various kinds of paths. Sometimes deliberately leave the path and then return; call attention to the change in surface, and note directionality.

The student should anticipate that a typical path is less predictable than a typical sidewalk. It probably curves continually. It may go uphill and downhill frequently. Its edges may not be clearly defined.

Talk with parents and camp counselors about paths. It is often assumed, for example, that a blind camper could not possibly proceed from a tent to a rest room or lodge unless there is a railing. Explain that a clearly-defined path is a reliable route.

EXAMPLE 5: *BOUNDARIES*
A child at a picnic may roam about while being watched by the adults. One way he can avoid going too far is to keep track of the voices of adults sitting nearby.

The child also may be shown boundaries within which he may roam. A fence takes care of this, but is not the only way. A driveway or path often provides a boundary. There may be a forest, or high grass that is unmowed. A play area may have sand underfoot, with grass beyond. The child can be told to stop at such boundaries.

Go with parents to a park, help the child demonstrate techniques, and call attention to boundaries the child should recognize.

The Modules, "Back Yard Boundaries," "Back Yard (Overall)," and "Playground" have detailed suggestions which apply here also.

EXAMPLE 6: *PARTIAL SIGHT*

A blind adult recalls: "I have always had usable vision. But I couldn't tell drop-offs. I ran into poles. I fell off steps. On vacations I dreaded caves and mountains....Now that I have a cane, I use it to supplement my vision, and I enjoy walking anywhere."

How sad for a child to dread interesting places like mountains and caves, just because cane travel instruction was not provided.

Barbara Cheadle comments,

> ...our son has some usable vision but he has little or no depth perception. He could never be sure if a change in shape, texture or composition of the surface he was on also meant a step-up, or a drop-down. He was also finding out that what appeared to be a smooth, flat surface – all of one color and composition – could mask unexpected drop-offs. He fell flat on his face once because he did not have his cane and he assumed that the concrete walk in front of him was flat. It was a walk-way into a church building and had several of those long steps of varying widths.
>
> –*Future Reflections*, March-May, 1984.

These anecdotes illustrate the importance of cane usage for students with partial, limited vision. Many times, instead of teaching good techniques, parents and educators lead the student into assuming, "I can't manage that by myself," or, "I didn't want to go there anyway." How sad. How unnecessary.

EXAMPLE 7: *CAVES, ETC.*

How can one avoid bumping one's head on a low ceiling or doorway? A simple, yet very effective aid is a hat with a brim which extends outward around the head. The brim will brush against an object or a surface, easily calling attention to it before the head is bumped. It also supplies a slight cushioning in case there is an actual bump.

(Note that a hat offers the same advantages with low-hanging tree branches.)

Reaching a hand upward is sensible when first entering a cave or when under a particularly low ceiling. But it should not be necessary to keep a hand up continually.

Cave floors are notoriously uneven. As described for steep mountain areas, the traveler should grip the cane loosely, shorten it up, and tap or slide it more than usual to examine the surface in detail.

A few large caves have readily discernible paths.

EXAMPLE 8: *WHERE TO PUT THE CANE*

If a person is actually "engaging in a sport," the cane is generally not used during the actual event. For example, a person ordinarily does not use the cane while actually swimming or playing football. (It *should* be used, however, when going to and from the site of the actual sport.)

It is a mistake, however, to extend this concept to hiking in a park or exploring a cave. Such activity is not "engaging in a sport" in the sense meant above. The hands are not being used to execute swimming strokes or to catch a ball. The legs and feet are basically walking normally. Obstructions and changes of terrain are present and need to be recognized.

Walking around in a park or cave should be regarded as a slight variation of regular walking, and the cane should be used to the normal extent (indeed, with extra diligence). Within this context, however, there may be some genuine examples of "engaging in a sport" in the sense of cane non-use. Also, of course, the cane is at rest when the person sits down.

With a young student, go to a park (or a park-like playground) and dramatize a family outing. Walk around over various uneven terrain. Bend down and pretend to explore a small cave. Set the cane down and play catch. Find a small gulch and reach across it with the cane; pretend it is a tiny creek, and jump across.

Assure your student that the fiberglass cane will not be harmed if it gets wet or dirty. (Be sure he knows how to clean it.)

If he is **fishing,** the cane should not be at the shelter house or in the car—it should be beside him or behind him at the river bank.

Even a young child can walk to a **swing or slide,** place the cane on the ground beside the equipment, proceed with play, and then retrieve the cane. Playmates should be taught to leave the cane alone.

Certain **amusement park rides** are not appropriate for keeping one's cane, depending on the dynamics of the ride and how the cane would be secured. The student should walk to the location with the cane (preferably to the actual seat). Then, if necessary, he should leave the cane with the attendant with instructions to return it immediately when the ride is over.

Getting into and out of a boat is easily managed. If the boat is large and has a gangplank, it is little different from walking into a somewhat unusual building. Without a gangplank, a typical approach is to extend the cane to examine the floor of the boat; grasp hold of the side with at least one hand; then step on in as anyone else would do. Most boats have enough room to accommodate the cane. (Again, the cane will not be harmed by water.) To get out of a boat, a similar procedure is used; emphasize checking one's path carefully to avoid falling off the dock.

It is possible to use the cane while **skating.** It is safer and more comfortable than non-use. With proper technique (including a shorter reach than usual), there is no unusual likelihood of tripping other people.

EXAMPLE 9: *GENERAL ORIENTATION*
Note the major characteristics of any particular park. For example, a grove of trees may extend across the south edge; a creek may flow through the middle from west to east; a moderately busy street, with a parking lot adjacent, may form the east boundary. Such characteristics not only provide valuable orientation when actually encountered, but often can be perceived even from a distance. Perhaps the trees murmur in the breeze and provide shade for some distance; the brook is audible, and has terrain sloping toward it; vehicles and voices can be heard from the parking lot and street.

Patterns of sun and shade provide clues. They indicate the presence of the object producing the shade, and also the direction of the sun.

A Braille compass can be helpful.

A few items should be mentioned as *not* being as helpful as a person may initially assume:

– Moss does *not* always grow on the north side of a tree. It depends on many factors, including moisture and shade.
– The direction of the wind is changeable, both in the general sense and because of diversion by objects.
– Although Braille signs can be an enjoyable source of information about natural features, they are of very limited value for orientation. One must anticipate that the sign is there, find it, and stop to read it, before gaining any information. Even then, it may be of little or no value in finding one's way.

If there are paths, the pedestrian may prefer to use them. However, often there is no path in the desired area. Also, there may be several paths which wind around and intersect. Overall orientation remains important.

RELATED PRACTICE: Some things that might be considered "physical education" may beneficially be included in mobility lessons:

– Climbing on playground equipment
– Walking on rough terrain
– Rappelling and other mountaineering

skills
- Clambering up and down a steep embankment
- Wading through deep snow
- Ice skating
- Roller-skating
- Sliding on ice without skates

REFERENCE(S):
David Walker. "Hook, Line, and Golf Balls."

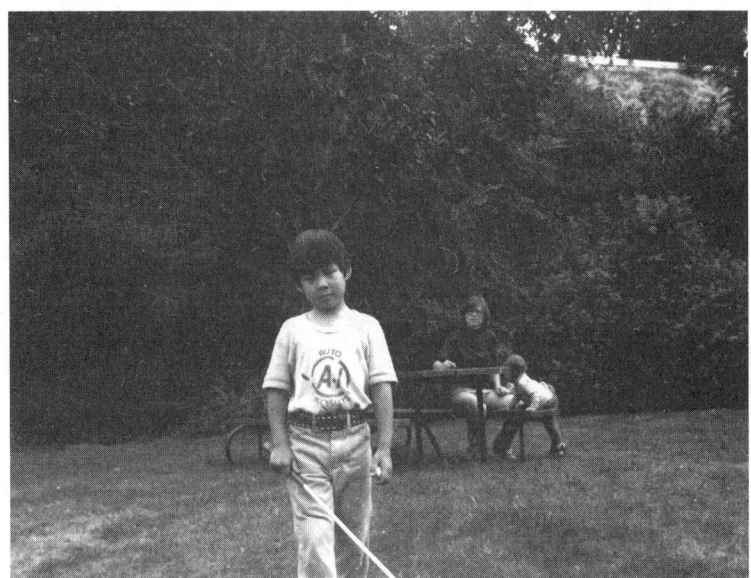

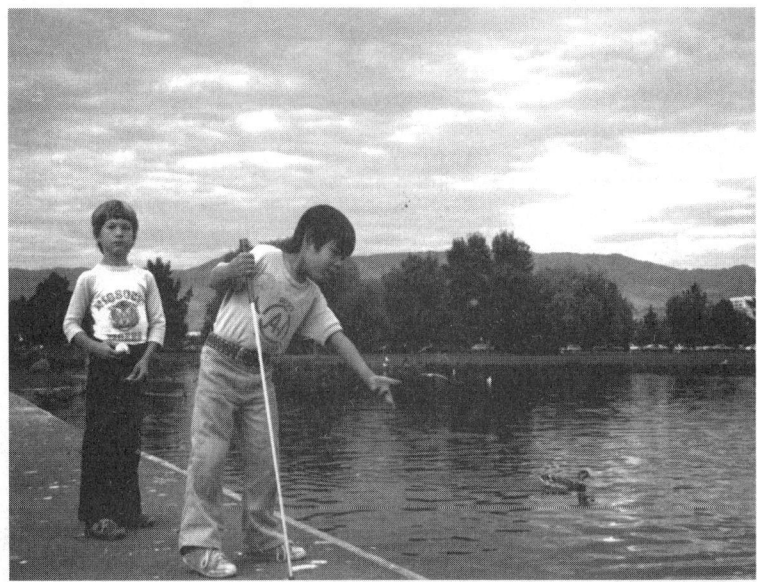

**Figure 87-2
The Great Outdoors**

MODULE 88
RURAL ENVIRONMENT

OBJECTIVE: The student will walk on varied surfaces, including sand, pebbles, and grassy hills.

OBJECTIVE: (*For a student who lives in a rural environment*) The student will walk independently to the following locations at his/her home, in any sequence: [list appropriate locations in individual setting–e.g., barn, machine shed, north boundary of south acres, etc.]

OBJECTIVE: (*For a student who does not live in a rural environment*) The student will tour a farm or other rural setting, walking independently on varied terrain while following the tour guide. He/she will discuss methods for independent travel in this setting.

AGE OF STUDENT: Preschool and up

FIGURE(S):

FIGURE 88-1: Loose Grip for Rough Terrain

PRIMARY SKILL EMPHASIS:
Varied terrain
Open space
Posture, grip, gait, and arc
Boundaries
Landmarks
Orientation overall
Air currents and echoes
Examining things tactually
Interpreting odors
Careers

ADDITIONAL SKILL EMPHASIS:
Compass directions
Flexibility and confidence
Hills and inclines
Overhanging objects
Sound direction and meaning
Walking in company with others
Barefoot walking
Detecting step-downs or drop-offs
Maps
Weather and temperature
Obstacles in path

SEE ALSO (Other Modules):
OUTDOOR LOCATIONS Modules
Rough Terrain
Compass Directions
Back Yard Boundaries
Back Yard (Overall)
What's Out There? (On the School Grounds)
Walking Across Open Space

ACTIVITIES: Many suggestions in the Module, "The Great Outdoors," apply here also. Refer to that Module for suggestions which are not repeated here.

Figure 88-1 illustrates the modified, looser grip recommended for rough terrain.

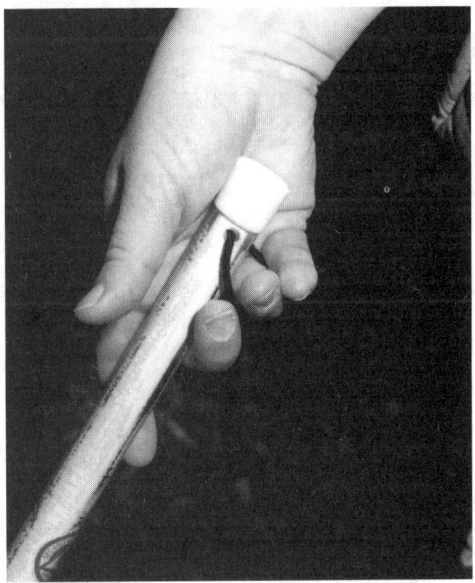

Figure 88-1
Loose Grip for Rough Terrain

EXAMPLE 1: *ROADS, FENCES, BOUNDARIES*

A road or highway is a major boundary and a landmark. In the quiet countryside, traffic can be heard a considerable distance away.

Similarly, a railroad track is easily recognized. Often there is a distinctive incline covered with gravel; tracks tend to be raised above the surrounding terrain. And a train whistle (as well as the sound of the moving train itself) can be heard for many miles.

Fences also are a major landmark. They may show boundaries between farms, between crops and pasture, around a feed lot, etc.

What kind of fences are in the area (barbed wire, electric, various kinds of wood construction, etc.)? Where do they run? Discuss according to compass directions—e.g., a barbed wire fence at the west boundary and an old wooden fence along the north.

Electric fences hum or snap continually, and can be heard some distance away.

EXAMPLE 2: *CREEKS AND PONDS*

As with roads and fences, any body of water is a major landmark and boundary.

The approach is downhill; walking away is uphill.

When a person crosses a creek, he should realize he must cross it again to return to where he started. The student should learn where the creek can be crossed easily. Is there a bridge? Where? Is the creek narrow enough to step across, and if so, where? For example, on the Monthei farm the creek is easily crossed on the western part of the property. If one finds a deep ravine instead, one is too far east.

How large is the pond? Is it possible to walk around it?

Note features and characteristics at various points—boat ramps, marshy areas, various kinds of vegetation, etc.

Especially with a large body of water, there are distinctive odors.

EXAMPLE 3: *SOUNDS AND ODORS*

Many **odors** (both pleasant and unpleasant!) aid in orientation in a rural area.

Prominent odors are associated with animals. It is easy to tell when the hog lot is near. Other animals have distinctive odors also, some more noticeable than others. Wind direction and other factors may vary the distance for detecting particular odors.

When fertilizer (especially manure) has been spread recently, the fields have a powerful odor. Other characteristics produce odors from fields and crops—newly plowed earth, blossoms, newly mowed hay, etc. Different fields (especially with different crops) will have different characteristics.

Marshes and bodies of water have distinctive odors.

Sounds can often be heard for a surprising distance in the country. Notable examples include:

- Animals: cattle, hogs, chickens, dogs, etc.
- Railroad trains
- Traffic on a road or highway
- Bodies of water (not only the water itself, but also related sounds such as geese, ducks, or boats).
- Electric fences which hum or snap continually
- Electrical substations or wires: sounds from within, or sounds from wind vibration
- A pump or generator
- Wind blowing the trees
- Tractors and other farm equipment

Consider more than one possible source for a sound or odor. Can we smell the neighbor's feed lot, as well as our own? Are there two roads within earshot?

EXAMPLE 4: *OTHER FEATURES*

Analyze land features, both natural and man-made. Do we find a large hill to the east and a small hill northwest? Where are the corn fields, the alfalfa fields, the soybean fields? (Even a young child can quickly learn to distinguish crops by touch.)

The ground leading to a creek or pond will slope downhill. A road, highway, or railroad is usually slightly above the surrounding terrain; in addition, there may be a depression or ditch just outside this rise.

In regions with irrigation, note the arrangements. Ditches and control gates are excellent landmarks.

Patterns of sunlight and shadow (which can be felt as well as seen), together with echoes and air currents, can be useful. They may indicate when one is approaching a grove of trees, a barn, a steep hill, etc.

Wind direction, while sometimes helpful, is too variable to be relied upon as a sole source of information. Likewise, moss (despite traditional lore) does *not* always grow on the north side of a tree.

Note distinctive features of various buildings. If the machine shed has metal siding and the old barn is wooden, one touch with the cane will distinguish between them.

EXAMPLE 5: *THE "BIG PICTURE"*

From the beginning, help your student build a mental map of the overall layout. Emphasize compass directions. Does the railroad run north and south? Is the pond in the southeast part of the property? Does the driveway go southeast to meet the road which runs east and west? Note the location and orientation of the road, fence, river, etc.

Make a simple tactual map and refer to it periodically. Consider making two maps – one of the whole farm and its immediate surroundings, and another showing the house and nearby outbuildings.

EXAMPLE 6: *EXPECTATIONS BY AGE*

There is much variation in rural living. The distance to the road may be long or short. A creek may be small and inconsequential, or deep and strong. Paths may be well-defined or nebulous. Each situation is somewhat different; but good training and opportunity should enable each rural youngster to achieve age-appropriate independence.

Below is an example of expectations on a typical Midwestern farm:

AGE SIX (using the cane, and walking independently except as noted):

- From the house, go to and from the swings in the side yard.
- Observe the boundaries of the side yard: machine shed, house, road, and fences. Roam freely within these boundaries (setting down the cane when actually playing).
- Go to and from a car parked in the driveway.
- Go to and from the school bus stop (at the road).
- Go to and from the mailbox (at the road).
- Walk with other people anywhere around the farm, using the cane and not necessarily holding someone's hand.
- Recognize each outbuilding (walking with someone else to reach those relatively far from the house).

AGE TEN (using the cane, and walking independently except as noted):

- Maintain all above skills.
- Walk from the house to each outbuilding, as desired (barn, machine sheds, chicken house, etc.), and hog lot. Walk between any two of these locations.
- Enter the chicken yard or chicken house; feed chickens and gather eggs.
- Walk independently to the hog lot; assist with hogs.
- Walk independently in and around the north fields. Note boundaries (fences and creek). Cross the creek appropriately.
- Play or roam as desired along the creek and in the north fields. Perform errands, including delivering things to family members working there.
- Walk up the road to the home of the nearest neighbor.

AGE FIFTEEN (using the cane, walking independently):

- Walk independently over the entire farm.

Perform age-appropriate chores.
- Walk to any of several neighbors' homes.
- Walk five miles to or from town as desired (including to or from school occasionally).

As always, parents and teachers should work together. Typically, the teacher instructs the student in the basic skills of cane usage in various locations. He or she comes to the home at least occasionally, demonstrating techniques and pointing out how and where to apply them. Parents follow through with continual practice in daily life.

The Module, "Back Yard (Overall)," discusses defining the boundaries of areas such as the "side yard" above.

The Module, "The Great Outdoors," offers ideas for defining and following paths.

As discussed in the Module, "Sidewalk Flawed or Obstructed," in some places there are no sidewalks. It is important to provide practice in walking on the grass near the edge of the street or road. Also, if there is little traffic, the student can readily walk along in the street at the edge (preferably on the left if possible). He should cane the curb or edge continually, to avoid drifting out into the middle of the road.

EXAMPLE 7: *A TOUR*
(For a student who does not live on a farm)

If a student frequently visits a particular farm, there should be regular instruction and practice comparable to what would be done if he lived there.

Otherwise, depending on the ease of making arrangements, the student should tour a farm occasionally if at all possible. Sooner or later he will need these techniques – if not on a farm, at least in a park.

During the tour, emphasize walking independently on varied terrain while following the tour guide. Use the human-guide technique very little, if at all.

If visiting is completely impossible, techniques should at least be discussed. If they are not even mentioned, the student and his family will tend to believe independence in a rural environment is impractical.

REMARKS: Visiting a farm is important for concept development. It also has vocational implications: many blind people are successful in farming and related occupations.

RELATED PRACTICE:
Maps
Vocational planning

MODULE 89
MORE IDEAS
For Lessons
In Outdoor Locations

AGE OF STUDENT: Preschool and up

ABOUT THIS LIST:

Following is a representative list of typical attractions. Examining different things at various times helps assure variety, interest, and a depth of experience. Many other suggestions appear in the Modules in this section and are not necessarily duplicated on this list.

Be alert to interesting things that are seasonal or temporary (e.g., water in a normally dry ditch). If something would be especially valuable for your particular student, plan ahead.

Help your student to examine what is accessible, and notice sounds and odors. Describe aspects that are not accessible.

CAUTION: Always be alert for possible hazards. These may be physical – dirty trash, deep water, sharp edges, etc. Or they may be in the form of persons, such as loiterers. If the student should not explore the area without an adult present, make this clear. Consider carefully beforehand whether you yourself can assure the student's safety.

Be careful to respect private property. If you wish to explore an area where the public would not ordinarily go, ask permission.

IDEAS:

- Drawbridge
- Cable car
- Passenger train
- Trolley
- Amusement park
- State fair
- Zoo
- Small "petting zoo"
- Rock garden or xeriscape
- Desert
- Real or model windmill
- Hills or mountains
- Cliff or bluff
- Beach or riverbank
- Boardwalk (as in Atlantic City): both on and under
- Fenced yard with unusual shape or characteristics
- Unusual vehicles on display – military tanks, parade floats, antique cars, etc.
- Houseboat, ferry boat, etc.
- Unusual stairways: wide and shallow, narrow and steep, spiral, brick, etc.
- Tree house or playhouse
- Local vegetation (e.g., palm tree)
- Local landmarks (e.g., the Dutch bell tower in Pella, Iowa)
- Lobster traps, fish nets, etc.
- Caves
- Prehistoric ruins
- "Living history" farm
- Rock formations to climb on and/or examine
- College or university
- Construction area (perimeter where the public may watch)
- Lighthouse, foghorn

PUBLIC TRANSPORTATION

MODULE 90
PUBLIC BUSES

OBJECTIVE: (*Upper elementary grades*) The student will ride a familiar route on a public bus, to a familiar destination. He/she will discuss methods of coping with various possible contingencies or problems.

OBJECTIVE: (*Junior high and above*) The student will follow directions to ride a city bus on an unfamiliar route, to an unfamiliar destination. He/she will discuss methods of coping with possible contingencies or problems, and will actually deal with at least two such situations (either unexpected or arranged by the teacher).

AGE OF STUDENT: Generally, children age 9 and up are ready to learn to use public transportation. The age for actually riding alone will vary with the community, individual ability, and practical needs. Certainly by the teen years a student should be able to ride alone.

This is a subject where comparison with sighted students may or may not be helpful. Certainly, if other students typically ride the bus at a given age, a blind student should also. But it does *not* follow that if sighted students do not ride the bus, a blind student should not. Sighted students may depend solely on automobile transportation – at first being driven by others, and expecting to drive themselves as soon as they are old enough. An important part of a blind student's equivalent is taking the bus, even if others do not.

FIGURE(S):
FIGURE 90-1: Understanding the Route

PRIMARY SKILL EMPHASIS:
Public transportation
Communication and instructions
Finding a seat
Purchase or transaction
Meeting the public
In a crowd or a line
Addresses
Stowing cane
Sound direction and meaning
Street patterns
Flexibility and confidence

ADDITIONAL SKILL EMPHASIS:
Emergency procedures
Etiquette
Understanding vision and partial vision
Responsibility and citizenship
Weather and temperature
Orientation overall
Street crossing

SEE ALSO (Other Modules):
School Bus
Walking In a Line of People
Asking Directions And Figuring It Out
Inclement Weather (Including Ice Underfoot)
Urban Rapid Transit

TEACHER PREPARATION: Many people today are so accustomed to traveling by car that a bus ride is an unfamiliar experience. Even if you are experienced with buses in general, it is wise to ride on the system in question before taking your student.

Consider logistics carefully. If you arrive in a car, where will you leave it, and how will you get back to it? (Usually the easiest way is to ride the bus back.)

Be sure that you and your student have enough fare, in the form required, for at least twice as many rides as you expect. Have change for a public phone. Be prepared for the possibility of lost tickets, missed connections, misunderstanding of schedules, etc.

If rules require you and the student to remain together, plan carefully for this. For example, even when "pretending to be just another passenger," as in Examples below, do not let yourself get far away from the student when waiting in line—you may have trouble getting both of you onto the same bus.

These lessons take time—certainly more than one class period. One solution is to work after school (possibly in combination with a last-period study hall). Otherwise, it may be necessary to make special arrangements to get two or more hours.

STUDENT BACKGROUND: Before a student rides alone, she needs to be able to climb steps, cross streets, and demonstrate an appropriate level of general maturity. The Example, "Readiness," below, discusses preparation and background. Other examples assume that someone will accompany the student at first, and give less and less help as ability increases.

CAUTION: With appropriate planning, riding the public bus is safe and enjoyable for student and teacher. Planning is essential, however. You and your student must think through what to do in case of various contingencies, such as a bus that never comes.

Is there any part of town that is genuinely unsafe?

Carry identification to prove you are a teacher of blind students. Kidnapping and other crimes are all too common. Someone may think you are a child snatcher, especially if you "suddenly" show up to help a student having difficulty.

See "Teacher Preparation," above, and "Anticipating Contingencies," below, for points about avoiding problems.

ACTIVITIES:

EXAMPLE 1: *READINESS*
For a child too young to ride independently, a trip on the public bus provides valuable readiness. If she has watched others analyze schedules, count fare, inquire about stops, etc., she will expect to do these things herself later. If she has already stepped on and off the bus, examined the fare box, sat in various seats, etc., these things will not be new. All this will make progress faster and easier when the time comes to learn independence.

The bus is a superb way to include variety in a routine lesson. Is the seven-year-old tired of crossing the streets near home and school? Is she rusty at going up and down unfamiliar steps? Does she need practice in locating a seat? A bus excursion provides practice with all of these and more, plus readiness for later instruction. At this time, the teacher takes responsibility for the bus ride itself. The student's official "lesson" is to step on and off the bus smoothly; seek and select a seat; and walk to and from bus stops with an appropriate degree of independence.

Encourage families to ride the bus with their young blind child.

The Module, "School Bus," has many suggestions relevant to a public bus.

EXAMPLE 2: *LEVELS OF INDEPENDENCE*
Beginning: Before the first instructional ride, discuss arrangements and determine what your student already knows. Build a background as needed.

Discuss where to board, where the fare box is located, and the arrangement of seats. Depending on the student's age and maturity, you may choose to assist her a good deal the first time—perhaps directly showing her how to proceed, without expecting real independence. With a relatively mature beginner, however, the student should receive little direct help even the first time.

Have the student go ahead of you and pay the fare, request announcement of the desired stop, and find a seat as she would if traveling alone. If the student follows behind the teacher, she will learn much less about how to do it alone.

For at least one trip, sit next to the student and talk with her about things she should be noticing. Examples include turns, inclines, and other landmarks which are audible or can be detected from the movement of the bus.

Increasing independence: Soon you should "pretend to be just another passenger." At this stage, you will ride the same bus as the student, and be prepared to help if needed. However, you will not converse with her, and you will select a seat as far away as practical. Explain this carefully ahead of time, so the student does not misunderstand and think she is abandoned.

Explain also that you may assert yourself as the teacher at any time, and may choose to join the student. If you do this unexpectedly, make it very clear who you are – introducing yourself quietly by name is the simplest. Otherwise, in a noisy public place, the student may be unsure whether it is the teacher or a stranger speaking.

Riding alone: If school rules permit, or if a parent is monitoring progress, the next step may be "riding alone but with someone checking at the other end." This is very natural when the ride is between school and home. If the youngster does not arrive as expected, someone will look for her. The same kind of thing can be arranged in visiting a friend or relative. Another approach is for the instructor to meet the student at the other end (perhaps at a store), but to go there by a different means. Or, the student might call home when she arrives.

Prepared in this way, the student becomes ready to travel entirely alone, when and where appropriate for her age and the locality.

Always discuss how the trip went, as soon as possible afterward.

EXAMPLE 3: *TO AND FROM THE RIGHT STOP*

Talk about the placement of bus stops in your city generally. Some routinely stop just before an intersection, some after the intersection, and some at random locations within a block. Some cities have buses that run up and down a street, so that by crossing the street, a bus going the other way can be caught. Some smaller bus systems or some less traveled routes have the bus circle back another direction, so that the rider gets off or on at the same point and circles around to get to destinations.

These things should be checked with the bus company. Have the student do this for practice. Getting route information is an important skill to teach. Encourage students to ask about stopping patterns, exact pickup points, etc.

Also, the student should be able to hand any sighted person a schedule and ask him or her to read certain items – and be prepared to instruct that person in *how* to read the schedule. For a beginner, introduce the format by providing at least a partial schedule in Braille or large print. Also, the student should practice eliciting information from you as you hold a written schedule.

Walking to and from the stop itself offers excellent opportunities to practice various skills. If the student rides only a familiar route, consider the variation of getting on or off at a different stop and walking a bit farther.

Tell hair-raising tales of buses barely missed, to impress your student with the importance of arriving *before* the bus is expected.

Review the skills of joining and following a line of people. (See the Module, "Walking In a Line of People.") There may be many or few people waiting, or no one at all.

Help the student use listening skills, together with good cane skills, to enter the bus. It may be immediately at the curb or some distance out in the street. The first step up is usually quite high. The bus (and its door) may be somewhat forward or back in relation to where it was expected. None of these variables should be a problem for an experienced and flexible traveler.

Practice locating a seat. The front seats usually face sideways; if they are occupied, the cane will readily encounter people's feet. As the traveler walks on back, she can slide the cane gently in front of each forward-facing seat to see if it is occupied. It is also possible to touch the back of each seat with the free hand and note whether someone is seated there; however, this brings the possibility of touching someone where he/she would rather not be touched. The student can also ask passengers about empty seats.

EXAMPLE 4: *ON AND OFF THE RIGHT BUS*

Getting on: At some stops only one route goes by. This can be determined by studying the schedule. The student needs only to be sure that she is indeed approaching the public bus, and not some other vehicle.

Often, however, more than one route will serve a given stop. If the various buses arrive reliably at widely separated times, this may be sufficient indication. Or, different buses may stop at slightly different places. Frequently, however, the only good way to distinguish buses is to ask the driver.

Ideally, each bus should stop, and the driver should announce the route number to the blind person. Alternatively, the passenger should approach the bus and ask.

Inquiring of other waiting passengers is sometimes practical, but may be unreliable. Good judgment about whom to ask must be developed. Also, even if another passenger says it is the right bus, the traveler should check with the driver also.

Sighted passengers may hail the bus (by waving at it). The blind traveler should stand attentively with the cane clearly visible, and the driver should then stop and announce the route.

When a bus pulls up, the doors open and can often be heard (though not always, if there is heavy traffic). Noting where other passengers go when getting on and off can be helpful, along with checking with the cane to find the door.

Getting off: Upon entering, the blind passenger should ask the driver to announce the desired stop. (Alternatively, the passenger may have a definite plan in mind for determining the stop, as described below.) Help your student develop skill in enhancing the request as needed. On a long, unfamiliar trip it may be wise to talk with the driver at judicious points, for a brief discussion of progress. (This helps the driver remember to announce the stop, and also adds to the knowledge of the passenger.) On a familiar trip, one learns to gauge progress by noting turns, railroad tracks, etc.

As was true at the bus stop, asking other passengers for information can be helpful but may not be reliable. The more information learned about the route, the better; but the mature person makes a judgment about the reliability of the source.

There are some circumstances when a blind passenger may not need individual help in knowing where to get off. In many cities, all stops – or all "major" stops and transfer points – are routinely announced. (With the *Americans With Disabilities Act*, this is becoming more and more common.) Or, there may be a very distinctive turn or other maneuver just before the stop. One should also estimate beforehand the approximate length of time the trip will take.

When some stops are routinely called, a good method is to wait until the driver announces the major stop which most closely precedes the desired street, and *then* ask the driver to call the individual stop. This avoids asking the driver to remember a request for a long period. Suppose, for example, that the driver routinely calls Mississippi, Arkansas, Colorado, Evans, Hampden, ... etc. Suppose that the traveler wishes to get off at Cornell, which is a minor street shortly after Evans. She listens attentively until Evans is called, and *then* approaches the driver to ask for Cornell to be called.

Encourage the driver to call the actual *street name*, rather than saying "This is your stop." Calling the street shows that the passenger takes the reponsibility for deciding where to get off. It also prevents possible confusion over whose stop is being called; more than one passenger (blind or sighted) might have asked for an individual announcement.

Partial vision is *not* reliable, and it is important to discuss this. Although students with some sight wear sleep shades during *lessons* on a bus, they also ride at other times when not wearing them. Emphasize that the same techniques are recommended when the eyes are not covered.

In case of difficulty: If there are difficulties regarding drivers' announcing stops, seek advice and help from the National Federation of the Blind.

EXAMPLE 5: *EXPANDING EXPERIENCE*

This Example lists factors which should be discussed, if not actually experienced. If they do not arise naturally in introductory lessons, the teacher should make a point of bringing them up.

General conduct: In many ways, the expected conduct for public transportation is comparable to that for a school bus. There are differences, however. If students on a school bus are rowdy, the driver will say something. On a public bus, however, probably no one will say anything to the offenders—but the driver and the other passengers will regard them as immature and possibly threatening. If the driver *does* say or do anything, it could be very serious—possibly even involving the police. Therefore, young passengers must discipline themselves.

What if your student is with friends or acquaintances who become rowdy? Discuss ways to handle this, including moving to a seat near the driver.

Eating and drinking anything may be prohibited.

Walking while the bus is in motion is one thing that *is* permitted (within reason) on a public bus. A passenger may change seats, or walk up to speak to the driver.

Understanding the route: Analyze the route the bus takes. Don't let your student view it as a nebulous passage comparable to the Star Trek™ Transporter!

Consider using a simple tactual map. While riding, watch for noticeable maneuvers or conditions that indicate location along the route. Examples include turns, railroad tracks, steep hills, passengers getting on or off, etc. The rider should think, for example, "We had a long stretch with no turns. Now we've made three turns in quick succession, and we're slowing down a lot. We must be downtown."

Analyze street patterns, especially if there is an alphabetical or numerical progression.

Ryan goes from West Des Moines High School to his job on the east side of Des Moines. (Figure 90-1) He boards the bus at 35th Street in West Des Moines. The bus turns east on Grand Avenue. The route crosses streets with decreasing numbers, until it reaches First Street, where railroad tracks provide a landmark. (It is important to understand that West Des Moines is a separate incorporated city; it is not the same thing as "the west side of Des Moines," the next area to be traversed.)

In the city of Des Moines, the route goes on from 62nd Street to First Street. After First Street in Des Moines, the bus crosses the river which divides the west side from the east side. Street numbers then increase, and are called East First Street, East Second Street, etc. Ryan's stop is at East 12th and Grand.

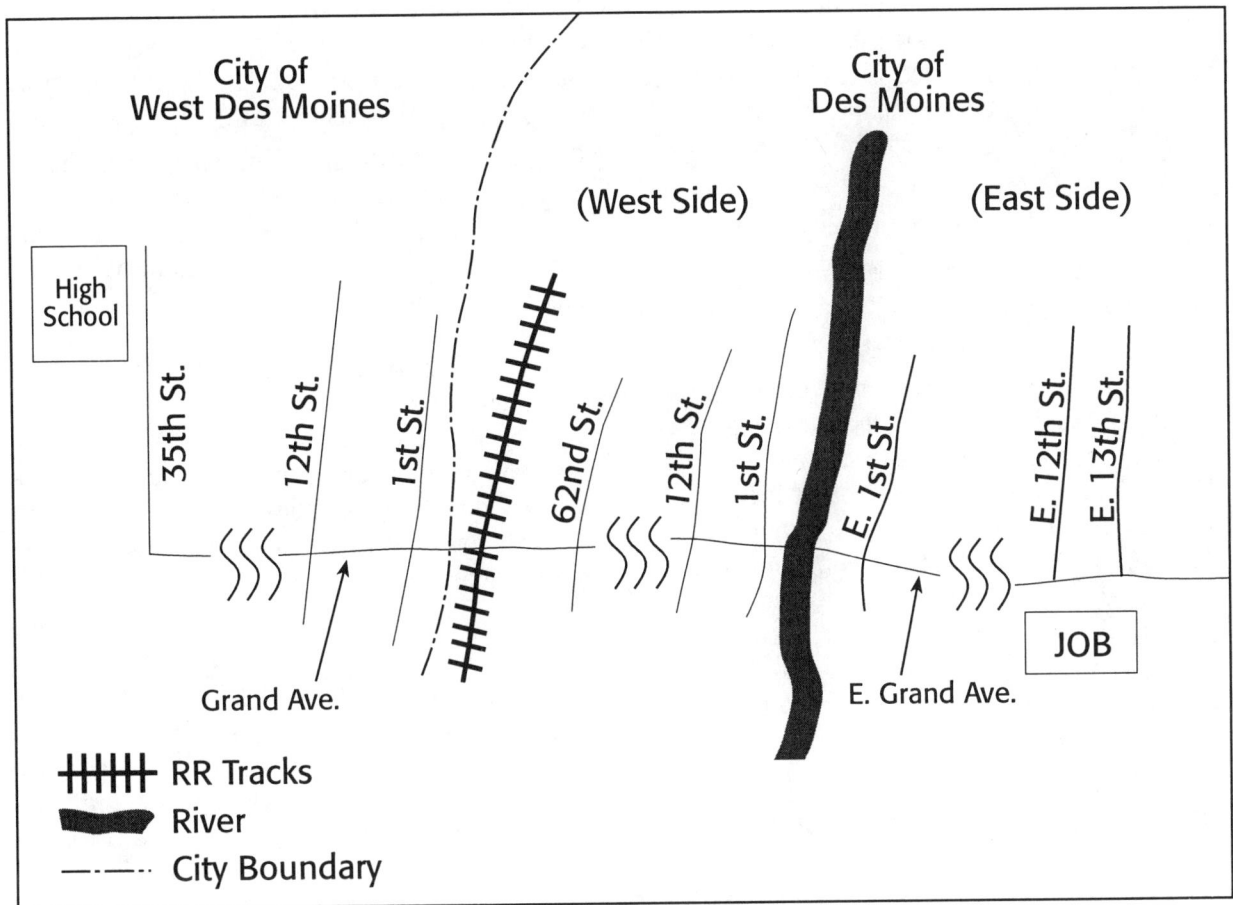

**Figure 90-1
Understanding the Route**

Had Ryan not grasped these patterns, there would have been confusion over *which* 12th Street he wanted. Also, in talking with the driver along the way, information about progress would not have been meaningful.

It is important for every traveler to understand the route, whether or not it is complicated.

Fare: Instruct your student not to allow the driver to take her money, since she needs to learn where and how to put it in the fare box. She must understand requirements and options in her present situation, and she should also know about common variations. The concept of a "transfer" ticket, and when it may be used, can be quite involved. Discuss tokens, weekly and monthly passes, student passes, "exact change only," etc.

My students are amused when I describe an incident from one of the Star Trek™ films. As I recall, Spock and Captain Kirk had traveled back into the 20th Century and were learning the quaint customs of the time. Among other things, they were exploring how to ride a city bus. They stepped onto a bus; the doors closed; then, almost immediately, the doors opened and the two travelers emerged as the bus left without them. As they stood there dumfounded, Spock asked in bewilderment, "What did he mean – 'exact change only'?" It was all quite hilarious.

The bus stop itself: Some bus stops have benches and/or shelters. But the traveler must not expect to find them everywhere. It is foolish to spend much energy in searching for a bench or shelter if there does not seem to be one. Even when they are present, it is sometimes best not to use them. While sighted passengers may hail the right bus, the blind traveler should stand attentively with the cane clearly visible, and the driver should stop and announce the route. Therefore, it is unwise for the blind traveler to be seated (or even inside a shelter) when the desired bus may be approaching; the driver will not realize that the traveler is blind.

In a large city, there may be a station comparable to depots for trains or intercity buses.

The bus itself: A young beginner unfamiliar with buses should examine an empty bus (perhaps a school bus) in detail.

The maturing student needs to be aware of variations. Typically, there are regular doors at the front and near the back, both on the same side. This is different from a school bus, which usually has only one regular door at the front, plus an emergency door in the back end (and perhaps elsewhere). On a public bus, passengers may enter at the front and exit at the back. A very large bus may have more than two doors; it may even have the body divided into two parts connected by a flexible middle.

Usually doors are opened and closed by the driver only. One can hear them open and close if the area is not too noisy. There may or may not be an audible signal (such as a chime) just before the doors close and the bus departs.

Transferring to a connecting route: Will the connecting bus stop in the same place, or must one walk to a different place? Can one get a transfer ticket on the first bus, to avoid paying fare again?

Outside your town: What if your locality has no city buses? Perhaps a trip to a nearby city can be arranged occasionally. Perhaps a summer program will include bus travel.

Regardless of whether you have local buses, acquaint your student with intercity bus travel (at least through discussion). Point out advantages and disadvantages in comparison with other modes of travel.

EXAMPLE 6: *ANTICIPATING CONTINGENCIES*

This may be the first time when the student is really alone in public, without having a parent or teacher directly controlling where she is. Help her gain control by planning how to handle common problems.

Below is a "discussion list" which I send home with each student. It includes summaries of general methods (e.g., how to know where to get off). It also asks questions that parents should help answer (e.g., from whom the student could accept a ride if offered). I find that some families have never discussed this kind of thing before—perhaps not consciously realizing that the student will be by herself in public more and more often. These concepts apply also when the student is out in public and not riding a bus.

DISCUSSION POINTS FOR RIDING THE PUBLIC BUS

(1) When getting onto the bus, always check with the driver to be sure the bus is the one you want. Think, however, about what you would do if you did find yourself on the wrong bus.

(2) The recommended method for knowing where to get off is: Ask the driver to announce your stop. (Your vision may be unreliable, even if you think you can see where you are. Your friends may forget to tell you, or they may even play tricks on you.)

(3) What general behavior is acceptable? (Example: How loud is it all right to laugh and talk with friends?)

(4) What if someone teases or bothers you?

(5) Some chatting with passengers is OK even if you do not know them. You might talk about the weather, for example. However, avoid giving personal information. Also, remember that you don't *have to* respond to what someone else may say.

(6) Is eating and drinking allowed on the bus?

(7) Is there anyone from whom you may accept a ride in a private car?

(8) What if something goes wrong with the bus route? For example: you miss your stop; you get off at the wrong place and get lost; the bus never comes; you lose your money or ticket.

(9) Memorize at least two phone numbers for use in case of emergency. If you are traveling during the school day, include the school telephone (_____).

Getting lost: This is the most obvious contingency. One might get on the wrong bus; get off at the wrong stop; or get lost after leaving the bus. Emphasize prevention, through careful planning and attention, and through good travel techniques. Also discuss at least one specific idea for righting a major confusion. For example:

- On the wrong bus: Ask the driver for detailed advice on what to do. At the very least, it should be possible to ride all the way around to the starting point (possibly requiring more fare).
- On the correct bus, but having traveled past the desired stop: Ask the driver for advice. If it is not far, you may decide to get off and walk back. If it is far, the driver can advise about transferring to a different bus or riding all the way around.
- It is important to understand how to get off one bus and proceed to board a bus coming from the opposite direction. This may seem obvious, but needs analysis.
- Off at the wrong stop: If the traveler has actually gotten off at the wrong place, it is no longer possible to get advice from the driver. (One option, however, is to wait for the next bus and ask *that* driver.) If the area is familiar (perhaps a block or two from the desired stop), it may easily be figured out. This contingency illustrates why it is important for the student to practice re-orienting herself in various situations.
- Note at least two public places along the route where one could seek help and/or make a phone call.
- These kinds of problems emphasize the importance of having extra cash.

Lost ticket and/or money: A traveler should have extra cash. On the other hand, carrying large amounts of money in public tempts thieves. "Twice as much cash as you think you will need" is a good rule. Also, "Always have enough cash to pay your fare in case something happens to your ticket."

Also discuss ideas to use in case one nevertheless does not have enough money and/or tickets.

Threats from other people: Review general principles about protecting oneself in public, as appropriate for the locality. If the route takes the student to a different area (e.g., from a quiet suburb to a busy downtown area with crime), emphasize any differences in precautions.

Discuss possible problems of harassment. For minor problems with other teenagers, it may be sufficient to ignore it or move to another seat. For more serious threats, the remedies are similar to those for being lost: talk to the driver, go to a public place and make a phone call, etc.

Controversial issues: There are a number of controversies concerning the balance between special accommodations for the handicapped vs. the right to be treated normally. Mention these issues to students and parents, especially any current local questions.

Most bus lines offer a **reduced fare** for "the handicapped." However, there are major disadvantages to accepting this on the basis of blindness. Blindness alone does not prevent one's boarding and riding in the normal way with only minor accommodations. Paying full fare asserts that one is a normal passenger, with normal rights and responsibilities. A special "handicapped" fare, on the other hand, tends to assert that one needs much special help. It makes it more likely that unwanted help (e.g., special seating) will be forced.

Each person must make his/her own decisions. There can be circumstances in which accepting a lowered fare is the best choice at the time. And in the case of a young student, there is usually a reduced "student" fare which has no problematic connotations.

Various forms of **"special transit"** are becoming increasingly available. This is usually in the form of small vehicles which transport eligible persons door-to-door by appointment. For persons with additional disabilities, and in areas where there is no regular public bus, this may be the best choice. However, for persons who are merely blind, and those with relatively mild additional disabilities, special transit is almost always a less desirable choice. Route-based (regular) transportation is more reliable and consistent, and its use maintains and emphasizes many important aspects of independent travel.

Another issue is that of **seating.** Front seats are often marked "For the handicapped and elderly." Sometimes sitting there is indeed helpful—among other things, for ease in talking with the driver about the route. But seating should be the passenger's choice. I tell my students that they should have the right to sit where they choose; if they find themselves forced into special seating, then parents and teachers will help them discuss it with the bus company later.

I recall an elderly Black man from the South, discussing this problem and saying, "I *never* thought—I *really* never thought—that someday I would be fighting for my right to sit at the *back* of the bus!!"

A related matter is the **right to stand.** If others stand in a crowded bus, a blind passenger should have the right to stand also.

Would the teacher help? Assure your student that in case of a severe problem you would indeed help. Nevertheless, the student needs to learn how to handle contingencies; you will not be around forever. If the student is mature enough to handle a given problem, you may choose not to intervene.

Consider a "secret signal" by which the student may indicate she wants help. This prevents the dilemma she would otherwise face when the teacher is watching but not assisting: "Should I call out the teacher's name and look foolish and helpless, or should I suffer along in silence?"

A confidential signal should look like normal behavior to other people but cause the teacher to come and speak to the student. Examples include: scratching one's head repeatedly; stretching twice in an exaggerated manner; placing the cane in a certain position; etc. If this option is overused, it is dealt with according to the student's maturity.

EXAMPLE 7: *"WHAT IF?"*

A good way to review and emphasize preparation is to ask questions from time to time—e.g., "What would you do if...?"

- the bus never comes?
- you lose your ticket?
- you realize you are on the wrong bus?
- a large teenager starts calling you bad names and poking you, hard?
- you realize you got off at the wrong stop?

RELATED PRACTICE:

- Maps
- Riding rapid transit, streetcars, intercity buses, etc.
- Reading and interpreting schedules
- Calling the bus company for information

REFERENCE(S):

Thomas Bickford. *Care and Feeding of the Long White Cane,* pp. 59-74

MODULE 91
TAXICABS

OBJECTIVE: The student will summon a taxicab, direct the driver, proceed to the destination, and pay.

AGE OF STUDENT: Fourth grade and above

PRIMARY SKILL EMPHASIS:
Public transportation
Communication and instructions
Purchase or transaction
Addresses
Stowing cane

ADDITIONAL SKILL EMPHASIS:
Attitudes toward blindness
Finding a person
Flexibility and confidence
Street patterns
Human guide

SEE ALSO (Other Modules):
  Meeting a Car
  School Bus
  Asking Directions And Figuring It Out
  Public Buses

TEACHER PREPARATION:
Determine whether taxi service is available in the community. If it is, study the fare structure, service boundaries, and other characteristics.

If taxi service is not available locally, consider a trip to a city that has it. In any event, make time to discuss taxi service.

REMARKS: Taxi usage varies greatly. In small communities, it is often not available. In some large cities it is used extensively. In many places it is hardly ever used by persons who have cars, and the student may not know such a service exists.

CAUTION: Usually, riding in a taxi is safe. However, local conditions should always be considered.

The student must be prepared to verify that the person is indeed a taxi driver.

ACTIVITIES:

EXAMPLE 1: *CONCEPTS AND DISCUSSION*
Review what the student already knows about various means of transportation, especially public transportation. Recall that a city bus travels a fixed route. Discuss the advantages and disadvantages of a taxicab as compared to a city bus:

Advantages of Taxi (vs. bus):

- Goes between any two chosen locations (within a certain area)
- Usually is not shared with other passengers
- Usually does not make other stops before your destination – hence is faster
- Available even when buses are not scheduled
- Less preparation required of passenger (e.g., studying bus routes)
- Personal attention

Disadvantages of Taxi (vs. bus):

- Much greater cost
- Usually not as reliable in respect to coming at a specific time
- Quality of vehicle often variable (may be dirty or in poor repair)

Compare taxi service with various other forms of public transportation, both fixed-route and individual. Include any special transportation for the disabled.

Compare advantages and disadvantages of owning a car, both for a sighted driver and for a blind person who hires a driver. People tend to assume that using taxis is much more expensive than owning a car, but often it is not – even with several trips per week.

As with any independent activity in the community, review safety considerations. Review ways for verifying that the vehicle is indeed a taxi. If the student were not pointedly practicing the use of a taxi, with whom (if anyone) might he accept a ride in a private car?

Discuss aspects of accepting help from the public and/or the driver. It is normal, for example, for a hotel doorman to summon a taxi for a guest, and for the driver to load bags for the customer. It is *not* appropriate for a passerby to grab the blind person, pull him to the door of the taxi, and tell the driver what he thinks the passenger wants.

Emphasize flexibility. A person should be informed about all kinds of transportation and choose intelligently according to the situation.

EXAMPLE 2: *TOUR*

Tour the taxi dispatch office. Examine radio equipment, and listen to the dispatching.

Enter a taxicab and talk with the driver. Examine the meter, radio, etc. What identification must the driver display? What training was needed? How is help provided if the driver is unfamiliar with an address?

EXAMPLE 3: *LOCAL TAXI*

If practical, arrange an actual ride in a taxi. An independent passenger should:

- Get the phone number of the taxi company, and make the call
- Describe the location for picking up the passenger (verifying the time frame)
- Meet the cab as arranged, get in, and direct the driver
- Pay (with a suitable tip)
- Obtain any appropriate information or help from the driver at the destination (e.g., finding the right door)
- Proceed with the errand

The passenger should estimate the fare (including appropriate tips). Discuss the fare beforehand, over the telephone and/or with the driver. This helps prevent being cheated or misunderstood. The rider must have enough money and should not assume the driver has change. The rider should also have at least a general idea of the route to the destination – again, to prevent cheating or misunderstanding.

Review personal safety considerations, as with any independent activity in the community.

EXAMPLE 4: *COMPARE OTHER COMMUNITIES*

Analyze ways of summoning a taxicab.

In many communities, taxis are almost always called by telephone.

When there are large numbers of potential customers (as, a hotel or airport), there often is a "lineup." The customer approaches this area (possibly assisted by a doorman) and takes the first cab in line. (See suggestions in "School Bus" for finding a vehicle in a lineup.)

The above instances are similar to the Module, "Meeting a Car." A taxi is clearly expected, and the customer verifies identity.

In large cities, taxis are often "hailed." A sighted customer may stand at the curb, watch for an empty taxi, and wave emphatically. Various options exist for a blind customer, including:

- Use a telephone and call a taxi to a specific location.
- Use assistance from a doorman or other individual
- In a busy location with many taxis passing, one choice is to signal continually (e.g., hold up one's hand) until a cab pulls over. This requires particular care in verifying that the vehicle is indeed a taxi. (It is usually *not* wise merely to ask, "Is this a taxi?" That makes misrepresentation too easy. It is better to ask a very general question, or one which would be irrelevant for a non-taxi – for example, "Hello, who's this?" or "What zones do you cover?")

MODULE 92
THE AIRPORT
And Air Travel

OBJECTIVE: [*Preschool through elementary grades*] The student will tour the airport and discuss procedures. He/she will use the cane appropriately while touring.

OBJECTIVE: [*Seventh grade and up*] The student will discuss methods used by mature travelers in intercity travel. He/she will travel independently in an airport–walking where other passengers walk, asking directions as necessary, and rarely using a human guide.

AGE OF STUDENT: See Examples

PRIMARY SKILL EMPHASIS:
Public transportation
Meeting the public
Communication and instructions
Purchase or transaction
Orientation overall
In a crowd or a line

ADDITIONAL SKILL EMPHASIS:
Flexibility and confidence
Attitudes toward blindness
Responsibility and citizenship
Stowing cane
Elevators
Escalators
Finding a seat
Human guide
General travel (indoors)
Careers

SEE ALSO (Other Modules):
PUBLIC TRANSPORTATION Modules
School Bus
Elevators
Escalators
Asking Directions And Figuring It Out
General Overview – Buildings
In a Crowd

TEACHER PREPARATION: If possible, arrange to enter a plane which is on the ground. This must be requested *before* going to the airport, and the same is true of any other activity which might require special permission. In some airports, non-passengers are ordinarily not permitted past the security check.

Study the layout of the airport beforehand, especially for an older student.

Study the current status of the rights of blind persons in air travel, along with any current controversies. Think about the student's maturity in understanding these matters.

STUDENT BACKGROUND: Beforehand, discuss what the student already knows about air transportation. Has she been on an airplane before? Also discuss transportation to the airport, both at home and at the destination. Mention taxis, limousines, public buses, etc., as alternatives to one's own car or a rental car.

Name a place to which the student would enjoy traveling by air. Plan to discuss this imagined trip with airline personnel.

Depending on the student's maturity, discuss the problems which blind passengers have often experienced – overprotection, discrimination, misunderstanding, etc. What can be done about it?

REMARKS: The airport is an exceptional opportunity to practice walking in a crowd, following directions in an unfamiliar environment, and many other skills. A trip to the airport is exciting and motivating at any age.

ACTIVITIES:

EXAMPLE 1: *TOUR*
(*Preschool through elementary grades*)
Entering the Terminal:
Listen to traffic and walk across the driveway.

Enter the terminal building. Is there an automatic door?

Discuss the overall layout of the airport. This is a good opportunity to include compass directions.

Ticket Counter:
Greet a ticket agent. Examine facilities for weighing and checking baggage. Ask about schedules and fares for the imagined trip. Consider the imagined route in regard to compass directions and the states which the route would pass over.

Discuss the monitor or board which lists arrivals and departures.

Security Check:
Discuss the Security checkpoint, and examine the facilities as much as practical. Think whether anything on the person of the student or teacher is likely to cause a "beep." (If the archway does "beep," the person may remove something and try again, or the attendant may use a hand scanner.) Place purse, bag, etc., on the conveyor for inspection.

Try to have the student walk through the archway independently with the cane. It is often helpful to touch the frame edge of the arch with one hand just before going through, to align oneself and avoid running into the frame while actually going through. (Touching it while going through may cause a "beep.")

Attendants tend to give too much help to a blind passenger. They may want to use a hand-scanner immediately instead of the arch. They may assume the cane will set off the alarm, and may try to take it away. (A fiberglass cane will not set off the alarm.) Help the student pass through Security with as little fuss as possible; discuss ways to minimize difficulties and maximize independence.

Discuss why the Security check is done.

Boarding Area:
Go to the waiting room near a gate. The student finds a seat independently. Listen to the announcements over the loudspeaker. Greet an employee and discuss the imagined trip.

The Aircraft:
If possible, tour an actual aircraft. Walking down a jetway can easily be done independently even by an inexperienced traveler.

Greet a crew member.

Touring the cockpit is exciting but may not be permitted. If it is permitted, help the student to examine the area meaningfully without disturbing delicate equipment.

Note the "galley" (food service area).

Examine the passenger area of the plane (as in the Module, "School Bus.") At a passenger seat, note the air vent, light controls, tray table, reclining seat back, attendant call button, etc. The cane may be stowed under the seats (aligned front-to-back and not extending into the aisle), or against the wall.

Where are the emergency exits? Count the number of rows (if any) between the chosen seat and the nearest exit.

Emphasize that aircraft are not all alike.

Other Areas in the Terminal:
Go to a snack bar and have a small treat. The student selects and pays for her own treat.

Practice using the elevator, escalator, and moving sidewalk, if available.

Note that when you go back out past Security, you do not go through an inspection. However, a guard watches so that no one goes *in* the exit and avoids inspection.

Baggage Claim:
Go to the "baggage claim" area. Is there a guard who would ask for claim slips? Is there a turnstile?

Examine the conveyor which brings luggage in.

(Caution: Safely touching a moving luggage conveyor is usually possible if it is done judiciously and carefully. Guide your student's hand if you decide this is appropriate. An immature student, however, should examine only a stopped conveyor.)

Discuss techniques a blind person can use to retrieve luggage, notably:

   Touch each piece of luggage as it passes by,

to identify one's own and pull it off. It is helpful to have a bag with a distinctive texture or some other notable tactual characteristic.

Ask for assistance from a sighted person (an airline employee, a congenial fellow passenger, etc.) Describe the visual characteristics of the bag.

It is useful to have a visually conspicuous characteristic; a large, bright sticker on each side, for example, can add distinctiveness to a common-looking bag. Remove any extra stickers, tags, or markings which could cause confusion.

It is important for the blind passenger to know the visual characteristics of each bag, even when she does not plan to ask for assistance. Any bag can be lost or misplaced; usually the first question asked is the color.

In any case, there should be a Braille label for certain verification. There also should be a print label giving name, address, and telephone number.

Features not directly examined:
Describe and discuss any key features at the airport which cannot be examined at this time. (Example: describe the interior of a plane if it is not possible to board.)

Describe features which are common at other airports, especially if the local airport is small.

Look for interesting and important aspects which might be missed without verbal description. Describe, for example, the people on the ground who direct planes to and from the gate. They use hand signals and wear ear protectors because of high noise levels.

Discuss concepts which a young student might not understand – e.g., how the traffic controllers in the Tower direct the pilots.

EXAMPLE 2: *OVERALL ORIENTATION*
(*Seventh grade and up*)

For this Example, it is important that the teacher be familiar with the overall layout of the airport.

Beforehand, discuss air transportation and the airport itself. If the student is extremely inexperienced, a detailed tour covering the points described in Example 1 may be in order before proceeding as below.

Select a flight which will depart soon. Go briskly through the sequence of procedures as a real passenger would.

Review techniques for walking in a crowd. In this Example, the student is accompanied by the teacher, but should rarely use the human-guide technique. Much of the time, the student should proceed ahead of the teacher. At other times, she might follow the teacher if it is not too hard to stay together.

A special motorized cart should *not* be used. (A blind traveler should not need such a cart except in a situation where a sighted passenger would – e.g., because of physical problems, extreme time pressure, etc.) However, if a shuttle vehicle is routinely used by everyone, it would be a desirable part of this experience.

Note that many airports are designed in similar ways – typically:

- Passengers walk in from the outside drive, following signs labeled with the name of the airline. There may be a curbside check-in.
- The main check-in desks are straight ahead.
- Go to the left or right of the check-in area to enter a concourse leading to gates. A very large airport will have more than one concourse, each with its own Security checkpoint.
- Larger restaurants and stores are likely to be near the check-in desks, outside Security. However, there may be other vendors in the concourse.
- Rest rooms are found in each major area.
- The baggage claim area is typically one floor below the level on which the passengers board and deplane.
- Near the baggage claim is a "ground transportation area." It includes rental car companies and public transportation. Taxis, buses, limou-

sines, and shuttles are found outside a nearby door.

Analyze the overall shape of the airport building, and mention other common arrangements. Some airports are shaped like a half moon, others like an H. Some have each concourse extending out like the spokes of a wheel. Some are so large that you must take a shuttle bus to different concourses. An arriving traveler can inquire about the overall shape of the airport, and use this to build an accurate mental picture.

Note amenities and conveniences such as:

- "Skycap" personnel who will move luggage (a tip is expected)
- Rental carts for moving one's own luggage
- Storage lockers
- Rest rooms
- Waiting areas with seats
- Snack bars, gift shops, etc.
- Automatic Teller Machines (ATM's) and other vending machines

EXAMPLE 3: *THE INDEPENDENT TRAVELER*
(*High school and adult*)

In this Example, the student proceeds as though she were alone. The teacher observes (and helps, if needed) to the appropriate degree according to circumstances. The student goes independently through the procedures, asking directions as needed. At check-in points, she may need to explain that she is practicing.

Pre-select a genuine flight number. At the check-in line, the student inquires about the selected flight. She asks directions as necessary and proceeds to the gate.

After reaching the gate, the student turns around and imagines she is an arriving passenger. She goes to the baggage claim area and the taxi stand, asking directions along the way as needed, but not using a human guide.

Afterward, discuss the experience. Analyze any problems encountered, and how they might be overcome in a future experience. Review the problems of discrimination and overprotection and how to counteract them. Review laws and regulations affecting the blind.

FOLLOW-UP: Invite a blind adult to talk about independence in intercity travel.

Even a young student can begin to discuss problems of overprotection, discrimination, misunderstanding, etc. What can be done about it?

Examine Braille maps of various areas and the world. Trace the planned trip and other imagined trips.

REFERENCE(S):

Willoughby and Duffy. *Handbook for Itinerant and Resource Teachers of Blind and Visually Impaired Students,* p. 174.

MODULE 93
URBAN RAPID TRANSIT
Subways and Elevated Trains
By Sharon L. Monthei

OBJECTIVE: 1. (*Upper elementary grades – where rapid transit is readily available*) The student will ride a familiar route on the [rapid transit] system, to a familiar destination. He/she will discuss methods of coping with various contingencies or problems.

OBJECTIVE: 2. (*Junior high and above – where rapid transit is readily available*) The student will follow directions to ride the [rapid transit] on an unfamiliar route to an unfamiliar destination. He/she will discuss how to deal with various contingencies or problems, and will actually deal with at least one such situation (either unexpected or arranged by the teacher).

OBJECTIVE: 3. (*High school – where rapid transit is not available locally*) The student will discuss methods for travel on rapid transit.

AGE OF STUDENT: Upper elementary grades and above

FIGURE(S):
FIGURE 93-1: Safe Entry

PRIMARY SKILL EMPHASIS:
Public transportation
Finding a seat
Escalators
Detecting step-downs or drop-offs
Communication and instructions
Purchase or transaction
Meeting the public
In a crowd or a line
Stowing cane
Addresses
Sound direction and meaning
Orientation overall
Flexibility and confidence

ADDITIONAL SKILL EMPHASIS:
Maps
Street patterns
Street crossing
Elevators
Emergency procedures
Responsibility and citizenship
Attitudes toward blindness
Stairs

SEE ALSO (Other Modules):
Public Buses
Asking Directions And Figuring It Out
In a Crowd
Escalators
Elevators
Unexpected Drop-off or Step-Down

REMARKS: Much of the information about subways and "el" (elevated) trains is the same as that for public buses. Therefore, almost everything in the Module, "Public Buses," applies here also and will not be repeated. The two Modules should be considered complementary.

CAUTION: For the prudent traveler with good preparation, riding rapid transit is safe and efficient. Emphasize, however, the vital importance of checking the platform edge with the cane, and of checking the floor of the car before stepping off the platform.

Also, consider safety in regard to high-crime areas.

TEACHER PREPARATION: As discussed in the Module, "Public Buses," the teacher must plan carefully to phase out help gradually. On the one hand, a beginner needs help with important safety issues and dealing with general confusion. On the other hand, the maturing student needs to learn to handle routine and contingency situations independently.

STUDENT BACKGROUND:
The student should be experienced with elevators, escalators, and unexpected step-downs. Urban Rapid Transit tends to be either raised above ground or down below ground (or some of each). The level of the tracks may be different from that of the station or platform.

ACTIVITIES:

EXAMPLE 1: *OVERVIEW OF ROUTE*
To ride the rapid transit trains, specific information about routes, the stations, the types of platforms, and the design of the cars should be given in advance. In addition to teaching how to ride the trains, it is valuable to teach where the trains go, and how to use the transit information service. A description of the train routes and a list of the stops will be useful.

The student must have a clear understanding of what route he wishes to take, and in which direction.

Many routes have trains that alternate between certain stops. For example, in Chicago the A train stops at some of the same stations as the B train, but not all. If you need a stop that is only on the B train, it may be necessary to ask a passenger which train you are getting onto. In case of a mistake, you need to get off at the next AB station and wait for the next train. (At an AB station, both kinds of trains stop in alternation. Therefore, the next train should be the other kind.) On weekends and late at night, all trains become the same, stopping at all stations. A definite, predictable pattern such as this makes trains easy to use independently.

EXAMPLE 2: *OVERVIEW: STATION LAYOUTS*
It is not possible for a student to go to every station, so general characteristics and types of station designs will be useful for a student in feeling comfortable when traveling in unfamiliar stations. Routes involving stations of various types should be given – stations with two or four exits, stations along the expressways, underground stations, elevated stations, center platform stations, and side platform stations.

Give very specific directions about how to get into a station, and ask students to repeat them until they have them worked out. Students are highly motivated to learn these directions. An overall description of the layout of the station is helpful, but maps may be of little use because of the various levels within stations. Some stations have as many as three levels – typically (a) ground level, (b) train level, and (c) a third level which may be exclusively for passengers to change to a different train by walking across a bridge.

On the first lesson, instructions about the stations, the trains, the platform arrangement, and how to get to the boarding area should be given on the spot to reinforce the verbal descriptions given before.

Because of the noise and crowds, riding rapid transit trains can be frightening to students who otherwise seem calm. Even being in the station can be unnerving at first. Spend considerable time talking with students in the station and on the train until they are over this fear. Remember that being in a noisy train station can be like becoming suddenly deaf and blind – the usual sensory input is blocked.

The student must understand and remember the direction in which he is traveling. Routes into stations are often quite complicated; in order to predict where to stand to get the right train, you need to know which direction you are facing.

For example, the Chicago "El" system consists of exclusively "right-handed" trains. This means that if you want to go in a specific direction, you should face that direction and take the train on your right.

A center-platform station is between two sets of tracks. Standing on the platform is like being in the median of a divided highway.

In a side-platform station, there is only one set of tracks for your platform. (If it is the wrong set of tracks, you will need to go up or down to get to another platform.) Again, if it is a "right-handed" station, if you face in the direction you wish to go, your train will be on your right.

Some stations may be "left-handed." This is rather like being in the median of a divided highway in England, where traffic keeps to the left as it moves along. If you face in the direction you wish to go, your train will be on your left.

There are large signs in the stations and on the platforms telling people which way to go to get on which train. A blind person can expect to get accurate information by asking another commuter: He can simply ask the person to read the signs and explain in which direction the arrows point.

EXAMPLE 3: SAFETY

The teacher should stay right beside the student the first few times in the station. This will ensure safety, and it will facilitate teaching the techniques for finding the platform edge and walking along the edge. If the platform is on the left, direct the student to put the cane in his left hand so he can walk as far from the edge as possible. If the platform is on the right, the cane should be in the right hand.

Edge of Platform
The student must locate the platform edge, keep track of it, move carefully, and not make assumptions.

Thomas Bickford says, "As I walk along subway platforms, I walk a little more slowly than usual, and I swing my cane a little wider than usual. I also slide the cane on the surface, the only time I use this otherwise poor technique. I want to know immediately if the cane drops over the edge." (*Care and Feeding of the Long White Cane*, p. 65.) It is vital to keep the cane *ahead* of oneself, and never to step sideways or backward.

Since underground stations and stations along the expressways are very noisy, orientation by sound is difficult.

Discuss the consequences of stepping off the platform. An inexperienced student may not fully appreciate the depth of the drop-off and the inability of trains to stop quickly.

Furthermore, the traveler needs to understand the "third rail." It carries high-voltage electricity and is almost certain death to anyone who touches it.

The third rail is usually located away from the platform edge. Therefore, should the worst happen, a person must be sure to move back *toward* the platform and try to climb back up. A person must not just wait for help, because a train may be coming. We know at least two blind people who fell off platforms and climbed back up safely, having known how to avoid the third rail.

On and Off the Car
To board the train, a student should listen for the doors opening or for people walking onto the train; or, if it is too noisy, he can touch the side of the train with the cane to find the doors.

CAUTION: The student must be sure to put the cane tip on the floor of the car before entering. Spaces between cars are similar in width to door openings. (See Figure 93-1.) Blind persons have fallen onto the tracks, mistaking these spaces for open car doors.

When entering, it is important to know where to look for something to hang onto. Trains often lurch before a person has a chance to sit down—if indeed there *is* a place to sit down. Poles are to be found to the left and right of doors, and at the backs of seats. There is also an overhead rail, as there is on a bus. Some cars also have individual straps hanging from the ceiling.

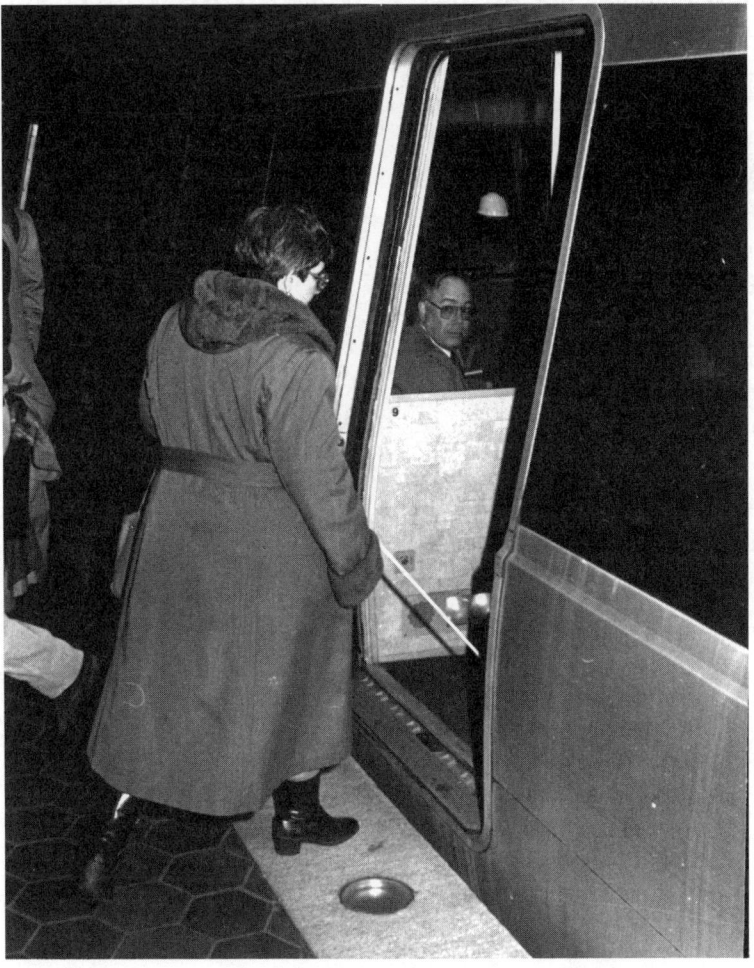

**Figure 93-1
Safe Entry**

EXAMPLE 4: *THE FARE*

Some transit systems have pay stations with attendants. Others have machines from which tickets are purchased. Often the passenger must put the ticket into a slot, go through a turnstile, and then pick up the stub out of another slot. Ticketing procedures should be explained in advance and also practiced with the teacher at the station.

The method of paying may vary according to day or time. For example, at less busy hours the passengers may pay on the train because there is no one at the pay station.

EXAMPLE 5: *INCREASING INDEPENDENCE*

Even during initial lessons, the student should generally precede the instructor, to maximize learning.

Because of the noise and general confusion, it is wise to have a student do the exact same route several times until it is really comfortable before moving on to other routes.

After a student becomes comfortable riding the trains, give a route and do not speak to the student again until it is completed. The teacher may ride on the same train or (if the school and parents permit) prearrange to meet somewhere to discuss how things went. To familiarize the student with using the transit information service, assign a route and request him to get directions from this service. The student will need to know how to use this service for his own travel needs.

As with bus travel, it is important to have something go wrong while the teacher is observing. The student needs to learn to handle unexpected situations before he travels alone. Overshooting a stop – the most common kind of error – is usually handled by simply crossing and taking the train in the opposite direction.

Train lines generally stop at prescribed locations which are announced aloud. Therefore, it is possible to count and anticipate stops. Different stops can be at different levels, and that can also be a clue about a specific stop. Note, however, that not all trains on a given route stop at every station.

The "Safety" example, above, includes vital information for the traveler who is learning independence.

EXAMPLE 6: *NO RAPID TRANSIT NEARBY*

If a subway or elevated train system exists in or near the community, it is desirable to teach its use even if the student does not presently live near the train. Someday he may live near it, and he will certainly want to use it in traveling about the city anyway. It is an excellent confidence builder as well.

REMARKS: The Module, "Public Buses," contains much information which applies here also.

REFERENCE(S):
Thomas Bickford. *Care and Feeding of the Long White Cane.*

APPENDIX

APPENDIX A

THE BLIND TRAVEL INSTRUCTOR
By Sharon L. Monthei
And Jennifer Dunnam

[Note: Sharon L. Monthei was formerly known as Sharon L. M. Duffy.]

If you are a blind person who wants to teach travel, keep the following things in mind:

A. In many ways, being a blind travel instructor is an effective teaching tool in and of itself. Make the most of it. Students can learn much through observation, and what a blind travel teacher does is excellent reinforcement for what she teaches.

B. Good basic teaching skills are important. Just because you are blind and a good cane traveler does not necessarily mean you will teach travel well.

C. Whether you are sighted or blind, a strong belief in yourself and in the ability of blind persons to travel safely is absolutely necessary to project confidence.

D. Most information about teaching travel in this book will apply to you in exactly the same way it applies to sighted teachers. Very much of it is common sense, and there is nothing mysterious about how a blind person teaches travel. Also, all of the following suggestions can be helpful to sighted teachers as well. Below are some suggestions:

(1) Stay close to beginners. Walk beside the student when she is not yet sensitive to the cane dropping off a curb, so that you will know exactly when the student is about to get there. You may or may not want to inform her about the curb, but you certainly want to know what she is going to encounter.

(2) Talk with students before each travel lesson in order to determine how they are feeling about life in general. It's good to know if a student is upset about something or is not feeling particularly well, since you will want to take these things into account in your teaching.

Talking things over after the lesson is essential also.

(3) Don't be afraid to touch your student—both to teach proper techniques and to see that the techniques are being practiced correctly. Of course, everyone should show courtesy and respect for another person's space. When touching a student, explain your purpose: "I want to show you how this technique is performed;" "I would like to see your hand position;" "Put your hand on mine, and I'll show you how this should feel."

(4) When walking behind a student on a hard surface, you will know that the student is arcing his cane wide enough if you can hear the cane on either side of his body. If the arc is not wide enough, the tap will be muffled. If one tap is muffled and the other is not, the student is skewing the arc. One possible reason for an arc that is wider on one side is that the student's hand may not be centered.

You can also tell that the arc is inadequate by the number of things that students hit with their bodies instead of their canes. Unfortunately, no matter how many times you correct a student about arcing, most students have to encounter a pole in an unpleasant way before they really figure out that they must arc wider.

(5) Frequent reminders about techniques are important. Remind students often of the following things during the early stages of training:

—Keep in step. When the right foot is forward, the cane should tap on the left side, and vice versa.

—Keep the cane centered. Right-handed people, if they don't center the cane, miss things on the left occasionally, and may also come too close to things in the center. Left-handed people tend to have the equivalent problem on the other side.

When the cane is centered, right-handed beginners may tend to arc widely enough on the left but not enough to the right, because they do not bend the wrist enough. (Again, if the person is left-handed, the equivalent tendency occurs on the other side.) The skewing occurs in the opposite direction if the cane is not centered.

Students follow the direction of their canes; therefore, an unequal arc may cause the student to drift toward the side on which the arc is widest.

—Tap the cane—don't slide it. Most beginners do not remain in step when sliding a cane.

—Before stepping onto a curb, be sure to sweep the cane across it to find any obstacles.

—Do not back up. Turn around and be sure the cane goes before each step you take.

—Do not use outstretched hands to find a door handle. Hold the cane vertically against the door, and slide the cane left or right until it comes in contact with the handle.

(6) Try to be familiar with a route before sending a student. When you do accompany a student to an unfamiliar area, it is helpful to be honest about it, because it allows an opportunity to demonstrate how an experienced traveler deals with unfamiliar situations. I usually say something like, "I've never been here either, so let's figure this out together."

Don't make assumptions. One inexperienced blind travel teacher went with a new student on a walk around the block where the student's house was located, but they did not arrive at her home after the fourth turn. The teacher had not walked around the block beforehand and didn't realize that this particular block had five corners!

(7) It is important to get a student to practice walking in step correctly from the very beginning. Have the student choose which foot will be forward first whenever she starts walking. If she is out of step, have her stop walking and then start again with the correct foot forward and the cane on the appropriate side. Have her show you how she starts—which way the cane moves with which foot. Reminders about being in step are enough for many students in the early stages. After a while, being out of step will "feel wrong" to the student.

(8) When teaching street crossings, remember not to stand where your body will obstruct sound. When crossing with a beginner, follow behind him and slightly closer to the parallel street so that you can judge if the student starts to drift into traffic.

If you need to intercede as in the case of a highway or other fast-moving street, remember to come up to the student on the street side and talk to him about the situation in a matter-of-fact fashion. You do not want to frighten your student. Being on the street side will keep the student from moving into traffic if he does panic at your approach.

(9) When teaching stair technique, stay very close in the beginning, climbing or descending the stairs at the same rate as the student. Be sure to show the student the proper techniques on more than one occasion, and check the student's technique whenever you feel it necessary.

(10) Remember that the best determinant whether a student is peeking under sleep shades has to do with behavior. If you suspect that a student is peeking, set up a situation in which she must negotiate a number of obstacles. You could also stand where she would touch you with her cane if she continued in the same path. Students who manage to avoid obstacles too often are suspect.

While looking for the entrance of a building, one student turned off of a sidewalk and walked through deep snow to a set of stairs which was visually conspicuous. It was clear that this student was peeking. The actual entrance to the building (about fifty feet further down the sidewalk) was preceded by a ramp which was completely free of snow; the stairway was a fire exit.

Mostly, you will know when a student is not using the sleep shades as directed. The real problem is convincing them that you know, without giving away how you know. It is better if they do not know all of your methods so they do not find ways around them. If you tell them you know they are peeking because they are walking faster than normal, they will simply walk more slowly the next time they decide to peek. [Note: See the Module, "Sleep Shades (Occluders)" for detailed discussion of the value of sleep shades. That Module and others include many examples of why the cane is useful even if the student walks quickly when using vision.]

Long discussions about adjusting to blindness, and about the value of sleep shades and the cane, help students to change peeking habits, especially if peeking is dealt with consistently and immediately.

(11) Sometimes it is desirable to follow a student quietly in order not to be a distraction. At times, a blind travel instructor may appear to the passer-by to be disoriented as she stands still to observe her student from a distance. When wishing to be present but inaccessible to my student, I am sometimes asked if I need help or directions, and therefore do not achieve my intent. This was a problem until I enlarged on the principle I always tell my students—that the more confident one appears, the less likely he/she is to be approached by helpful passers-by. When I began to adopt a more self-assured and slightly unapproachable manner, the problem diminished significantly.

NOTE: As with other parts of this book, if the student is very young or has special problems, general principles need to be adapted. For example, a very immature student may not yet be able to keep in step and should not be continually urged to do so.

REFERENCE(S):

Binder and Boone. "Orientation and Mobility: The Need for Reason."

Maria Morais, et al. *Techniques Used by Blind Cane Travel Instructors—A Practical Approach: Learning, Teaching, Believing.*

REFERENCES

(*NOTE: Many entries contain notations describing the topic or other characteristics of the reference. Also note that many items are available in Braille, large print, and/or recorded form. Some are also available in Spanish and/or other languages.*)

BOOKS AND PERIODICALS

For Parents and Educators

(1) Benson, Stephen O. *So What About Independent Travel.* Baltimore, MD: National Federation of the Blind.

(2) Bickford, Thomas. *Care and Feeding of the Long White Cane: Instructions in Cane Travel for Blind People.* Baltimore: National Federation of the Blind, 1993.

(3) Binder, George M., and Douglas C. Boone. "Orientation and Mobility: The Need for Reason." *Braille Monitor* (November 1994): 626-631.

(4) Blasch, Bruce B., and William R. Wiener. *Foundations of Orientation and Mobility, Second Edition.* New York: AFB Press, 1997.

(5) Castellano, Carol. "Serena Can Wait at the Bottom of the Hill." *Future Reflections* 14, no. 1 (1995): 34-36.
(*A parent resists the school's belief that the blind child cannot safely wait for her mother at the same place where others wait.*)

(6) Cheadle, Anna. "Making Sense of a Simulation Exercise." *Braille Monitor* (January 1995): 18-20.

(7) Cheadle, Barbara S., and Douglas C. Boone. "Linda Gets a Cane: Parents Prevail in Due Process Hearing." *Future Reflections* 13, no. 2 (1994): 3-20.

(8) Chong, Peggy. "Crossing for Blind Signs Crossed Out." *Braille Monitor* (January 1996): 31-34.

(9) Chong, Peggy. "I'm Partially Sighted, and I Use a White Cane." *Future Reflections* (Fall 1997): 5-8.

(10) Cutter, Joe. "O&M: A Process Toward Independence." *Future Reflections* 12, no. 2 (1993): 32-34.

(11) Cutter, Joe. "Parents: Blind Children's First Mobility Teachers." *Future Reflections* 13, no. 4 (1994): 11-23.

(12) Cutter, Joe. "Valuing the Blind Child's Independent Movements and Travel." *Braille Monitor* (May 1997): 318-320.

(13) D'Mello, Susie. "My Cane Is Helpful to Me in Many Ways." *Braille Monitor* (January 1998): 53-54.

(14) Drouillard, Richard, & Sherry Raynor. *Move It!!! (A Guide for Helping Visually Handicapped Children Grow).* Mason, MI: Ingham Intermediate School District.

(15) Foy, Christian J. *English/Spanish Basics for Orientation and Mobility Instructors.* New York: American Foundation for the Blind Press, 1991.

(16) Hartz, Deborah. "A Different View of the Grand Canyon." *Future Reflections* 12, no. 2 (1993): 11-12.
(*A young child hiking with her family*)

(17) Isaacs, Bill J. "No Cane, No Dog!" *Braille Monitor* (January 1995): 46-48.
(*Problems encountered in trying to travel without a cane or a dog.*)

(18) Jernigan, Kenneth. *Blindness: Handicap or Characteristic.* Baltimore, MD: National Federation of the Blind.

(19) Katona, Gail. "Going Camping." *Future Reflections* 13, no. 2 (1994): 25-27.

(20) Matson, Floyd. *Walking Alone and Marching Together: A History of the Organized Blind Movement in the United States, 1940-1990.* Baltimore, MD: National Federation of the Blind, 1990.

(21) Mettler, Richard. *Cognitive Learning Theory and Cane Travel Instruction: A New Paradigm.* Lincoln, NE: Nebraska Services for the Visually Impaired, 1995.

(22) Morais, Maria, Paul Lorensen, Roland Allen, Edward C. Bell, Arlene Hill, and Eric Woods. *Techniques Used by Blind Cane Travel Instructors – A Practical Approach: Learning, Teaching, Believing.* Baltimore, MD: National Federation of the Blind, 1997.

(23) National Federation of the Blind. "Around the Block, to the Mall, and Beyond." *Braille Monitor* (November 1997): 715-719.
(*Presentations by a panel of blind youngsters, ranging in age from nine years old to high school.*)

(24) National Federation of the Blind. *Braille Monitor.* Baltimore, MD: National Federation of the Blind.
(*A monthly magazine on topics related to blindness*)

(25) National Federation of the Blind. "Focus on Infants and Toddlers: Encouraging Independent Mobility." *Future Reflections* (Convention Report Issue 1997): 43-44.

(26) National Federation of the Blind. *Future Reflections.* Baltimore, MD: National Federation of the Blind.
(*Magazine for parents and educators of blind children. Four or more issues per year.*)

(27) National Federation of the Blind. *Model White Cane Law.* Baltimore, MD: National Federation of the Blind.

(28) National Federation of the Blind. "Walking Alone and Marching Together in Alamogordo." *Braille Monitor* (February 1994): 94-96.
(*A marathon walk.*)

(29) National Federation of the Blind. *White Cane Safety Day Proclamation.* Baltimore, MD: National Federation of the Blind.

(30) Neddo, Dawn. "But Will He Be Safe?" *Future Reflections* (Winter-Spring 1998): 8-10.

(31) Nichols, Allan D. "Does Your Horse Have a Broken Leg?" *Future Reflections* 13, no. 3 (1994): 38-40.
(*Description, with humor, about the use and maintenance of the white cane*)

(32) Olson, Carl. *The Encounter.* Baltimore, MD: National Federation of the Blind.
(Originally produced by the Nebraska Services for the Visually Impaired.)
(*In humorous cartoon format, common misconceptions about blindness and independence are analyzed and dispelled in this booklet.*)

(33) Pierce, Barbara. "Cane Do." *Dialogue* XXVII, No. 1 (Spring 1988): 60-65.

(34) Raynor, Sherry, & Richard Drouillard. *Get a Wiggle On (A Guide for Helping Visually Handicapped Children Grow).* Mason, MI: Ingham Intermediate School District.
(*This book is primarily about infants.*)

(35) Redington, Robert. "Walking With the Cane on Country Roads." *Dialogue* XXVIII, No. 2 (Summer 1989): 212-225.

(36) Ryles, Ruby. "Needed: Blind Individuals for University Training as Orientation and

Mobility Instructors." *Braille Monitor* (March 1997): 148-149.

(37) Scanlan, Joyce. "Accepting Help: How to Break the Cycle." *Future Reflections* 13, no. 3 (1994): 43-45.

(38) Simmons, Susan S., & Sharon O'Mara Maida. *Reaching, Crawling, Walking...Let's Get Moving* (Orientation and Mobility for Preschool Children). Los Angeles, CA: Blind Childrens Center, 1992.

(39) Walhof, Ramona. "Blindness—What it Means in the Mind of a Blind Child." *Future Reflections* (Spring 1996): 13-20.

(40) Walker, David. "Hook, Line, and Golf Balls." *Braille Monitor* (July 1995): 390-393.
(*Travel in an outdoor recreational setting.*)

(41) White, Loretta. "Parents Group Forms Children's Cane Bank." *Future Reflections* 12, No. 2 (1993): 34-35.

(42) Willoughby, Doris M., & Sharon L. M. Duffy. *Handbook for Itinerant and Resource Teachers of Blind and Visually Impaired Students.* Baltimore, MD: National Federation of the Blind, 1989.
(NOTE: In the text of MODULAR INSTRUCTION FOR INDEPENDENT TRAVEL, sometimes this book is referred to as simply the HANDBOOK. Also note: The co-author of MODULAR INSTRUCTION FOR INDEPENDENT TRAVEL, Sharon L. Monthei, was formerly known as Sharon L. M. Duffy and is also the co-author of the HANDBOOK.)

Publications for Children and Young People

(43) American Brotherhood for the Blind [now known as American Action Fund for Blind Children and Adults]. *Questions Kids Ask About Blindness.* Baltimore, MD: American Brotherhood for the Blind.
Now being distributed through the National Federation of the Blind.

(44) Litchfield, Ada B. *A Cane In Her Hand.* Morton Grove, IL: Albert Whitman & Co., 1977.
(*A young girl learns to use and appreciate her cane.*)

(45) National Federation of the Blind of Idaho. *Julie and Brandon, Our Blind Friends.* Boise, ID: National Federation of the Blind of Idaho, 1995.
(*Activity book for children about blindness*)

(46) Willoughby, Doris M. "Recess!" *Future Reflections* (Special Issue, 1995): 11-12.

VIDEOTAPES, DRAMAS, FILMS

(47) *Avoiding an IEP Disaster.* National Federation of the Blind (edited by Myra Adler Lesser), 1997. Videocassette.
(*Part 6 emphasizes Orientation and Mobility in the IEP.*)

(48) *It's OK To Be Blind.* National Federation of the Blind (edited by Myra Adler Lesser), 1996. Videocassette.

(49) *The Kids on the Block.* (*A puppet show about disabilities.*) The Kids on the Block, Inc.

(50) *Kids With Canes.* Produced by Nebraska Services for the Visually Impaired; now being distributed through the National Federation of the Blind. Videocassette.

(51) *What's It Like To Be a Kid Who's Blind?* Tucson, AZ: Myra Adler Lesser, 1995. Videocassette.

(52) *White Canes for Blind Kids.* National Federation of the Blind (edited by Myra Adler Lesser), 1997. Videocassette.

ADDRESSES

American Action Fund for Blind Children and Adults
1800 Johnson Street
Baltimore, MD 21230
(*Formerly known as American Brotherhood for the Blind*)

American Council of the Blind (ACB)
1155 15th Street NW
Washington, DC 20005

American Foundation for the Blind (AFB)
11 Penn Plaza
Suite 300
New York, NY 10001

American Printing House for the Blind (APH)
1839 Frankfort Avenue
PO Box 6085
Louisville, KY 40206-0085

Association for the Education and Rehabilitation
Of the Blind and Visually Impaired (AER)
4600 Duke Street, Suite 430
Alexandria, VA 22304

BLIND, Inc.
100 East 22nd Street
Minneapolis, MN 55404
(*"Blindness – Learning In New Dimensions."
Instruction and resources for blind children and teenagers,
as well as adults.*)

Blind Childrens Center
4120 Marathon Street
Los Angeles, CA 90029

Blinded Veterans Association
477 H Street NW
Washington, DC 20001-2694

Canadian National Institute for the Blind (CNIB)
1929 Bayview Avenue
Toronto, ON M4G 3E8

Colorado Center for the Blind (CCB)
1830 South Acoma
Denver, CO 80223
(*Instruction and resources for blind children and teenagers
as well as adults.*)

REFERENCES

Council for Exceptional Children (CEC)
1920 Association Drive
Reston, VA 20191-1589

Delta Gamma Foundation
3250 Riverside Drive
PO Box 21397
Columbus, OH 43221-0397
(*Civic projects emphasize work with blind people*)

Helen Keller National Center
For Deaf-Blind Youths and Adults
111 Middle Neck Road
Sands Point, NY 11050

The Kids on the Block
9385 Gerwig Lane #C
Columbia, MD 21046-1583
(*Producers of a puppet show about disabilities*)

Myra Adler Lesser
137 Lesser Lane
Chicora, PA 16025
(*Editor and producer of videotapes; parent of a blind child*)

Lions Clubs International
300 22nd Street
Oak Brook, IL 60521
(*Civic projects emphasize work with people who are blind and/or deaf*)

Louisiana Center for the Blind
101 South Trenton Street
Ruston, LA 71270
(*Instruction and resources for blind children and teenagers as well as adults.*)

National Federation of the Blind (NFB)
National Center for the Blind
1800 Johnson Street
Baltimore, MD 21230

NFB Committee on Concerns of the Deaf-Blind
1800 Johnson Street
Baltimore, MD 21230

National Organization of Parents of Blind Children
(NOPBC)
1800 Johnson Street
Baltimore, MD 21230

Nebraska Services for the Visually Impaired
4600 Valley Road
Suite 100
Lincoln, NE 68510

Rainshine Canes
P.O. Box 5615
Madison, WI 53705
(*Solid, unbreakable fiberglass canes*)

Royal National Institute for the Blind (RNIB)
P.O. Box 173
Peterborough, PE2 6XU
England, UK

INDEXES

INDEX 1

INDEX OF SKILLS

NOTE: This Index is based on the Skills List, which is given in Chapter A, "How to Use This Book." It calls attention to the skills that are most obviously involved in a particular Module. Note that *Module numbers* are given, and *not* page numbers. For each skill, first the Modules which give it "primary" emphasis are given in bold type; then the Modules which give it lesser emphasis ("additional skill emphasis") are listed in lighter type.

To convert Module numbers into page numbers, see the Table of Contents at the front of the book. Also see the "Index of Chapter and Module Titles," which follows this "Index of Skills." The "Index of Chapter and Module Titles" gives the names of the Chapters and Modules in alphabetical order, with page numbers.

Addresses, Modules **22, 64, 90, 91, 93**, 16, 48, 59, 63, 81, 84

Air currents and echoes, Modules **52, 88**, 6, 16, 17, 23, 31, 42, 43, 50, 56, 58, 63, 85, 86, 87

Attitudes toward blindness, Modules **1, 2, 4, 7, 8, 57, 84**, 30, 35, 41, 44, 46, 82, 91, 92, 93

Barefoot walking, Modules 11, 19, 20, 23, 85, 86, 87, 88

Boundaries, Modules **19, 20, 21, 42, 60, 85, 87, 88**, 16, 43, 45, 86

Careers, Modules **84, 88**, 70, 74, 76, 77, 78, 79, 80, 81, 82, 83, 85, 92

Carrying things, Modules **12, 33, 34, 36, 77, 79**, 16, 25, 31, 32, 35, 46, 58, 71, 73, 74, 81, 82

Climbing, clambering, crawling, etc., Modules **42**, 11, 17, 86, 87

Communication and instructions, Modules **14, 30, 36, 41, 44, 48, 67, 70, 74, 77, 80, 82, 90, 91, 92, 93**, 9, 10, 27, 35, 38, 46, 54, 59, 61, 64, 65, 72, 79, 81

Compass directions, Modules **10, 29, 37, 38, 43, 45, 47, 48, 66, 67, 74**, 5, 9, 14, 16, 19, 20, 24, 28, 49, 54, 55, 61, 63, 64, 65, 68, 80, 87, 88

Corners, turns, and angles, Modules **9, 14, 15, 17, 20, 28, 29, 45, 47, 48, 54, 61, 63, 65, 66, 67, 70**, 3, 5, 6, 10, 16, 19, 21, 24, 27, 31, 32, 33, 37, 43, 52, 60, 64, 71, 72, 73, 74, 76

Correcting a path, Modules **5, 20, 33, 43, 46, 49, 54, 56, 60, 61, 62, 66**, 6, 19, 28, 29, 31, 37, 53, 55, 58, 63, 65, 68

Daily living skills, Modules **12, 25, 82, 83, 84**, 29, 33, 34, 35, 36, 40, 51, 58, 67, 70, 72, 74, 77, 78, 79

Detecting step-downs or drop-offs, Modules **1, 3, 8, 11, 17, 21, 23, 44, 49, 53, 57, 59, 71, 76, 85, 86, 87, 93**, 2, 5, 7, 12, 40, 43, 73, 88

Doors and doorways, Modules **1, 16, 28, 29, 30, 31, 32, 40, 70, 72, 75, 80, 81**, 12, 14, 15, 19, 23, 24, 27, 34, 36, 37, 42, 44, 45, 51, 59, 60, 74, 77, 78, 82

Elevators, Modules 70, 72, 80, 81, 16, 84, 92, 93

Emergency procedures, Modules 30, 44, 75, 16, 32, 37, 72, 85, 90, 93

Escalators, Modules 1, 73, 74, 80, 93, 70, 71, 92

Etiquette, Modules 35, 4, 33, 34, 36, 42, 67, 82, 90

Examining things tactually, Modules 21, 23, 25, 34, 42, 88, 7, 11, 14, 15, 19, 20, 36, 43, 72, 78, 79, 83, 85, 86, 87

Finding a person, Modules 6, 35, 36, 41, 77, 78, 81, 82, 84, 8, 13, 33, 34, 46, 51, 67, 80, 83, 91

Finding a seat, Modules 27, 33, 34, 40, 76, 78, 82, 90, 93, 8, 23, 71, 80, 84, 92

Flexibility and confidence, Modules 5, 7, 8, 11, 12, 30, 37, 44, 52, 57, 58, 59, 60, 61, 62, 64, 75, 90, 93, 4, 13, 17, 32, 33, 35, 41, 56, 65, 66, 67, 68, 74, 76, 88, 91, 92

Floor plans, Modules 14, 15, 16, 17, 24, 27, 28, 30, 31, 33, 37, 38, 45, 70, 75, 76, 79, 80, 81, 25, 29, 32, 71, 72, 73, 74, 78

General travel (indoors), Modules 14, 15, 28, 29, 34, 36, 37, 38, 74, 80, 31, 71, 75, 92

General travel (outdoors), Modules 11, 22, 41, 43, 48, 51, 58, 63

General travel, Modules 1, 2, 3, 4, 5, 6, 7, 8, 16, 23, 25, 46, 50, 52, 67, 77, 81, 84, 9, 10, 57

Hills and inclines, Modules 19, 86, 87, 11, 20, 23, 42, 43, 45, 47, 56, 58, 59, 85, 88

Human guide, Modules 4, 13, 78, 79, 84, 12, 33, 35, 46, 76, 81, 91, 92

In a crowd or a line, Modules 13, 30, 33, 34, 35, 36, 38, 40, 44, 46, 74, 76, 79, 80, 82, 90, 92, 93, 4, 6, 8, 29, 31, 41, 42, 70, 72, 73, 77, 81, 83, 85

Interpreting odors, Modules 25, 51, 74, 83, 88, 17, 23, 33, 34, 43, 58, 63, 78, 79, 85, 86, 87

Landmarks, Modules 1, 5, 6, 19, 20, 21, 27, 28, 34, 36, 42, 43, 45, 50, 51, 74, 85, 87, 88, 2, 9, 10, 15, 16, 24, 31, 32, 52, 53, 60, 64, 73, 86

Maps, Modules 10, 22, 45, 5, 19, 20, 25, 42, 43, 48, 55, 63, 64, 65, 66, 87, 88, 93

Meeting the public, Modules 35, 67, 90, 92, 93, 13, 70, 72, 76, 77, 78, 79, 80, 81, 82, 85

Moving straight ahead, Modules 1, 5, 6, 20, 43, 47, 49, 54, 60, 61, 66, 3, 13, 19, 57, 65, 68

Obstacles in path, Modules 1, 2, 3, 5, 13, 20, 27, 32, 33, 34, 42, 43, 52, 53, 56, 62, 83, 7, 19, 46, 47, 57, 58, 76, 87, 88

Open space, Modules 19, 20, 21, 42, 43, 60, 87, 88, 6, 11, 21, 34, 57, 74, 85

Orientation overall, Modules 5, 16, 19, 20, 24, 28, 30, 32, 36, 37, 38, 42, 43, 45, 56, 60, 63, 64, 70, 74, 86, 87, 88, 92, 93, 9, 10, 21, 31, 48, 50, 51, 65, 71, 90

Orientation within a room, Modules 14, 15, 27, 29, 33, 34, 60, 36, 37, 76, 82

Overhanging objects, Modules 17, 5, 19, 20, 43, 83, 86, 87, 88

Parallel and perpendicular, Modules 6, 53, 54, 55, 61, 65, 66, 68, 37, 41, 48, 49, 62, 64, 86

Posture, grip, gait, and arc, Modules 1, 2, 3, 4, 5, 13, 31, 32, 47, 58, 59, 71, 73, 87, 88, 7, 12, 57, 72

Public transportation, Modules 90, 91, 92, 93, 84

Purchase or transaction, Modules 33, 34, 35, 36, 74, 77, 79, 81, 82, 83, 85, 90, 91, 92, 93, 12, 13, 51, 67, 73, 76, 80

Responsibility and citizenship, Modules 30, 43, 84, 8, 12, 25, 33, 35, 36, 44, 74, 75, 77, 81, 90, 92, 93

Right and left, Modules **9, 14, 19, 20, 28, 29, 37, 47, 48, 54, 67, 74,** 2, 3, 5, 6, 10, 12, 15, 16, 21, 24, 27, 31, 32, 43, 45, 49, 53, 55, 60, 61, 63, 64, 65, 66, 68, 73, 80

Sidewalk, Modules **21, 22, 43, 47, 53, 56, 58, 63,** 2, 41, 46, 48, 49, 51, 59

Sound direction and meaning, Modules **6, 21, 35, 41, 46, 49, 50, 52, 53, 54, 55, 58, 62, 65, 68, 74, 76, 83, 90, 93,** 2, 7, 16, 17, 23, 24, 28, 33, 34, 40, 42, 43, 48, 61, 63, 66, 72, 73, 77, 78, 79, 85, 86, 87, 88

Stairs, Modules **1, 2, 12, 16, 23, 30, 40, 44, 71, 73, 76, 80,** 5, 14, 28, 38, 46, 57, 59, 70, 72, 75, 81, 93

Stowing cane, Modules **12, 33, 34, 40, 42, 76, 78, 84, 85, 90, 91, 93,** 2, 14, 15, 27, 29, 35, 43, 87, 92

Street crossing, Modules **6, 21, 49, 53, 54, 55, 58, 61, 62, 63, 64, 65, 66, 68,** 40, 41, 48, 59, 90, 93

Street patterns, Modules **22, 54, 55, 61, 63, 64, 65, 66, 86, 90,** 48, 53, 62, 68, 91, 93

Structure of buildings, Modules **15, 17, 24, 25, 45,** 16, 21, 23, 28, 30, 31, 32, 37, 38, 70, 71, 72, 75, 76

Techniques, Modules **See specific topics**

Traffic movement, Modules **6, 22, 41, 49, 54, 55, 61, 62, 65, 66, 68,** 16, 25, 48, 53, 64, 83

Understanding vision and partial vision, Modules **7, 8, 22, 57, 84,** 41, 90

Varied terrain, Modules **11, 17, 19, 20, 21, 42, 43, 46, 56, 57, 58, 85, 86, 87, 88,** 3, 24, 45, 53, 59, 60, 63

Walking in company with others, Modules **4, 12, 13, 46, 78, 79, 84,** 6, 76, 80, 87, 88

Weather and temperature, Modules **58,** 8, 11, 17, 19, 20, 25, 42, 43, 50, 52, 56, 79, 83, 85, 86, 87, 88, 90

INDEX 2

INDEX OF CHAPTER AND MODULE TITLES

NOTE: This Index gives the Modules in alphabetical order. It is similar to the Table of Contents in that it shows the page number where each Module begins. However, the reader looking for a particular Module title will find it more quickly here.

To some degree, this Index is "permuted" – that is, an entry can be found by looking for a significant word. For example, the Module "Description of Basic Techniques" is also listed as "Techniques, Description of Basic."

Also note that the Index of Skills, preceding this Index, is based on the Skills List given in Chapter A ("How to Use This Book").

ADDRESS, HOME	Module 22 Page 120
ADULT, BLIND...VISITING AT HIS/HER WORKPLACE	Module 84 Page 332
AIR CURRENTS, ECHOES AND (Including "Facial Vision")	Module 52 Page 219
AIRPORT, THE, and Air Travel	Module 92 Page 366
ALLEYS (DRIVEWAYS ... AND STREETS)	Module 63 Page 261
ALTERNATE ROUTES WITHIN A BUILDING	Module 37 Page 164
APARTMENT HOUSE OR CONDOMINIUM	Module 16 Page 98
ARC (POSTURE, GAIT, AND ARC, Level Surface)	Module 3 Page 39
AROUND THE BLOCK	Module 48 Page 206
ASKING DIRECTIONS AND FIGURING IT OUT	Module 67 Page 279
ATTIC, UNFINISHED BASEMENT, "CRAWL SPACE"	Module 17 Page 103
AUDITORIUM OR THEATER, AN	Module 76 Page 312
BACK YARD BOUNDARIES	Module 19 Page 108
BACK YARD (OVERALL)	Module 20 Page 114
BANK, THE	Module 77 Page 317
BASEMENT, UNFINISHED, "CRAWL SPACE," OR ATTIC	Module 17 Page 103
BEACH, SWIMMING POOL OR	Module 85 Page 336
BLIND ADULT, VISITING...AT HIS/HER WORKPLACE	Module 84 Page 332
BLIND TRAVEL INSTRUCTOR, THE (Monthei and Dunnam)	Appendix A Page 377
BLOCK, AROUND THE	Module 48 Page 206
'BLOCKS,' NON-SQUARE	Module 64 Page 265
BOUNDARIES, BACK YARD	Module 19 Page 108
BRIDGES AND OVERPASSES	Module 86 Page 339

BUILDING, AN OFFICE	Module 81 Page 326
BUILDINGS (GENERAL OVERVIEW)	Module 70 Page 288
BUILDINGS, STAIRS IN UNFAMILIAR	Module 71 Page 293
BUS, SCHOOL	Module 40 Page 180
BUSES, PUBLIC	Module 90 Page 354
CABS, TAXI	Module 91 Page 364
CAR, MEETING A	Module 41 Page 182
CARRYING THINGS	Module 12 Page 84
CLASSROOM, ORIENTATION INSIDE NEW	Module 27 Page 132
Community, Outdoors – MORE IDEAS for Lessons	Module 69 Page 285
COMPASS DIRECTIONS	Module 10 Page 78
COMPLICATED STREET CROSSINGS	Module 66 Page 272
CONDOMINIUM, APARTMENT HOUSE OR	Module 16 Page 98
CROWD, IN A	Module 13 Page 88
CURB, FROM HOUSE TO	Module 21 Page 117
CURBSIDE, WALKING AT	Module 53 Page 221
DECK, PORCH OR	Module 23 Page 121
DESCRIPTION OF BASIC TECHNIQUES (Including Stairway Technique)	Module 1 Page 24
Dim Light (POOR LIGHTING CONDITIONS)	Module 8 Page 69
DIRECTIONS, ASKING, AND FIGURING IT OUT	Module 67 Page 279
DIRECTIONS, COMPASS	Module 10 Page 78
DISTINCTIVE ODORS	Module 51 Page 217
DISTINCTIVE SOUNDS	Module 50 Page 214
DOCTOR'S OFFICE, A	Module 78 Page 319
DOORS AND DOORWAYS	Module 31 Page 143
DOORS CLOSED OR OPEN	Module 32 Page 147
DRIVEWAYS, ALLEYS, AND STREETS	Module 63 Page 261
DROP-OFF OR STEP-DOWN, UNEXPECTED	Module 59 Page 243
ECHOES AND AIR CURRENTS (Including "Facial Vision")	Module 52 Page 219
(Elevated Trains, Subways and) URBAN RAPID TRANSIT	Module 93 Page 370
ELEVATORS	Module 72 Page 297
EMERGENCY EXITS In Various Buildings	Module 75 Page 310
ERRANDS	Module 36 Page 161
ESCALATORS	Module 73 Page 300
EXITS, EMERGENCY (In Various Buildings)	Module 75 Page 310
EXTERIOR FIRE ESCAPE	Module 44 Page 194
["Facial Vision"] ECHOES AND AIR CURRENTS	Module 52 Page 219
FIGURING IT OUT, ASKING DIRECTIONS AND	Module 67 Page 279
FIRE DRILLS	Module 30 Page 140
FIRE ESCAPE, EXTERIOR	Module 44 Page 194

Index of Chapter and Module Titles

FOLLOWING SOMEONE, WALKING INDEPENDENTLY WHILE	Module 46 Page 200
FROM HOUSE TO CURB	Module 21 Page 117
GAIT (POSTURE, GAIT, AND ARC, Level Surface)	Module 3 Page 39
Gas Station (See SERVICE STATION, A)	Module 83 Page 330
GENERAL OVERVIEW – BUILDINGS	Module 70 Page 288
GENERAL PRINCIPLES AND OVERALL PLANNING	Chapter B Page 9
Glare (POOR LIGHTING CONDITIONS)	Module 8 Page 69
GREAT OUTDOORS, THE	Module 87 Page 341
GROCERY STORE, A	Module 79 Page 321
GUIDE, HUMAN	Module 4 Page 45
HOME ADDRESS	Module 22 Page 120
Home, Indoors, MORE IDEAS for Lessons	Module 18 Page 105
Home, Outdoors, MORE IDEAS for Lessons	Module 26 Page 128
HOME – CONTENTS OF ROOM	Module 14 Page 92
HOTELS AND MOTELS	Module 80 Page 324
HOUSE, OUTSIDE AND INSIDE THE	Module 24 Page 123
HOUSE TO CURB, FROM	Module 21 Page 117
HOW TO USE THIS BOOK (Scope and Style)	Chapter A Page 3
HUMAN GUIDE	Module 4 Page 45
(Ice Underfoot, Including) INCLEMENT WEATHER	Module 58 Page 240
IDEAS, MORE, For Lessons at Home, Indoors	Module 18 Page 105
IDEAS, MORE, For Lessons at Home, Outdoors	Module 26 Page 128
IDEAS, MORE, For Lessons at School, Indoors	Module 39 Page 176
IDEAS, MORE, For Lessons in Outdoor Locations	Module 89 Page 351
IDEAS, MORE, For Lessons in the Community, Outdoors	Module 69 Page 285
IN A CROWD	Module 13 Page 88
INCLEMENT WEATHER (Including Ice Underfoot)	Module 58 Page 240
Index of Chapter and Module Titles	Index 2 Page 393
Index of Skills	Index 1 Page 389
INTERSECTIONS, UNCONTROLLED	Module 68 Page 283
INTRODUCING THE CANE (Including Stairway Techniques)	Module 2 Page 30
INTRODUCTION (Sharon L. Monthei)	Chapter C Page 19
IRREGULAR STREETS	Module 65 Page 269
KITCHEN, LUNCHROOM AND: Overall Layout and Procedures	Module 34 Page 154
LEFT, RIGHT AND	Module 9 Page 73
Level Surface (POSTURE, GAIT, AND ARC)	Module 3 Page 39
LIGHTING, POOR CONDITIONS	Module 8 Page 69
LIGHTS, STREET CROSSING WITH (Basic Skills)	Module 54 Page 223
LINE OF PEOPLE, WALKING IN A	Module 35 Page 156
LUNCHROOM AND KITCHEN: Overall Layout and Procedures	Module 34 Page 154

LUNCHTIME	Module 33 Page 151
MALLS	Module 74 Page 302
MEETING A CAR	Module 41 Page 182
MORE IDEAS For Lessons at Home, Indoors	Module 18 Page 105
MORE IDEAS For Lessons at Home, Outdoors	Module 26 Page 128
MORE IDEAS For Lessons at School, Indoors	Module 39 Page 176
MORE IDEAS For Lessons in Outdoor Locations	Module 89 Page 351
MORE IDEAS For Lessons in the Community, Outdoors	Module 69 Page 285
NEW BUILDINGS AND NEW CLASSROOMS, ROUTES FOR	Module 38 Page 170
Night (POOR LIGHTING CONDITIONS)	Module 8 Page 69
NON-SQUARE 'BLOCKS'	Module 64 Page 265
OBSTACLES: NOTING THEM AND PROCEEDING	Module 5 Page 50
OBSTRUCTED, SIDEWALK FLAWED OR	Module 56 Page 234
OBSTRUCTION, STREET CROSSING WITH	Module 62 Page 257
Occluders (SLEEP SHADES)	Module 7 Page 60
ODORS, DISTINCTIVE	Module 51 Page 217
OFFICE BUILDING, AN	Module 81 Page 326
OPEN SPACE, WALKING ACROSS	Module 60 Page 246
ORIENTATION INSIDE NEW CLASSROOM	Module 27 Page 132
Outdoor Locations (MORE IDEAS for Lessons)	Module 89 Page 351
OUTDOORS, THE GREAT	Module 87 Page 341
OUTSIDE AND INSIDE THE HOUSE	Module 24 Page 123
OUTSIDE AND INSIDE THE SCHOOL	Module 45 Page 196
OVERPASSES, BRIDGES AND	Module 86 Page 339
PLANNING, GENERAL PRINCIPLES AND OVERALL	Chapter B Page 9
PLAYGROUND	Module 42 Page 185
POOL, SWIMMING ... OR BEACH	Module 85 Page 336
POOR LIGHTING CONDITIONS (At Night, in Dim Light, and With Glare)	Module 8 Page 69
PORCH OR DECK	Module 23 Page 121
POSTURE, GAIT, AND ARC (Level Surface)	Module 3 Page 39
PRINCIPLES, GENERAL ... AND OVERALL PLANNING	Chapter B Page 9
PUBLIC BUSES	Module 90 Page 354
Railroad Crossing	Module 66 Page 272
Railroad (URBAN RAPID TRANSIT)	Module 93 Page 370
REFERENCES	Page 381
REST ROOMS AT SCHOOL	Module 29 Page 137
RESTAURANT, A	Module 82 Page 328
RIGHT AND LEFT	Module 9 Page 73
ROOM, CONTENTS OF (HOME)	Module 14 Page 92
ROOM, WHAT IS A	Module 15 Page 94

ROUGH TERRAIN	Module 11	Page 81
ROUTES FOR NEW BUILDINGS AND NEW CLASSROOMS	Module 38	Page 170
ROUTES FOR NEW CLASSROOM (Early Elementary Grades)	Module 28	Page 134
RURAL ENVIRONMENT	Module 88	Page 347
SCHOOL BUS	Module 40	Page 180
(School Grounds, On the) WHAT'S OUT THERE?	Module 43	Page 190
Scope and Style (HOW TO USE THIS BOOK)	Chapter A	Page 3
SERVICE STATION, A	Module 83	Page 330
SIDEWALK FLAWED OR OBSTRUCTED	Module 56	Page 234
SIDEWALKS	Module 47	Page 203
Sighted Guide (See HUMAN GUIDE)	Module 4	Page 45
SLEEP SHADES (Occluders)	Module 7	Page 60
SOUND, WALKING TOWARD A	Module 6	Page 57
SOUNDS, DISTINCTIVE	Module 50	Page 214
STAIRS IN UNFAMILIAR BUILDINGS	Module 71	Page 293
Stairway (DESCRIPTION OF BASIC TECHNIQUES)	Module 1	Page 24
Stairway Technique (INTRODUCING THE CANE)	Module 2	Page 30
STEP-DOWN, UNEXPECTED DROP-OFF OR	Module 59	Page 243
STOP SIGNS	Module 55	Page 229
STORE, A GROCERY	Module 79	Page 321
STREET CROSSING (Developing Flexibility and Competence)	Module 61	Page 250
STREET CROSSING WITH LIGHTS (Basic Skills)	Module 54	Page 223
STREET CROSSING WITH LITTLE TRAFFIC	Module 49	Page 209
STREET CROSSING WITH OBSTRUCTION	Module 62	Page 257
STREET CROSSINGS, COMPLICATED	Module 66	Page 272
STREETS (DRIVEWAYS, ALLEYS, AND)	Module 63	Page 261
STREETS, IRREGULAR	Module 65	Page 269
(Subways and Elevated Trains) URBAN RAPID TRANSIT	Module 93	Page 370
SWIMMING POOL OR BEACH	Module 85	Page 336
TAXICABS	Module 91	Page 364
TECHNIQUES, DESCRIPTION OF BASIC (Including Stairway)	Module 1	Page 24
TERRAIN, ROUGH	Module 11	Page 81
THEATER, AN AUDITORIUM OR	Module 76	Page 312
TRAFFIC, STREET CROSSING WITH LITTLE	Module 49	Page 209
Trains, Elevated (URBAN RAPID TRANSIT: Subways and ...)	Module 93	Page 370
TRANSIT, RAPID URBAN: Subways and Elevated Trains	Module 93	Page 370
TRASH, UTILITIES AND	Module 25	Page 125
UNCONTROLLED INTERSECTIONS	Module 68	Page 283
UNEXPECTED DROP-OFF OR STEP-DOWN	Module 59	Page 243
UNFINISHED BASEMENT, "CRAWL SPACE," OR ATTIC	Module 17	Page 103
URBAN RAPID TRANSIT: Subways and Elevated Trains	Module 93	Page 370

UTILITIES AND TRASH	Module 25	Page 125
VISITING A BLIND ADULT AT HIS/HER WORKPLACE	Module 84	Page 332
VISUALLY CONFUSING APPEARANCE	Module 57	Page 237
WALKING ACROSS OPEN SPACE	Module 60	Page 246
WALKING AT CURBSIDE	Module 53	Page 221
WALKING IN A LINE OF PEOPLE	Module 35	Page 156
WALKING INDEPENDENTLY WHILE FOLLOWING SOMEONE	Module 46	Page 200
WALKING TOWARD A SOUND	Module 6	Page 57
WEATHER, INCLEMENT (Including Ice Underfoot)	Module 58	Page 240
WHAT IS A "ROOM"?	Module 15	Page 94
WHAT'S OUT THERE? (On the School Grounds)	Module 43	Page 190
WORKPLACE, VISITING A BLIND ADULT AT HIS/HER	Module 84	Page 332
YARD (BACK YARD, OVERALL)	Module 20	Page 114